Vascular Disasters

Editors

ALEX KOYFMAN
BRIT LONG

EMERGENCY MEDICINE CLINICS OF NORTH AMERICA

www.emed.theclinics.com

Consulting Editor
AMAL MATTU

November 2017 • Volume 35 • Number 4

ELSEVIER

1600 John F. Kennedy Boulevard • Suite 1800 • Philadelphia, Pennsylvania, 19103-2899

http://www.theclinics.com

EMERGENCY MEDICINE CLINICS OF NORTH AMERICA Volume 35, Number 4
November 2017 ISSN 0733-8627, ISBN-13: 978-0-323-54875-5

Editor: Colleen Dietzler

Developmental Editor: Casey Potter

Emergency Medicine Clinics of North America (ISSN 0733-8627) is published quarterly by Elsevier Inc., 360 Park Avenue South, New York, NY, 10010-1710. Months of issue are February, May, August, and November. Business and Editorial Offices: 1600 John F. Kennedy Boulevard, Suite 1800, Philadelphia, PA 19103-2899. Customer Service Office: 6277 Sea Harbor Drive, Orlando, FL 32887-4800. Periodicals postage paid at New York, NY, and additional mailing offices. Subscription prices are $100.00 per year (US students), $323.00 per year (US individuals), $608.00 per year (US institutions), $220.00 per year (international students), $455.00 per year (international individuals), $747.00 per year (international institutions), $220.00 per year (Canadian students), $389.00 per year (Canadian individuals), and $747.00 per year (Canadian institutions). International air speed delivery is included in all *Clinics*' subscription prices. All prices are subject to change without notice. **POSTMASTER:** Send address changes to *Emergency Medicine Clinics of North America*, Elsevier Periodicals Customer Service, 11830 Westline Industrial Drive, St. Louis, MO 63146. Customer Service (orders, claims, online, change of address): Elsevier Periodicals **Customer Service, 11830 Westline Industrial Drive, St. Louis, MO 63146. Tel: 1-800-654-2452 (U.S. and Canada); 314-453-7041 (outside U.S. and Canada). Fax: 314-453-5170. E-mail: journalscustomerservice-usa@elsevier.com (for print support); journalsonlinesupport-usa@elsevier.com (for online support).**

Reprints. For copies of 100 or more of articles in this publication, please contact the Commercial Reprints Department, Elsevier Inc., 360 Park Avenue South, New York, NY 10010-1710. Tel.: 212-633-3874; Fax: 212-633-3820; E-mail: reprints@elsevier.com.

Emergency Medicine Clinics of North America is covered in *MEDLINE/PubMed (Index Medicus), Current Contents/Clinical Medicine, EMBASE/Excerpta Medica, BIOSIS, SciSearch, CINAHL, ISI/BIOMED,* and *Research Alert.*

Contributors

CONSULTING EDITOR

AMAL MATTU, MD
Professor and Vice Chair, Department of Emergency Medicine, University of Maryland School of Medicine, Baltimore, Maryland

EDITORS

ALEX KOYFMAN, MD
Clinical Assistant Professor, Department of Emergency Medicine, Parkland Hospital, The University of Texas Southwestern Medical Center, Dallas, Texas

BRIT LONG, MD
Staff Physician, San Antonio Uniformed Services Health Education Consortium, Department of Emergency Medicine, San Antonio Military Medical Center, JBSA Fort Sam Houston, Texas

AUTHORS

STEPHEN ALERHAND, MD
Instructor and Ultrasound Fellow, Department of Emergency Medicine, Icahn School of Medicine at Mount Sinai, New York, New York

COURTNEY R. CASSELLA, MD
Department of Emergency Medicine, Icahn School of Medicine at Mount Sinai, New York, New York

ROBERT COONEY, MD, MSMedEd, RDMS, FACEP, FAAEM
Program Director, Emergency Medicine Residency Program, Geisinger Medical Center, Danville, Pennsylvania

ANDY JAGODA, MD, FACEP
Professor and Chair Emeritus, Department of Emergency Medicine, Icahn School of Medicine at Mount Sinai, New York, New York

ALEX KOYFMAN, MD
Clinical Assistant Professor, Department of Emergency Medicine, Parkland Hospital, The University of Texas Southwestern Medical Center, Dallas, Texas

CAPPI LAY, MD
Assistant Professor, Departments of Emergency Medicine and Neurocritical Care, Icahn School of Medicine at Mount Sinai, New York, New York

CHRISTIE LECH, MD
Faculty, Department of Emergency Medicine, NYU Langone Medical Center, Bellevue Hospital Center, New York, New York

BRIT LONG, MD
Staff Physician, San Antonio Uniformed Services Health Education Consortium, Department of Emergency Medicine, San Antonio Military Medical Center, JBSA Fort Sam Houston, Texas

MARK OLAF, DO, FACEP
Assistant Regional Dean and Medical Student Clerkship Director, Geisinger Commonwealth School of Medicine, Department of Emergency Medicine, Geisinger Medical Center, Danville, Pennsylvania

JENNIFER J. ROBERTSON, MD, MSEd
Assistant Professor, Emory University School of Medicine, Atlanta, Georgia

MICHAEL S. RUNYON, MD, MPH
Professor of Emergency Medicine, Chief of Academic Affairs and Faculty Development, Department of Emergency Medicine, Carolinas HealthCare System, Charlotte, North Carolina

JAMIE R. SANTISTEVAN, MD
Faculty, Department of Emergency Medicine, University of Wisconsin School of Medicine and Public Health, Madison, Wisconsin; Staff Physician, Emergency Department, Beloit Health System, Beloit, Wisconsin

ERICA MARIE SIMON, DO, MHA
Emergency Medicine Resident, San Antonio Uniformed Services Health Education Consortium, San Antonio Military Medical Center, JBSA Fort Sam Houston, Texas

MANPREET SINGH, MD
Faculty, Department of Emergency Medicine, Harbor-UCLA Medical Center, Assistant Professor of Emergency Medicine, David Geffen School of Medicine at UCLA, Torrance, California

RICHARD SLAMA, MD, LT
Emergency Medicine Resident, Naval Medical Center Portsmouth, Portsmouth, Virginia

REUBEN J. STRAYER, MD
Department of Emergency Medicine, Maimonides Medical Center, Brooklyn, New York

SHANE MATTHEW SUMMERS, MD
Emergency Medicine Program Director, San Antonio Uniformed Services Health Education Consortium, San Antonio Military Medical Center, JBSA Fort Sam Houston, Texas

ANAND SWAMINATHAN, MD, MPH
Assistant Professor, Assistant Residency Director, Department of Emergency Medicine, NYU Langone Medical Center, Bellevue Hospital Center, New York, New York

FRANK VILLAUME, MD, LCDR
NMCP Attending Physician, Portsmouth, Virginia

Contents

Foreword: Vascular Emergencies xiii

Amal Mattu

Preface: Time-Critical Vascular Disasters xv

Alex Koyfman and Brit Long

Thoracic Aortic Syndromes 713

Reuben J. Strayer

Aortic dissection (AD) is a lethal, treatable disruption of the aortic vessel wall. It often presents without classic features, mimicking symptoms of other conditions, and diagnosis is often delayed. Established high-risk markers of AD should be sought and indicate advanced aortic imaging with CT, MRI, or TEE. Treatment is immediate surgical evaluation, aggressive symptom relief, and reduction of the force of blood against the aortic wall by control of heart rate, followed by blood pressure.

Extracranial Cervical Artery Dissections 727

Jennifer J. Robertson and Alex Koyfman

Cervical artery dissections (CeAD) include both internal carotid and vertebral artery dissections. They are rare but important causes of stroke, especially in younger patients. CeAD should be considered in patients with strokelike symptoms, a new-onset headache and/or neck pain, and/or other risk factors. Early imaging with computed tomography (CT) or MRI is key to making the diagnosis. Treatment may vary depending on the extent of the dissection, timing of the dissection, and other comorbidities. The overall prognosis is good, but does depend on the initial severity of symptoms.

Deep Venous Thrombosis 743

Mark Olaf and Robert Cooney

Deep venous thrombosis (DVT) is a frequently encountered condition that is often diagnosed and treated in the outpatient setting. Risk stratification is helpful and recommended in the evaluation of DVT. An evidence-based diagnostic approach is discussed here. Once diagnosed, the mainstay of DVT treatment is anticoagulation. The specific type and duration of anticoagulation depend on the suspected etiology of the venous thromboembolism, as well as risks of bleeding and other patient comorbidities. Both specific details and a standardized approach to this vast treatment landscape are presented.

Vascular Access Complications: An Emergency Medicine Approach 771

Erica Marie Simon and Shane Matthew Summers

Millions of central venous and arterial catheters are placed across the United States annually as mechanisms of obtaining advanced

hemodynamic monitoring and facilitating acute resuscitation. Although presumably life-saving or sustaining in many circumstances, current literature identifies the preprocedural and postprocedural complications of infection, thrombosis, embolism, and iatrogenic injury as resulting in patient morbidity and mortality. Today, through the application of aseptic technique, performance of operator training, and the utilization of ultrasound, emergency physicians may limit vascular access complications and improve patient outcomes.

Penetrating Vascular Injury: Diagnosis and Management Updates **789**

Richard Slama and Frank Villaume

Penetrating vascular injury is becoming increasingly common in the United States and abroad. Much of the current research and treatment is derived from wartime and translation to the civilian sector has been lacking. Penetrating vascular injury can be classified as extremity, junctional, or noncompressible. Diagnosis can be obvious but at other times subtle and difficult to diagnose. Although there are numerous modalities, computed tomography angiography is the diagnostic study of choice. It is hoped that care will be improved by using an algorithmic approach integrating experience from military and civilian research.

Subarachnoid Hemorrhage: Updates in Diagnosis and Management **803**

Brit Long, Alex Koyfman, and Michael S. Runyon

Subarachnoid hemorrhage (SAH) is a neurologic emergency due to bleeding into the subarachnoid space. Mortality can reach 50%. The clinical presentation is most often in the form of headache, classically defined as maximal at onset and worst of life. The most common cause is traumatic; approximately 80% of nontraumatic SAHs are due to aneurysmal rupture, with the remainder from idiopathic peri-mesencephalic hemorrhage or other less common causes. Noncontrast brain computed tomography (CT) performed within 6 hours of symptom onset has sensitivity approaching 100%. Lumbar puncture may be considered after this period for definitive diagnosis if initial CT is normal.

Spontaneous Intracerebral Hemorrhage **825**

Stephen Alerhand and Cappi Lay

Although commonly arising from poorly controlled hypertension, spontaneous intracerebral hemorrhage may occur secondary to several other etiologies. Clinical presentation to the emergency department ranges from headache with vomiting to coma. In addition to managing the ABCs, the crux of emergency management lies in stopping hematoma expansion and other complications to prevent clinical deterioration. This may be achieved primarily through anticoagulation reversal, blood pressure, empiric management of intracranial pressure, and early neurosurgical consultation for posterior fossa hemorrhage. Patients must be admitted to intensive care. The effects of intracerebral hemorrhage are potentially devastating with very poor prognoses for functional outcome and mortality.

surgery consultation. The decision for endovascular thrombolysis or standard surgery depends on etiology, duration, and location of vascular occlusion. This article evaluates the diagnostic approach and management for acute limb ischemia.

Ischemic Stroke: Advances in Diagnosis and Management **911**

Courtney R. Cassella and Andy Jagoda

Acute ischemic stroke carries the risk of morbidity and mortality. Since the advent of intravenous thrombolysis, there have been improvements in stroke care and functional outcomes. Studies of populations once excluded from thrombolysis have begun to elucidate candidates who might benefit and thus should be engaged in the process of shared decision-making. Imaging is evolving to better target the ischemic penumbra salvageable with prompt reperfusion. Availability and use of computed tomography angiography identifies large-vessel occlusions, and new-generation endovascular therapy devices are improving outcomes in these patients. With this progress in stroke treatment, risk stratification tools and shared decision-making are fundamental.

EMERGENCY MEDICINE CLINICS OF NORTH AMERICA

FORTHCOMING ISSUES

February 2018
Trauma
Christopher Hicks and
Andrew Petrosoniak, *Editors*

May 2018
Pediatric Emergency Medicine
Sean M. Fox and Dale Woolridge, *Editors*

August 2018
Hematology Oncology Emergencies
Colin G. Kaide and Sarah B. Dubbs, *Editors*

RECENT ISSUES

August 2017
Observation Medicine
R. Gentry Wilkerson and
Christopher Baugh, *Editors*

May 2017
Wilderness and Environmental Medicine
Eric A. Weiss and Douglas Sward, *Editors*

February 2017
Severe Sepsis Care in the Emergency Department
Jack Perkins and Michael E. Winters, *Editors*

RELATED INTEREST

Interventional Cardiology Clinics, July 2017 (Vol. 6, Issue 3)
Interventional Heart Failure
Srihari S. Naidu, *Editor*

PROGRAM OBJECTIVE

The goal of *Emergency Medicine Clinics of North America* is to keep practicing emergency medicine physicians and emergency medicine residents up to date with current clinical practice in emergency medicine by providing timely articles reviewing the state of the art in patient care.

LEARNING OBJECTIVES

Upon completion of this activity, participants will be able to:

1. Review thoracic outlet syndromes, among other vascular disasters.
2. Recognize the dangers of ischemia and hemorrhages in emergency situations.
3. Discuss the risk of deep vein thrombosis in emergency medicine.

ACCREDITATION

The Elsevier Office of Continuing Medical Education (EOCME) is accredited by the Accreditation Council for Continuing Medical Education (ACCME) to provide continuing medical education for physicians.

The EOCME designates this enduring material for a maximum of 15 *AMA PRA Category 1 Credit*(s)™. Physicians should claim only the credit commensurate with the extent of their participation in the activity.

All other healthcare professionals requesting continuing education credit for this enduring material will be issued a certificate of participation.

DISCLOSURE OF CONFLICTS OF INTEREST

The EOCME assesses conflict of interest with its instructors, faculty, planners, and other individuals who are in a position to control the content of CME activities. All relevant conflicts of interest that are identified are thoroughly vetted by EOCME for fair balance, scientific objectivity, and patient care recommendations. EOCME is committed to providing its learners with CME activities that promote improvements or quality in healthcare and not a specific proprietary business or a commercial interest.

The planning committee, staff, authors and editors listed below have identified no financial relationships or relationships to products or devices they or their spouse/life partner have with commercial interest related to the content of this CME activity:

Stephen Alerhand, MD; Courtney R. Cassella, MD, FACEP; Robert Cooney, MD, MSMedEd, RDMS, FACEP, FAAEM; Anjali Fortna; Alex Koyfman, MD; Cappi Lay, MD; Christie Lech, MD; Leah Logan; Britt Long, MD; Amal Mattu, MD; Mark Olaf, DO, FACEP; Katie Pfaff; Jennifer J. Robertson, MD, MSEd; Jamie R. Santistevan, MD; Erica Marie Simon, DO, MHA; Manpreet Singh, MD; Richard Slama, MD, LT; Reuben J. Strayer, MD; Shane Matthew Summers, MD; Anand Swaminathan, MD, MPH; Frank Villaume, MD, LCDR; Vignesh Viswanathan.

The planning committee, staff, authors and editors listed below have identified financial relationships or relationships to products or devices they or their spouse/life partner have with commercial interest related to the content of this CME activity:

Andy Jagoda, MD is on the speakers' bureau for Pfizer Inc.; Janssen Global Services, LLC; and Johnson & Johnson Services, Inc., and is a consultant/advisor for Brain Trauma Foundation and EB Medicine.

Michael S. Runyon, MD, MPH has research support from Janssen Global Services, LLC; Emergency MCG Inc; Siemens Medical Solutions USA, Inc; Boehringer Ingelheim GmbH; Trinity Biotech; and BRAHMS GmbH, and receives royalties/patents from Wolters Kluwer.

UNAPPROVED/OFF-LABEL USE DISCLOSURE

The EOCME requires CME faculty to disclose to the participants:

1. When products or procedures being discussed are off-label, unlabelled, experimental, and/or investigational (not US Food and Drug Administration [FDA] approved); and
2. Any limitations on the information presented, such as data that are preliminary or that represent ongoing research, interim analyses, and/or unsupported opinions. Faculty may discuss information about pharmaceutical agents that is outside of FDA-approved labelling. This information is intended solely for CME and is not intended to promote off-label use of these medications. If you have any questions, contact the medical affairs department of the manufacturer for the most recent prescribing information.

TO ENROLL

To enroll in the *Emergency Medicine Clinics* Continuing Medical Education program, call customer service at 1-800-654-2452 or sign up online at http://www.theclinics.com/home/cme. The CME program is available to subscribers for an additional annual fee of $235 USD.

METHOD OF PARTICIPATION

In order to claim credit, participants must complete the following:

1. Complete enrolment as indicated above.
2. Read the activity.
3. Complete the CME Test and Evaluation. Participants must achieve a score of 70% on the test. All CME Tests and Evaluations must be completed online.

CME INQUIRIES/SPECIAL NEEDS

For all CME inquiries or special needs, please contact elsevierCME@elsevier.com.

Foreword
Vascular Emergencies

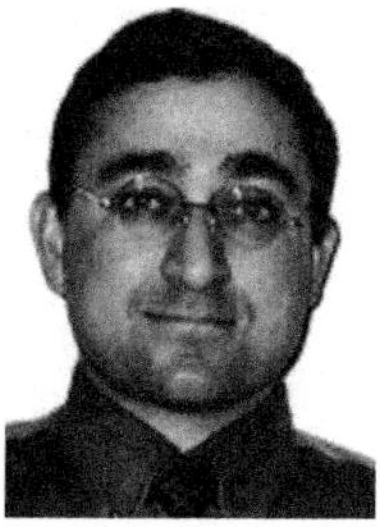

Amal Mattu, MD
Consulting Editor

Cardiovascular disease is the number 1 cause of death in the United States and other first-world countries around the globe. It's no surprise, therefore, that a great deal of attention in emergency medicine is paid to the recognition and treatment of cardiovascular diseases. However, when the term "cardiovascular" is used in this context, most providers and laypersons only hear the first part of that word, "cardio." Emergency "cardio" seems to get the bulk of attention, and "vascular" often takes a back seat. It's important to remember, though, that a huge number of patients in the United States suffer morbidity and mortality from noncardiac vascular conditions. Granted, some of these conditions do certainly get their fair share of attention, including stroke, intracranial bleeds, venous thromboembolism, and aortic disease. But there are other conditions that are equally dangerous, yet they are often given at most only a passing thought...until too late.

Drs Alex Koyfman and Brit Long have assembled an outstanding set of authors and topics in this issue of *Emergency Medicine Clinics of North America* to remind us of these noncardiac vascular conditions that are highly morbid or lethal. As expected, they provide updates on some of the "big ticket" entities such as ischemic and hemorrhagic stroke, deep venous thrombosis, and aortic syndromes (thoracic and abdominal), but they also give us outstanding updates on other high-risk vascular conditions that we must not forget. Cervical artery dissection, an increasingly recognized cause of stroke in young patients, is addressed in an early article. Penetrating vascular injury is addressed as well as vascular access complications. Later, the authors provide us with updates on two uncommon but catastrophic conditions, cerebral venous thrombosis and mesenteric ischemia. They also address vascular limb ischemia, the often-forgotten vascular disaster of the lower extremities.

For anyone who loves to learn about high-risk entities (Isn't that all of us in Emergency Medicine?), you will love this issue of *Emergency Medicine Clinics of North America*. This issue is certain to provide timely updates on common conditions and

Emerg Med Clin N Am 35 (2017) xiii–xiv
http://dx.doi.org/10.1016/j.emc.2017.08.002
0733-8627/17/© 2017 Published by Elsevier Inc.

to heighten your awareness of less common deadly conditions. We owe our thanks to Dr Koyfman, Dr Long, and the many excellent authors for providing us with some much-needed reading that is certain to help us save more lives in the Emergency Department.

Amal Mattu, MD
Department of Emergency Medicine
University of Maryland School of Medicine
110 South Paca Street
6th Floor, Suite 200
Baltimore, MD 21201, USA

E-mail address:
amalmattu@comcast.net

Preface
Time-Critical Vascular Disasters

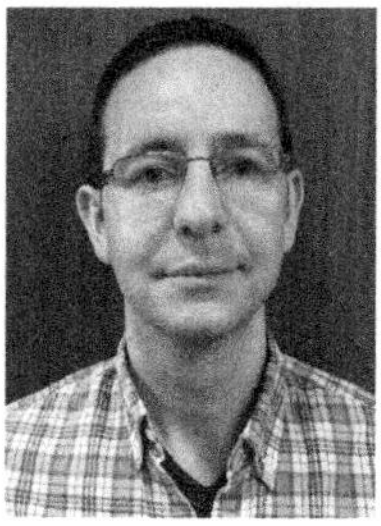

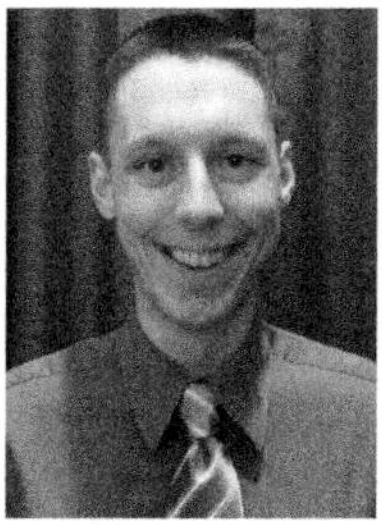

Alex Koyfman, MD   Brit Long, MD
Editors

The body's highway for oxygen and nutrients is the vascular system, ranging from the aorta to small capillaries. This system interacts with every organ system in the body, with a myriad of pathology that must be considered.

Emergency physicians specialize in recognizing and managing critical conditions, and vascular disasters include several diseases that may result in significant morbidity and mortality. From subarachnoid hemorrhage to aortic dissection, vascular emergencies can be deadly. Unfortunately, these conditions are rare and present similarly to other, more common conditions that are less critical. Emergency physicians are tasked with considering these deadly diseases, while appropriately utilizing resources for the evaluation and management of vascular emergencies. This issue of *Emergency Medicine Clinics of North America* investigates vascular disorders. Our intent is to provide physicians with the most current literature and evidence on conditions, including subarachnoid hemorrhage, deep vein thrombosis, mesenteric ischemia, vascular access complications, stroke (ischemic and hemorrhagic), and many others.

It is our pleasure to edit for *Emergency Medicine Clinics of North America*, and we thank all of the authors involved in construction of this issue. We greatly appreciate the assistance of Dr Amal Mattu and the staff at Elsevier. We also extend our gratitude to our families and colleagues for their amazing support and patience during the writing and editing phases. We hope this issue improves your clinical knowledge and practice, and thanks for reading!

Alex Koyfman, MD
The University of Texas
Southwestern Medical Center
Department of Emergency Medicine
5323 Harry Hines Boulevard
Dallas, TX 75390, USA

Emerg Med Clin N Am 35 (2017) xv–xvi
http://dx.doi.org/10.1016/j.emc.2017.08.001

Brit Long, MD
San Antonio Military Medical Center
Department of Emergency Medicine
3841 Roger Brooke Drive
Fort Sam Houston, TX 78234, USA

E-mail addresses:
Akoyfman8@gmail.com (A. Koyfman)
Brit.long@yahoo.com (B. Long)

Thoracic Aortic Syndromes

Reuben J. Strayer, MD

KEYWORDS

• Aortic dissection • Aortic intramural hemorrhage • Penetrating aortic ulcer

KEY POINTS

- Aortic dissection is an uncommon disease that often presents with varied and atypical findings suggestive of more frequently encountered conditions; therefore, it poses an exceptional diagnostic challenge to emergency providers.
- Mortality associated with aortic dissection is significant at presentation and advances with every hour the lesion is left untreated.
- Although almost all patients who have symptoms possibly caused by aortic dissection will not have aortic dissection, key features of the disease, including risk factors, pain characteristics, physical examination findings, and routine ancillary studies, allow clinicians to develop a rational approach to diagnostic testing.
- When the diagnosis is sufficiently likely to indicate definitive testing, computed tomography angiography is the advanced imaging test of choice in most centers, but transesophageal echocardiography and MRI may be appropriate alternatives in certain circumstances.
- Patients with diagnosed or strongly suspected aortic dissection require expeditious surgical evaluation, aggressive analgesia and anxiolysis, and treatment with rapid-acting, titratable agents to first lower heart rate, and then blood pressure, to specific targets.

INTRODUCTION

Aortic dissection (AD) is among the most immediately lethal diseases in medicine, with a mortality of 1% per hour,[1] and has effective temporizing medical therapies and a surgical cure. AD is, therefore, among the disorders of greatest interest to emergency physicians, yet is not diagnosed on its initial presentation in up to half of cases.[2–4] In fact, 1 expert asserts that “difficulty in diagnosis, delayed diagnosis or failure to diagnose are so common as to approach the norm for this disease, even in the best hands…”[5] This article explains why AD poses a diagnostic dilemma, proposes a strategy for its rational evaluation, and describes the principles of treatment.

Disclosure Statement: No funding or conflicts.
Department of Emergency Medicine, Maimonides Medical Center, 4821 Fort Hamilton Parkway, Brooklyn, NY 11219, USA
E-mail address: emupdates@gmail.com

Emerg Med Clin N Am 35 (2017) 713–725
http://dx.doi.org/10.1016/j.emc.2017.06.002
0733-8627/17/

PATHOPHYSIOLOGY

AD occurs when the innermost layer of the aortic vessel wall is torn, creating a false lumen that transmits a longitudinal column of blood. It is sometimes referred to as a dissecting aortic aneurysm; however, this term is discouraged because it is both inaccurate and conflates AD with aortic aneurysm, a distinct clinical entity. AD is thought to result from the hydrostatic pressure accumulated as blood is pumped through the aorta, as well as movement of the aorta itself, with every cardiac cycle. Histologically, AD is associated with characteristic changes in the vessel wall known as medial degeneration. The former term, cystic medial necrosis, has fallen out of favor because the observed lesion demonstrates neither cysts nor necrosis.

Conditions that increase the pressure exerted by blood on the vessel wall predispose patients to AD. These include hypertension, pregnancy, stimulant use (eg, cocaine), weight-lifting, and pheochromocytoma. AD is more likely in conditions that weaken the vessel and accelerate medial degeneration, such as large-vessel vasculitides and congenital connective tissue disorders, including Marfan, Loeys-Dietz, Ehlers-Danlos, and Turner syndromes. Finally, AD may be caused by lesions of the aortic valve itself, such as bicuspid aortic valve, aortic valve instrumentation or aortic surgery, and syphilitic aortitis.

The Stanford classification designates type A dissections as lesions involving the ascending aorta, whereas type B dissections are confined to the descending aorta. Type A dissections are more common and much more dangerous, which drives differences in the therapeutic approach. Variants of AD include aortic intramural hemorrhage, which is a hematoma completely contained within the vessel wall, and penetrating aortic ulcer, which is a disruption in the vessel wall that usually leads not to dissection but to aneurysm. These lesions are both treated similarly to AD.

AD causes morbidity and mortality by several mechanisms. Type A dissections can progress proximally to cause pericardial effusion with tamponade, as well as acute aortic valve insufficiency. Both types of dissections can breach the outer adventitial layer of the vessel, leading to free rupture and exsanguination into the chest or abdomen. Most sequelae of AD, however, result from the false lumen extending across ostia of branch arteries, leading to acute ischemia of potentially any organ in the body.

CLINICAL FEATURES AND EPIDEMIOLOGY

AD is an uncommon disease, with prevalence estimates ranging from 3.5 to 6.0 per 100,000 patient-years in the general population.[6] Untreated, AD carries a devastating mortality of 40% on presentation and an additional 1% rate of death per hour, to a 1-year mortality of 90%.[1] In a center where postmortem CT is routinely performed on patients with out-of-hospital cardiac arrest of uncertain cause, AD was determined to be the cause in 7% of cases.[7]

Approximately 1 in 10,000 emergency department (ED) patients will have AD, a number so small that emergency providers may only see several cases in their career. Only one-quarter of patients with AD present with a combination of classic features (pain of sudden onset or ripping or tearing quality, blood pressure differential, and widened mediastinum on chest xray [CXR]); 1 in 25 patients diagnosed with AD has none of the classic features.[1] Furthermore, AD can cause myriad symptoms localizing to any organ system or body part, and each of these symptoms can be explained by more common conditions, often by more common dangerous conditions that quite reasonably establish the focus of care but ultimately turn out to be distractors.[8]

Emergency clinicians are thus confronted with innumerable patients whose symptoms could be caused by AD but almost certainly are not. AD could, therefore, be said to represent not just a needle in a haystack but a needle in a haystack that is disguised as a blade of hay. Consequently, physicians evaluating patients whose symptoms may be caused by AD must understand the clinically relevant risk factors and clinical manifestations of this condition and develop a risk stratification strategy that identifies as many patients with the disease as possible without overusing advanced imaging studies that subject patients to important harms.

Despite the rarity of the disease, good data are available on clinical features of AD, owing to the International Registry of Acute Aortic Dissection (IRAD) and a variety of other longitudinal studies.[9] Pain is more likely to be abrupt and most severe at onset than to be tearing or ripping. Pain location is a reflection of the site of the lesion and includes chest pain radiating to the neck, jaw, or classically, the back; thoracic or lumbar back pain; and abdominal pain. Although chest pain is the most common presenting symptom, 1 study found that of ED subjects diagnosed with AD, more than 40% did not have chest pain on presentation.[10] Another study found 1 subject diagnosed with AD for every 980 subjects presenting with atraumatic chest pain.[11] Seventeen percent of subjects in 1 series had painless AD. These subjects presented predominantly with transient or persistent disturbance of consciousness or focal neurologic deficits.[12]

Constitutional symptoms are often marked and include nausea, diaphoresis, and (classically) extreme apprehension with a (justified) sense of impending doom. Patients with AD present with focal neurologic symptoms in 17% and syncope in 9% of cases. Though scenarios classically associated with AD, such as migratory pain, chest pain with neurologic deficits, and chest pain of sudden onset or with pulse deficit, occur in only a minority of cases, their presence strongly suggests the disease. It is commonly believed that patients with AD must be very ill or distressed with abnormal vitals, but ambulatory mode of arrival is an important risk factor for missing the disease at initial presentation.[13]

Many patients with AD will present with acute on chronic hypertension and AD is a cardinal hypertensive emergency. Hypotension is ominous in the setting of AD because it often indicates either proximal extension with cardiac tamponade or free or contained rupture. Pseudohypotension, peripheral hypotension with central normotension, may be caused by dissection across the subclavian arteries. Subclavian or iliac artery embarrassment may also lead to a pulse deficit or blood pressure differential across limbs; this classic finding is present in only 20% to 30% of cases; its absence should not be reassuring.[14] The murmur of aortic regurgitation, or signs of cardiac tamponade, may be present. If the dissection involves the left or (more commonly) right coronary artery, acute myocardial infarction (AMI) and its attendant signs and symptoms can result. A variety of neurologic deficits, including weakness or even coma, may be caused by AD, depending on the cerebral or spinal branch arteries affected. Distal AD can cause ischemia to either kidney, lower extremity ischemia, mesenteric ischemia, and resulting abdominal pain, back pain, or diarrhea.

DIAGNOSIS

Routine laboratory testing is not helpful for ruling in or ruling out AD. Troponin positivity is much more likely to represent primary cardiac pathology condition but is common in AD.[15] Therefore, when clinical features suggest dissection, a positive troponin should not dissuade the practitioner from ruling out the diagnosis of AD.

The use of serum quantitative D-dimer testing has been proposed as a strategy to rule out AD because blood in the false lumen activates the clotting cascade, generating fibrin degradation products detected by modern D-dimer assays with high sensitivity.[16–20] Unfortunately, further work has demonstrated an unacceptably high false-negative rate, and the ACEP clinical policy recommends that clinicians "not rely on D-dimer alone to exclude the diagnosis of aortic dissection."[21] In 1 study, D-dimer was falsely negative in 9 of 113 confirmed AD cases,[22] perhaps due to an AD variant in which the thrombosed lumen does not communicate with circulating blood, isolating the clot from detection by serum testing.[23] Furthermore, although a decision analysis of D-dimer and computed tomography (CT) angiography testing thresholds has been performed,[24] there is no evidence that D-dimer testing can be incorporated into a larger risk stratification strategy that would allow clinicians to sensitively exclude AD without greatly expanding the number of patients who receive advanced imaging studies. Given the experience with D-dimer testing to rule out pulmonary embolism, which has increased the number of advanced imaging studies ordered without increasing the number of pulmonary embolism diagnoses,[25] a comprehensive approach that accounts for false negatives and false positives should be validated before D-dimer testing is used routinely in the diagnosis of AD.

Plain CXR is indicated in patients with chest pain of uncertain cause and whenever AD is considered. The CXR is most useful when it provides an alternative explanation for the patient's symptoms. A variety of CXR abnormalities are associated with AD (**Box 1**), the most important being mediastinal widening, which is present in more than half of cases but is nonspecific.[26] The absence of suggestive CXR findings makes AD less likely. However, 10% to 20% of patients with AD have a normal CXR; therefore, a negative study cannot exclude the disease and should not play a decisive role in the decision to pursue advanced imaging.[27]

The electrocardiogram in AD is used to evaluate the differential diagnosis and usually demonstrates nonspecific findings but may also indicate acute myocardial ischemia.[28] This presents a clinical challenge because not only do the symptoms of AD overlap with the symptoms of myocardial ischemia, AD can *cause* myocardial ischemia when the dissection flap involves the ostium of the left or right coronary artery. When myocardial infarction complicates AD, treatment is directed at AD. Furthermore, usual therapies for AMI may directly worsen outcomes of patients with AD. The clinician caring for a patient whose symptoms may be caused by either diagnosis must, therefore, have a strategy for managing their possible convergence (see later discussion).

Transthoracic echocardiography (TTE) poorly visualizes much of the aorta and is limited by patient, operator, and machine characteristics. AD cannot be excluded

Box 1
Signs of aortic dissection on chest radiography

Mediastinal widening

Disruption of normally distinct contour of aortic knob

Calcium sign: separation of intimal calcification from the vessel wall greater than 5 mm

Double-density appearance within aorta

Tracheal deviation to the right

Deviation of nasogastric tube to the right

by TTE.[21] However, point-of-care ultrasound by emergency physicians is recommended for all patients with suspected AD and should be considered for all patients with chest or abdominal pain of uncertain cause. In addition to evaluating alternative diagnoses, an intimal flap at either the aortic root or descending aorta may be distinguished by TTE, especially when augmented by suprasternal notch views, and is diagnostic.[29] TTE also reliably identifies complications of AD such as pericardial effusion and aortic regurgitation.[30–32]

Transesophageal echocardiography (TEE) is very accurate in both ruling in and ruling out AD and can be performed in a critical care area as resuscitative efforts are ongoing, which is a distinct advantage compared with CT and MRI, the 2 other definitive imaging modalities. However, TEE is uncommonly performed by emergency clinicians and not widely available on a consultative basis in many EDs. Invasive echocardiography may play a more prominent role in the emergency evaluation of AD as the technique sees broader application by emergency providers.[33]

Intravenous (IV) contrast-enhanced CT reliably confirms and excludes AD and may elucidate alternative diagnoses, including pulmonary embolism and obstructive coronary artery disease. Contemporary CT scanning is rapid and widely available. Therefore, CT is the most common definitive imaging study used in patients with suspected AD. Beyond the concerns raised by moving a potentially critically ill patient to the radiology suite, drawbacks of CT include the risks of IV contrast and ionizing radiation, as well several diagnostic pitfalls (**Box 2**). Though CT angiography is an excellent test for AD, these harms are underappreciated by both physicians and patients.[34,35]

MRI also accurately rules in and rules out AD,[36] and is free of contrast and radiation risk. However, limited availability and relatively long image acquisition times relegate MRI to a secondary imaging modality in most scenarios. MRI has a role in managing stable patients with an equivocal CT or TEE, or patients with known severe IV contrast allergy.

THE DECISION TO IMAGE

For emergency clinicians and other providers who manage patients with undifferentiated symptoms, the central challenge in the evaluation of AD is determining which patients require advanced imaging. Many reviews recommend that AD be considered in any patient presenting with chest pain, abdominal pain, back pain, or malperfusion of any organ, but this encompasses a set of patients so large as to be almost meaningless.

In 2010, the American College of Cardiology (ACC) Foundation and American Heart Association (AHA) published a multidisciplinary guideline on the diagnosis and management of patients with thoracic aortic disease, including AD.[37] This document

Box 2
Harms of computed tomography

Radiation or oncogenesis

Contrast harms (kidney injury, allergy, extravasation, volume overload)

False negatives, false positives

Incidental findings (may lead to further testing and therapies)

Overdiagnosis (true positives that would not have harmed patient)

Resource utilization (time, monetary cost, opportunity cost)

presents an evaluation pathway that guides clinicians in deciding which patients require advanced imaging to exclude the disease. The pathway hinges on AD risk markers from past medical history, history of present illness, and physical examination (**Box 3**). Patients with risk markers from more than 1 risk category are classified as high risk and assumed to have AD until proven otherwise. Patients with risk markers from 1 category are intermediate risk and should receive expedited aortic imaging. Finally, patients with no risk markers only require aortic imaging if no alternative diagnosis is identified and the patient has unexplained hypotension or widened mediastinum on CXR.

The ACC/AHA evaluation pathway was found by its authors to have a sensitivity of 95.7%: 1 out of 23 patients diagnosed with AD had zero risk markers.[2] An external validation confirmed that the evaluation pathway accurately risk stratified patients' likelihood of having AD (more risk markers are associated with higher risk). However, in this cohort, 1 out 11 subjects with AD had zero risk markers, and subjects with 5 risk markers were still as likely to not have AD as to have the disease.[38] The ACC/AHA pathway can, therefore, be used to inform the decision to image, but the absence of risk markers does not exclude the disease and the presence of risk markers does not mandate aortic imaging. Patient-specific factors must ultimately guide management. These factors include the results of ancillary testing and likelihood of an alternative diagnosis, how likely that patient is to be harmed by advanced imaging (eg, radiation harms are inversely proportional to age), candidacy for surgery if AD is diagnosed, and the patient's preferences.

Though many patients with AD do not have classic symptoms or signs, given the low prevalence of the disease, routinely excluding AD with CT angiography in

Box 3
American College of Cardiology and American Heart Association aortic dissection high-risk markers

High-risk conditions

Marfan syndrome

Family history aortic disease

Known aortic valve disease

Recent aortic manipulation

Known thoracic aortic aneurysm

High-risk pain features

Chest, back, or abdominal pain, described as any of the following:
- Abrupt onset
- Severe intensity
- Ripping or tearing

High-risk examination features

Evidence of perfusion deficit
- Pulse deficit
- Systolic blood pressure differential
- Focal neurologic deficit (in conjunction with pain)

Murmur of aortic insufficiency (new and with pain)

Hypotension or shock state

patients without typical features would cause more harm than good. Efforts are underway to develop an accurate diagnostic test with a favorable benefit-to-harm profile that may allow practitioners to safely exclude AD in patients who present with the broad range of symptoms that could be due to dissection but almost always are not.[39] Until these efforts are successful, a sound approach to AD uses a knowledge of the risk factors for and clinical findings suggestive of the disease to indicate advanced imaging, understanding that with rational application of current diagnostic paradigms and technology, missing the diagnosis on initial presentation will remain the standard of care.

AORTIC DISSECTION AND ST-SEGMENT ELEVATION MYOCARDIAL INFARCTION

For patients who present with symptoms consistent with both AD and myocardial ischemia, if the electrocardiogram demonstrates evidence of ST-segment elevation myocardial infarction (STEMI), management should be directed at AMI unless other evidence of AD is present. This recommendation is based on estimates of primary AMI occurring more than 1000 times more frequently than AMI resulting from AD,[40] and the benefit of timely reperfusion in STEMI. When STEMI is present on electrocardiogram and clinical features raise concern for AD, patients who can receive immediate on-site percutaneous intervention (PCI) may be transferred to cardiac catheterization with the plan to perform aortic angiography before coronary artery angiography.[41,42] If PCI is not immediately available, CT aortic angiography may be performed to exclude dissection as preparations are made for usual STEMI reperfusion care (eg, thrombolysis or transfer) (**Fig. 1**). Given the benefit-harm profile associated with usual antiplatelet or anticoagulant agents, in STEMI patients being evaluated for AD, it is reasonable to administer aspirin and hold other treatments until the diagnosis is clarified.

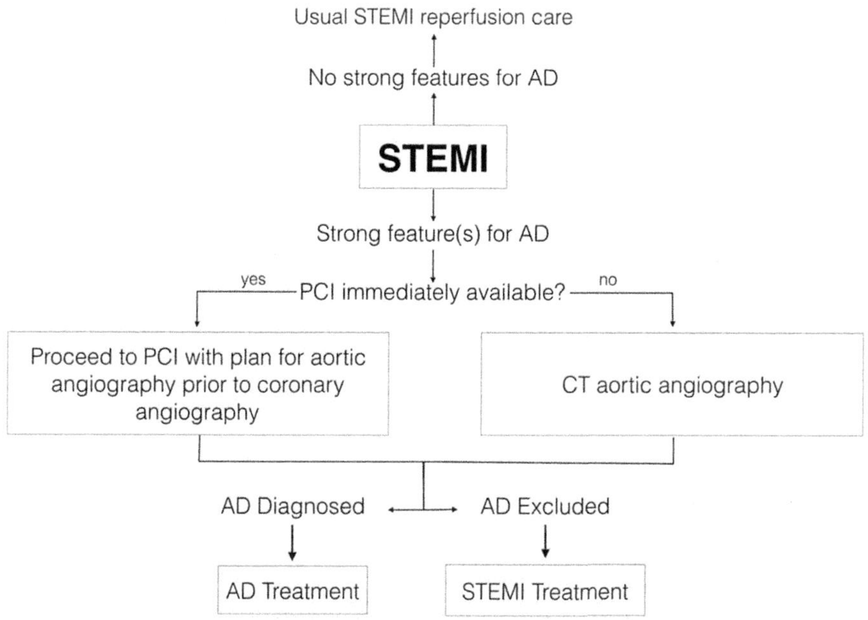

Fig. 1. Relationship between AD and STEMI.

TREATMENT

The primary concern for emergency physicians managing confirmed or highly suspected AD is to arrange for immediate surgical consultation. Though Stanford B dissections may ultimately be managed nonsurgically, all patients with AD should receive prompt surgical evaluation regardless of anatomic location[37] (**Fig. 2**).

The goal of medical therapy in the normotensive or hypertensive patient with AD is to reduce the frequency and magnitude of force bloodflow exerts on the aortic wall. Symptom control is the first priority and is easily overlooked. Patients with AD may have severe pain and anxiety, both of which merit attending to in their own right, but also produce a catecholamine response that directly undermines treatment objectives. Fortunately, unlike the underlying lesion, pain and anxiety are easily managed, and IV opioids (or similarly effective agents but not ketamine, which is catecholaminergic) should be immediately and aggressively titrated to relief of pain as soon as dissection is diagnosed or strongly suspected.

The cornerstone of medical management is beta blockade, titrated to a heart rate of 60 beats per minute. Widely available agents well suited to this purpose include metoprolol and esmolol, with esmolol offering the benefit of minute-to-minute titration. This is particularly advantageous in AD patients who may experience dramatic swings in blood pressure as the lesion evolves and, for example, causes pericardial tamponade or acute aortic insufficiency. Labetalol is widely recommended and is an acceptable alternative; however, labetalol tends to lower blood pressure more reliably than heart

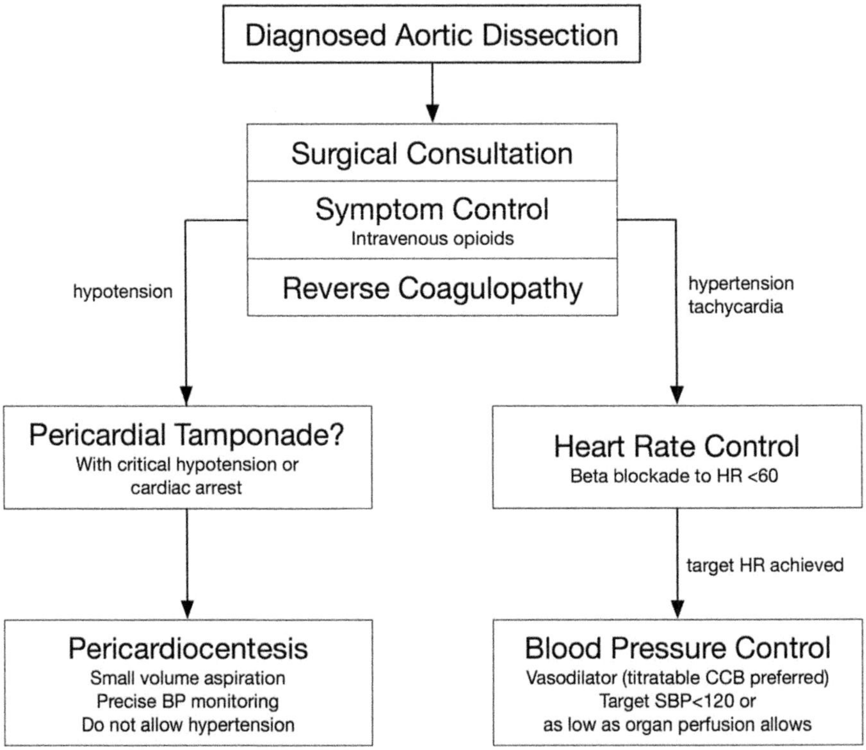

Fig. 2. Management of AD. BP, blood pressure; CCB, calcium channel blocker; HR, heart rate; SBP, systolic blood pressure.

rate.[43] Patients with a strong contraindication to beta blockade should receive IV diltiazem or verapamil for rate control.

When beta blockade has achieved its goal heart rate, blood pressure is the next therapeutic target. If, once heart rate is at or below target, systolic blood pressure is greater than 120 mm Hg, an additional agent should be added to lower blood pressure with a goal of less than 120 mm Hg, ideally titrated to as low a blood pressure as end organs (eg, mentation, skin perfusion) allow. Blood pressure should be measured in both arms and treatments directed at the highest reading. Nicardipine (or its more titratable cousin clevidipine), a parenteral dihydropyridine calcium channel blocker, has emerged as the first-line vasodilator infusion in many centers and is recommended in this context. Nitroprusside is effective and classically used for AD but is more difficult to manage and is associated with adverse effects such as cerebral blood vessel vasodilation[44] and cyanide or thiocyanate toxicity.[45] Fenoldopam, a peripheral dopamine agonist, and enalaprilat, an IV angiotensin-converting enzyme inhibitor, are variously recommended as vasodilator therapies and are both acceptable choices but less easily titratable than the alternatives.[44] Phentolamine, hydralazine, and nifedipine should be avoided in AD if possible. Vasodilator agents should not be administered before control of the heart rate is established with beta receptor or calcium channel blockade because this may result in reflex tachycardia and an increase in aortic wall stress (**Box 4**).

Medical therapies for patients with AD who are hypotensive are of minimal utility and limited to IV crystalloid and vasopressor support, pending surgical management.

Box 4
Medical therapies in aortic dissection (analgesia, heart rate control, blood pressure control)

Preferred therapies

Fentanyl[a]: 1 mcg/kg bolus, then 1 mcg/kg/h

Esmolol[b]: 500 mcg/kg bolus, then 50 mcg/kg/min (repeat bolus if titrating up infusion)

Nicardipine[c]: 5 mg/h, titrated every 5 to 10 minutes, maximum 15 mg/h

Clevidipine[c]: 2 mg/h, titrated every 1 to 2 minutes

Alternative therapies

Morphine[a]: 0.1 mg/kg bolus, then 0.1 mg/kg/h

Labetolol[b]: 0.4 mg/kg bolus, then 1 mg/min

Metoprolol[b]: 0.05 mg/kg every 5 to 10 minutes, maximum 15 mg

Propranolol[b]: 1 mg IV every 5 to 10 minutes, maximum 0.15 mg/kg

Diltiazem[b]: 0.2 mg/kg bolus, then 0.2 mg/kg/h

Verapamil[b]: 0.075 mg/kg bolus, then 0.075 mg/kg/h

Nitroprusside[c]: 0.3 mcg/kg/min, maximum 2 mcg/kg/min

Fenoldopam[c]: 0.1 mcg/kg/min, titrated every 10 to 15 minutes, max 1.6 mcg/kg/min

Enalaprilat[c]: 1.25 mg over 5 minutes every 4 to 6 hours, maximum 5 mg every 6 hours

Nitroglycerine[c]: 20 mcg/min, titrated every 3 to 5 minutes

Doses indicated are starting doses, titrate to effect
[a] Analgesia
[b] Heart rate control
[c] Blood pressure control

Pericardial tamponade is a common cause of hypotension in these cases and small-volume pericardiocentesis, with careful attention not to precipitate hypertension, is an appropriate ED therapy in the arrested or critically hypotensive dissection patient with tamponade.[46,47] Otherwise, all efforts should be focused on expeditious transfer of the patient to the operating theater.

SUMMARY

AD is an uncommon disease that often presents with varied and atypical findings suggestive of more frequently encountered conditions. Therefore, it poses an exceptional diagnostic challenge to emergency providers. Mortality associated with AD is significant at presentation and advances with every hour the lesion is left untreated. Although almost all patients who have symptoms possibly caused by AD will not have AD, key features of the disease, including risk factors, pain characteristics, physical examination findings, and routine ancillary studies, allow clinicians to develop a rational approach to diagnostic testing. When the diagnosis is sufficiently likely to indicate definitive testing, CT angiography is the advanced imaging test of choice in most centers, but TEE and MRI may be appropriate alternatives in certain circumstances. Patients with diagnosed or strongly suspected AD require expeditious surgical evaluation, aggressive analgesia and anxiolysis, and treatment with rapid-acting, titratable agents to first lower heart rate, and then blood pressure, to specific targets.

REFERENCES

1. Klompas M. Does this patient have an acute thoracic aortic dissection? JAMA 2002;287(17):2262–72.
2. Rogers AM, Hermann LK, Booher AM, et al, IRAD Investigators. Sensitivity of the aortic dissection detection risk score, a novel guideline-based tool for identification of acute aortic dissection at initial presentation: results from the international registry of acute aortic dissection. Circulation 2011;123(20):2213–8.
3. Hansen MS, Nogareda GJ, Hutchison SJ. Frequency of and inappropriate treatment of misdiagnosis of acute aortic dissection. Am J Cardiol 2007;99(6): 852–6.
4. Sullivan PR, Wolfson AB, Leckey RD, et al. Diagnosis of acute thoracic aortic dissection in the emergency department. Am J Emerg Med 2000;18(1):46–50.
5. Elefteriades JA, Barrett PW, Kopf GS. Litigation in nontraumatic aortic diseases–a tempest in the malpractice maelstrom. Cardiology 2008;109(4):263–72.
6. Mussa FF, Horton JD, Moridzadeh R, et al. Acute aortic dissection and intramural hematoma: a systematic review. JAMA 2016;316(7):754–63.
7. Tanaka Y, Sakata K, Sakurai Y, et al. Prevalence of type A acute aortic dissection in patients with out-of-hospital cardiopulmonary arrest. Am J Cardiol 2016; 117(11):1826–30.
8. Grock A, Weinstock MB, Jhun P, et al. Aortic dissection! Or is it? Sigh. Ann Emerg Med 2016;68(5):640–2.
9. Hagan PG, Nienaber CA, Isselbacher EM, et al. The International Registry of Acute Aortic Dissection (IRAD): new insights into an old disease. JAMA 2000; 283(7):897–903.
10. Fan KL, Leung LP. Clinical profile of patients of acute aortic dissection presenting to an emergency department without chest pain. Am J Emerg Med 2017;35(4): 599–601.

11. Alter SM, Eskin B, Allegra JR. Diagnosis of aortic dissection in emergency department patients is rare. West J Emerg Med 2015;16(5):629–31.
12. Imamura H, Sekiguchi Y, Iwashita T, et al. Painless acute aortic dissection. - Diagnostic, prognostic and clinical implications. Circ J 2011;75(1):59–66.
13. Kurabayashi M, Miwa N, Ueshima D, et al. Factors leading to failure to diagnose acute aortic dissection in the emergency room. J Cardiol 2011;58(3):287–93.
14. Pape LA, Awais M, Woznicki EM, et al. Presentation, diagnosis, and outcomes of acute aortic dissection: 17-year trends from the international registry of acute aortic dissection. J Am Coll Cardiol 2015;66(4):350–8.
15. Vrsalovic M. Acute aortic dissection associated troponin leak. Am J Emerg Med 2017;35(4):655–6.
16. Akutsu K, Sato N, Yamamoto T, et al. A rapid bedside D-dimer assay (cardiac D-dimer) for screening of clinically suspected acute aortic dissection. Circ J 2005;69(4):397–403.
17. Eggebrecht H, Naber CK, Bruch C, et al. Value of plasma fibrin D-dimers for detection of acute aortic dissection. J Am Coll Cardiol 2004;44(4):804–9.
18. Sodeck G, Domanovits H, Schillinger M, et al. D-Dimer in ruling out acute aortic dissection: a systematic review and prospective cohort study. Eur Heart J 2007;28(24):3067–75.
19. Suzuki T, Distante A, Zizza A, et al. Diagnosis of acute aortic dissection by D-dimer: the international registry of acute aortic dissection substudy on biomarkers (irad-bio) experience. Circulation 2009;119(20):2702–7.
20. Weber T, Högler S, Auer J, et al. D-Dimer in acute aortic dissection. Chest 2003;123(5):1375–8.
21. Diercks DB, Promes SB, Schuur JD, et al. Clinical policy: critical issues in the evaluation and management of adult patients with suspected acute nontraumatic thoracic aortic dissection. Ann Emerg Med 2015;65(1):32–42.e12.
22. Hazui H, Nishimoto M, Hoshiga M, et al. Young adult patients with short dissection length and thrombosed false lumen without ulcer-like projections are liable to have false-negative results of D-dimer testing for acute aortic dissection based on a study of 113 cases. Circ J 2006;70(12):1598–601.
23. Sutherland A, Escano J, Coon TP. D-Dimer as the sole screening test for acute aortic dissection: a review of the literature. Ann Emerg Med 2008;52(4):339–43.
24. Taylor RA, Iyer NS. A decision analysis to determine a testing threshold for computed tomographic angiography and D-dimer in the evaluation of aortic dissection. Am J Emerg Med 2013;31(7):1047–55.
25. Kabrhel C, Matts C, McNamara M, et al. A highly sensitive ELISA D-dimer increases testing but not diagnosis of pulmonary embolism. Acad Emerg Med 2006;13(5):519–24.
26. Zhan S, Hong S, Shan-Shan L, et al. Misdiagnosis of aortic dissection: experience of 361 patients. J Clin Hypertens (Greenwich) 2012;14(4):256–60.
27. Harris KM, Strauss CE, Eagle KA, et al, International Registry of Acute Aortic Dissection (IRAD) Investigators. Correlates of delayed recognition and treatment of acute type A aortic dissection: the International Registry of Acute Aortic Dissection (IRAD). Circulation 2011;124(18):1911–8.
28. Pourafkari L, Tajlil A, Ghaffari S, et al. Electrocardiography changes in acute aortic dissection-association with troponin leak, coronary anatomy, and prognosis. Am J Emerg Med 2016;34(8):1431–6.

29. Sparks SE, Kurz M, Franzen D. Early identification of an atypical case of type A dissection by transthoracic echocardiography by the emergency physician. Am J Emerg Med 2015;33(7):985.e1-3.
30. Evangelista A, Flachskampf FA, Erbel R, et al. Echocardiography in aortic diseases: EAE recommendations for clinical practice. Eur J Echocardiogr 2010; 11(8):645–58.
31. Fojtik JP, Costantino TG, Dean AJ. The diagnosis of aortic dissection by emergency medicine ultrasound. J Emerg Med 2007;32(2):191–6.
32. Perkins AM, Liteplo A, Noble VE. Ultrasound diagnosis of type A aortic dissection. J Emerg Med 2010;38(4):490–3.
33. Blaivas M. Transesophageal echocardiography during cardiopulmonary arrest in the emergency department. Resuscitation 2008;78(2):135–40.
34. Lumbreras B, Vilar J, González-Álvarez I, et al. Evaluation of clinicians' knowledge and practices regarding medical radiological exposure: findings from a mixed-methods investigation (survey and qualitative study). BMJ Open 2016; 6(10):e012361.
35. Lee CI, Haims AH, Monico EP, et al. Diagnostic CT scans: assessment of patient, physician, and radiologist awareness of radiation dose and possible risks. Radiology 2004;231(2):393–8.
36. Laissy JP, Blanc F, Soyer P, et al. Thoracic aortic dissection: diagnosis with transesophageal echocardiography versus MR imaging. Radiology 1995;194(2): 331–6.
37. Hiratzka LF, Bakris GL, Beckman JA, et al. 2010 ACCF/AHA/AATS/ACR/ASA/SCA/SCAI/SIR/STS/SVM guidelines for the diagnosis and management of patients with thoracic aortic disease: a report of the American College of Cardiology Foundation/American Heart Association Task Force on Practice Guidelines, American Association for Thoracic Surgery, American College of Radiology, American Stroke Association, Society of Cardiovascular Anesthesiologists, Society for Cardiovascular Angiography and Interventions, Society of Interventional Radiology, Society of Thoracic Surgeons, and Society for Vascular Medicine. Circulation 2010;121(13):e266–369.
38. Nazerian P, Giachino F, Vanni S, et al. Diagnostic performance of the aortic dissection detection risk score in patients with suspected acute aortic dissection. Eur Heart J Acute Cardiovasc Care 2014;3(4):373–81.
39. Ranasinghe AM, Bonser RS. Biomarkers in acute aortic dissection and other aortic syndromes. J Am Coll Cardiol 2010;56(19):1535–41.
40. Hermann L. Current guidelines for diagnosis and management of thoracic aortic disease in the emergency department. EM Pract Guidel Update 2010; 2(6):1–12.
41. Lentini S, Perrotta S. Aortic dissection with concomitant acute myocardial infarction: from diagnosis to management. J Emerg Trauma Shock 2011;4(2):273–8.
42. Ramanath VS, Eagle KA, Nienaber CA, et al. The role of preoperative coronary angiography in the setting of type A acute aortic dissection: insights from the International Registry of Acute Aortic Dissection. Am Heart J 2011;161(4):790–6.e1.
43. Silke B, Nelson GI, Ahuja RC, et al. Comparative haemodynamic dose response effects of propranolol and labetalol in coronary heart disease. Br Heart J 1982; 48(4):364–71.
44. Haas AR, Marik PE. Current diagnosis and management of hypertensive emergency. Semin Dial 2006;19(6):502–12.
45. Nelson N. Nitroprusside toxicity. Emerg Med 2000;32(10):71–5.

46. Cruz I, Stuart B, Caldeira D, et al. Controlled pericardiocentesis in patients with cardiac tamponade complicating aortic dissection: experience of a centre without cardiothoracic surgery. Eur Heart J Acute Cardiovasc Care 2015;4(2): 124–8.
47. Adler Y, Charron P, Imazio M, et al, European Society of Cardiology (ESC). 2015 ESC Guidelines for the diagnosis and management of pericardial diseases: the Task Force for the Diagnosis and Management of Pericardial Diseases of the European Society of Cardiology (ESC) Endorsed by: the European Association for Cardio-Thoracic Surgery (EACTS). Eur Heart J 2015;36(42):2921–64.

Extracranial Cervical Artery Dissections

Jennifer J. Robertson, MD, MSEd[a], Alex Koyfman, MD[b,*]

KEYWORDS

• Dissection • Stroke • Carotid • Vertebral • Cervical

KEY POINTS

- Cervical artery dissections (CeAD) are rare but important causes of stroke, especially in the younger population.
- Consider CeAD in patients with new-onset headache and neck pain with or without strokelike symptoms.
- Imaging is key to diagnosis, with several options available.
- Management involves treating acute stroke with thrombolysis or surgical therapy for eligible candidates. All others may be candidates for anticoagulation or antiplatelet therapy to reduce the risk of potential or worsening stroke symptoms. Either agent may be used.
- Prognosis remains good with low morbidity and mortality rates.

INTRODUCTION

The cervical arteries comprise bilateral internal carotid and vertebral arteries. These arteries are important structures of the neck, as they carry the main blood flow to the brain. Any thrombosis or damage to these vessels, including dissection, can lead to complications, such as cerebral ischemia, stroke, blindness, or death.[1,2] Although cervical artery dissections (CeADs) are rare causes of stroke overall, they are important causes of stroke in the younger population.[3–5] Unfortunately, given its rarity and nonspecific symptoms, CeAD is a difficult diagnosis to make. Affected patients can remain completely asymptomatic or asymptomatic for long periods of time. Patients may sustain delayed-onset stroke, which can contribute to difficulty in making the diagnosis.[3,6,7] Long-term, severe morbidity, such as stroke with loss of independence, can occur, and, thus, it is important to avoid missing this diagnosis.[8]

Conflict of Interest Disclosure: None. Institutional review board approval not required.
[a] Department of Emergency Medicine, Emory University School of Medicine, 1648 Pierce Drive Northeast, Atlanta, GA 30307, USA; [b] Department of Emergency Medicine, University of Texas-Southwestern, Parkland Hospital, 5323 Harry Hines Boulevard, Dallas, TX 75390, USA
* Corresponding author.
E-mail address: akoyfman8@gmail.com

Emerg Med Clin N Am 35 (2017) 727–741
http://dx.doi.org/10.1016/j.emc.2017.06.006

Although patients with CeAD may deny history of trauma, the reality is that most patients tend to have a history of trauma, albeit very mild.[9,10] In addition, spontaneous extracranial CeAD and extracranial CeADs that develop due to minor trauma are more commonly discussed in the literature.[11–14] This is opposed to pure intracranial CeADs and those due to major trauma and blunt aortic dissection.[3] This article focuses on the epidemiology, pathophysiology, diagnosis, and management of spontaneous extracranial CeADs and extracranial CeADs due to negligible trauma.

EPIDEMIOLOGY

The estimated incidence of CeAD is 2.6 to 5.0 per 100,000 per year, but recent epidemiologic studies are lacking.[5,14–16] An epidemiologic study in 2014 demonstrated that of nearly 1400 patients with stroke, CeAD accounted for only 2% of cases.[16] Most recently, a study in Vancouver found that of 438 patients with transient ischemic attack (TIA) or ischemic stroke, approximately 5.9% were due to CeAD. This percentage included both internal carotid artery dissection (ICAD) and vertebral artery dissection (VAD), but 1 patient did have an intracranial dissection.[17]

Compared with thrombosis, ischemic strokes due to CeAD are rare, approximating a total of only 1% to 2% of all ischemic stroke cases.[15] However, CeAD accounts for a much larger percentage of ischemic strokes in the younger population.[1,3,15] CeAD is most common in the fifth decade of life, and is rare in patients older than 65.[14,18] In the Vancouver study, the mean age of patients with stroke/TIA due to CeAD was 49.1 years.[17] In the 2014 study by Bejot and colleagues,[16] a mean age of 49.1 years also was observed. Overall, the incidence of ICAD is approximately twice that of VAD.[14] VAD tends to occur more commonly in younger women, whereas ICAD is more prevalent in older men.[19,20] Importantly, most epidemiologic studies on CeAD are observational and based on European and American populations, and, thus, the incidence of CeAD is estimated and patterns may differ in other populations.[3,14,16]

PATHOPHYSIOLOGY

The pathogenesis of CeAD is not well delineated. However, as will be mentioned in a subsequent section, CeAD is thought to be caused by minor trauma. It also may occur spontaneously in patients with predisposing arterial defects.[3] CeAD is characterized as a hematoma within the wall of the internal carotid artery or vertebral artery.[3,21] Initially, a tear occurs in the artery where blood enters the wall under pressure and causes separation of the layers. A false lumen develops, resulting in a hematoma. This narrows the arterial lumen, increasing risk of occlusion by the hematoma.[22] The hematoma or thrombus can lead to cerebral thromboembolism, decreased blood flow, and subsequent ischemic stroke.[21,23] The hematoma may also cause a mass effect on surrounding structures, leading to Horner syndrome (ptosis, anhidrosis, and miosis, though anhidrosis may not be present).

Thromboembolism, rather than hypoperfusion, has been found to cause most ischemic strokes in CeAD.[24]

CeAD is likely a multifactorial process that is not well understood but may be related to underlying risk factors, such as genetics, connective tissue diseases, and prior trauma.[3,9,25] It is estimated minor trauma plays a role in approximately 40% of cases of spontaneous extracranial CeAD.[9] In 2013, Engelter and colleagues[9] compared patients with CeAD who had sustained known neck trauma, patients with ischemic stroke with other etiologies, and healthy subjects. Overall, the investigators found that prior mechanical trauma was more common in patients with CeAD than in patients with ischemic stroke from other causes. In addition, neck pain was more common in patients with CeAD than in patients with other causes of stroke.

Despite the suspected role of minor trauma, it is not typical for minor traumas such as whiplash to cause CeAD in most individuals. Thus, it is hypothesized that patients who sustain CeAD with or without minor trauma likely have an underlying arteriopathy, inflammatory process, or structural instability of the arteries.[3,7,25,26] In fact, a 2011 study by Volker and colleagues[25] demonstrated biopsy-proven structural differences in the arterial walls of patients with spontaneous CeAD and those patients who sustained major trauma. There also seems to be a positive association with underlying kinking and coiling of the internal carotid artery and dissection, which suggests an underlying predisposition.[27,28] Of note, the underlying arteriopathy may or may not be permanent, may or may not be genetic, and may be due to inflammation, infection, or other unknown causes.[3]

Other reported underlying risk factors for CeAD include a history of migraine headaches,[29] pregnancy and postpartum states,[30,31] and a history of hypertension.[11] Manual strangulation can lead to CeAD but is considered to be uncommon.[32,33] The diagnosis should be pursued in strangulation victims only if they arrive unconscious, demonstrate physical evidence of neck trauma, have voice changes, or if they show any other unilateral neurologic signs.[33] Finally, even if patients deny trauma, the injury can be minor and may be something as simple as whiplash or stretching.[34,35] Therefore, it is important that CeAD be considered in patients who have risk factors for CeAD with concerning symptoms.

PRESENTATION

Diagnosis of CeAD is challenging, as presentations vary, including asymptomatic, mild cranial nerve deficit, and medullary ischemia leading to respiratory depression.[1,3,7,36] Patients may present with headache only, whereas others may demonstrate disorientation, seizures, back pain, or visual changes.[37–39] Case reports demonstrate some interesting manifestations of CeAD, including tongue swelling,[40] vocal cord paralysis,[41] and cervical radicular nerve pain.[42,43] However, the most common symptoms of CeAD include unilateral headache and/or neck pain, which occur in up to 80% of patients.[14,38,44] The characteristic presentation of ICAD is a partial Horner syndrome without anhidrosis, unilateral head and/or neck pain, and cerebral or retinal ischemia. VAD should be considered in patients with CeAD risk factors and new-onset headache with vertigo or ataxia. Typically, ICAD manifests as a frontal headache, whereas occipital headaches are more common in VAD.[45] Many other neurologic signs can be present.[38,44]

The International Headache Society (IHS) has developed diagnostic criteria called the International Classification of Headache Disorders (ICHD) that clinicians can refer to when considering CeAD.[38] According to the ICHD criteria, CeAD is commonly seen in patients who have sudden-onset headache with facial and/or neck pain that is ipsilateral to the dissected vessel. The pain can be isolated or as a warning sign of impending stroke.[38] Unfortunately, CeAD can mimic benign causes of headache, such as migraines, and therefore, it is important for providers to differentiate patients' "typical" headache symptoms from any new symptoms that could be concerning for CeAD.[38]

Another challenge in making the diagnosis of CeAD is that some patients can remain completely asymptomatic or asymptomatic for long periods of time.[3,7] When symptoms do occur, they typically occur within minutes to hours after the dissection, but may occur up to 1 month after the onset of the dissection.[9,10,12] The average time from the event to onset of symptoms is 2 to 3 days[46] (**Box 1**).

Box 1
Concerning symptoms prompting cervical artery dissection investigation

1. New unilateral headache or neck pain in patients with underlying risk factors, such as a personal history of connective tissue disease, hypertension, or neck trauma
2. Neck pain or a unilateral headache in any patient, but especially young patients, with neurologic deficits on examination
3. A patient with a history of neck trauma with focal neurologic deficits or visible evidence of neck trauma

Data from Refs.[14,38,44]

DIAGNOSIS

As previously mentioned, CeAD can have a wide variety of presentations, mimic benign headaches, and even be asymptomatic for up to 1 month after the actual dissection occurs.[10,12,26,45] Thus, it is not uncommon for diagnostic delays to occur. Although appropriate imaging can help make the diagnosis, patients may require more than 1 study if high clinical suspicion remains and the initial imaging study is normal.[38,45,47] There are several options to image CeAD. These include digital subtraction angiography, ultrasound with or without Doppler, computed tomography angiography (CT-A), and MRI with angiography (MRI/MRA).[45,47,48]

Digital Subtraction Angiography

Digital subtraction angiography (DSA) is considered the gold standard for imaging CeAD due to its capability to determine luminal abnormalities.[49] DSA has limitations, however, in that it is costly, invasive, and inferior in detecting vessel wall abnormalities such as hematomas.[45,48–51] In addition, DSA does not tend to identify the classic features of an intimal flap, double lumen, or dissecting aneurysms.[45,52,53] Thus, angiography may actually be read as normal in certain cases, especially if the hematoma does not cause any disruption of the arterial lumen.[45] DSA also has an associated risk of iatrogenic damage, vascular injury, contrast-induced kidney injury, and radiation exposure.[51]

DSA is quite accurate in finding an intraluminal thrombus and assessing collateral circulation. Thus, it can be considered as a diagnostic modality when other imaging studies are negative, but the diagnosis is still highly considered.[54]

Ultrasound

Ultrasound is a useful screening test, especially because it lacks ionizing radiation, does not require contrast dye, and is noninvasive. It is also helpful for monitoring patients with known CeAD, as serial imaging helps detect possible recanalization or progression to occlusion.[55]

Ultrasound has been reported to be quite sensitive, but may not be reliable for those with only local symptoms and those who have dissections above the angle of the mandible.[3,45,56–58] Ultrasound may be initially interpreted as normal, especially if the mural hematoma results in only small lumen abnormalities or if the dissection is in a specific segment, such as above the angle of the mandible, which is not accessed well by ultrasound.[59] Typically, confirmatory tests with CT-A or MRI/MRA are required, especially if clinical suspicion remains high or the dissection is suspected to be above the angle of the mandible.[3,45,56,58]

Signs of dissection on ultrasound include direct visualization of an intimal flap or mural hematoma as a thickened hypoechoic wall or an increase in the external caliber of the artery.[45,52] Occasionally, stenosis or occlusion can be seen when Doppler is used.[45] It is recommended that Doppler be used if there is a concern for hemodynamic impairment as a cause for the ischemia, even though thromboembolism is the most common cause of stroke from dissection.[24] The main limitation of ultrasound is that it cannot evaluate the entire length of the arteries due to some areas being impenetrable to the ultrasound beam. These areas include the sub and intrapetrous internal carotid artery and the vertebral artery within the bony foramen.[45,56] If CeAD occurs in these areas, ultrasound may not detect abnormalities.[59] Thus, unless there is a very low clinical suspicion for dissection, other tests, such as CT-A or MRI/MRA, should be obtained.[3] In addition, any positive findings on ultrasound should be confirmed with additional imaging studies, as false positives do occur.[58]

MRI/Magnetic Resonance Angiography

The American Heart Association (AHA)/American Stroke Association (ASA) recommends MRI/MRA as one of the first-line imaging studies for diagnosing CeAD.[38,56] Common findings on MRI/MRA include vessel wall thickening, acute ischemic stroke, and direct visualization of intramural hematomas.[44,45] This modality better evaluates for intramural hematomas with less reliance on luminal irregularities.[45,60] Dissections can be evaluated with cross-sectional T1, T2, or protein-density weighted images with MRA methods. This will visualize the intramural hematoma as well as directly evaluate the blood vessels without invasive angiography.[61] MRA also can be combined with MRI to demonstrate acute ischemic lesions.[53] This is especially important with concern for posterior fossa stroke.[50,62]

An acute intramural hematoma can be hypointense on T1-weighted and T2-weighted images and therefore may be hard to detect within the first 48 hours of onset.[53] Thus, a false-negative reading may occur with MRI at early stages, and if there is a high suspicion for CeAD, a different modality or repeat imaging is needed.[53]

Reported sensitivities of MRI/MRA for ICAD range from 78% to 100% and 20% to 94% for VAD.[63–67] Specificities of MRA/MRI for ICAD range from 99% to 100% and 29% to 100% for VAD.[64–67]

Computed Tomography Angiography

CT-A tends to rely on irregularities of the arterial lumen.[60] Signs of dissection on CT-A include increased wall thickening and wall diameter.[52] There are very few other direct findings of CeAD on CT-A.[45] However, CT-A does seem to be superior in demonstrating spatial resolution for severely narrowed vessels and may show intimal flaps better than MRI/MRA.[50] CT-A may also be better than MRI/MRA in diagnosing VAD because of the tortuous course of the VA, its close proximity to bone, and the typically smaller size of the mural hematoma.[62] Another concern with MRI/MRA in the diagnosis of VAD is that sometimes the perivertebral venous plexus can mimic similar intensity of a mural hematoma and thus, can falsely diagnose VAD.[62] CT-A may be less accurate if heavy calcifications are present.[47,68] Sensitivities of CT-A range from 47% to 100% for ICAD and 40% to 100% for VAD.[63,64,69,70] Specificities range from 88% to 99% for ICAD and 90% to 99% for VAD.[64,69–72] CT-A is recommended by the AHA, the ASA, and the IHS as an initial test for CeAD.[38,56] Based on several studies, CT-A is preferential in the diagnosis of VAD.[50,52,69]

Drawbacks to the use of CT-A in the diagnosis of dissection include exposure to ionizing radiation and decreased ability to directly visualize a mural hematoma.[45,73] Despite its superiority in detecting VAD, CT-A is unable to adequately detect posterior fossa ischemic lesions, so if concern for posterior circulation stroke is present, additional imaging with MRI should be obtained.[50,62] CT-A also cannot be used in patients with renal impairment or in those who have allergies to CT contrast.

TREATMENT

Because CeAD can cause stroke and significant disability, the major goals of treatment are twofold[1]: acutely save at-risk brain tissue and[2] prevent further ischemia and strokes from occurring.[74] Typically, antithrombotic treatment is recommended to reduce the risk of stroke within the first few days of dissection.[12] However, there are other options for treatment, including intravenous and intra-arterial thrombolysis and surgical or endovascular repair.[12,47,56,75–80]

Until recently, no randomized controlled trials (RCTs) had been conducted solely comparing anticoagulation versus antiplatelet agents.[13,21,74] There have been no known RCTs on thrombolysis or surgical therapy, but based on available data, these do remain options for eligible patients.[3,13,48,56,74–78,81–84] Treatments have been mostly based on case series, meta-analyses, case reports, and clinician discretion.[3,74] Although the focus of this article is on extracranial CeAD, some of the treatment regimens discussed as follows do not differentiate between intracranial and extracranial CeAD.

Thrombolysis

Stroke in patients with CeAD is most commonly caused by thrombosis.[21,23,24,85] Thrombolysis treats acute ischemic stroke through recanalization of an occluded artery.[78,83] It may include intra-arterial or intravenous thrombolysis. So far, no RCT has exclusively evaluated thrombolysis as a treatment for CeAD.[76,86] The original trials on the use of intravenous thrombolysis in acute stroke included those patients with CeAD,[78,83] so it still remains an option for those patients with CeAD who meet thrombolysis criteria.[74–76,78,82,83,87] Unfortunately, the AHA/ASA does not directly address the use of thrombolysis in CeAD, and there are no known specific guidelines available.[47,56]

The major risk of thrombolysis in any patient is spontaneous intracranial hemorrhage.[47] In theory, thrombolysis may promote worsening perfusion by leading to more intramural bleeding.[75,82] In addition, thrombolytics may potentially lyse the thrombus within the wall of the artery, leading to increased wall forces and dissection expansion.[76] However, it is thought that thrombolysis may improve flow by diminishing the size of the thrombus.[76] In the past 10 years, several nonrandomized studies have evaluated the use of both intravenous and intra-arterial thrombolysis in CeAD. Some included both intravenous and intra-arterial, and others evaluated one.[75,76,82,87–93] Based on these studies, both intra-arterial and intravenous thrombolysis have shown safety outcomes in patients with CeAD similar to those patients with nondissection stroke.[75,76,86,88,90,93] On the other hand, the actual efficacy of thrombolysis remains in question.[76,82,88] A 2012 multicenter study comparing patients with extracranial CeAD stroke who received intra-arterial and/or intravenous thrombolysis or no thrombolysis found essentially no difference in favorable 3-month outcomes, defined as a modified Rankin score (mRS) of 0 to 2.[94] Similarly, in a retrospective database study by Qureshi and colleagues,[76] no differences in in-hospital mortality and minimal disability were found between patients with CeAD stroke treated with thrombolysis and patients with CeAD not treated with thrombolysis. In a 2012 prospective observational study by Fuentes and colleagues,[88] patients with extracranial ICAD treated with thrombolysis tended to have similar 3-month outcomes (mRS) as those patients with

ICAD not treated with thrombolysis. A 2011 meta-analysis of both intra-arterial and intravenous thrombolysis in CeAD essentially demonstrated similar findings and concluded that both intra-arterial and intravenous thrombolysis in patients with CeAD show similar safety and overall outcomes compared with patients with stroke without CeAD.[75]

Most recently, there have been more studies on the safety and efficacy of intravenous and intra-arterial thrombolysis in cervical artery dissection and continue to confirm prior studies' results.[87,92,93] A 2015 prospective multicenter study and meta-analysis evaluated the safety and efficacy of intravenous thrombolysis in CeAD.[93] In the investigators' prospective study of 39 patients with dissection-related stroke, the rate of spontaneous intracranial hemorrhage was 0% and in-hospital mortality was 10%, whereas full recanalization and favorable functional outcome (mRS of 0–1) were 55% and 61%, respectively.[93] In their meta-analysis of 10 case series with a total of 234 patients, the investigators found pooled rates of spontaneous intracranial hemorrhage to be 2%, with a mortality rate of 4%. The pooled complete recanalization rate was 45%, whereas the favorable functional outcome rate was 41%. Based on this case series and meta-analysis, the investigators conclude that intravenous thrombolysis is just as safe in patients with CeAD stroke as in patients with nondissection ischemic stroke. In addition, the rates of favorable functional outcomes did not differ between patients with nondissection stroke and patients with stroke due to CeAD.[93] Similar results have been found in other studies evaluating intra-arterial thrombolysis.[87,92] Based on the current data, intravenous thrombolysis should not be withheld in those eligible patients with stroke due to CeAD.[93]

Antiplatelet/Anticoagulant Medications

In most patients with CeAD, the arterial lumen will heal on its own with a mean healing time of 3 months.[45] The main goal of treating these patients is preventing stroke in the acute phase of CeAD via anticoagulation or antiplatelet agents.[3,12,13,56] The 2011 AHA/ASA guidelines recommend treatment with either an anticoagulant, such as heparin or warfarin, or a platelet inhibitor, such as aspirin or clopidogrel, for at least 3 to 6 months.[56]

The AHA/ASA does not specify a preferred regimen. Several nonrandomized studies and meta-analyses showed no significant differences between the 2 agents, leaving the decision up to clinicians.[95–98]

Until recently, no RCT had been conducted on comparing antiplatelet versus anticoagulation for CeAD.[12,13] In 2007, a multicenter RCT, named the Cervical Artery Dissection in Stroke Study (CADISS), evaluated the efficacy of antiplatelet agents versus anticoagulation therapy in acute (within 7 days of onset) extracranial CeAD.[12]

In CADISS, antiplatelet agents included aspirin, dipyridamole, and/or clopidogrel, and anticoagulation agents included heparin followed by warfarin for at least 3 months. The investigators excluded intracranial dissections, those with symptom onset of more than 7 days, those already on an antiplatelet or anticoagulation agents, pregnant patients, and those with contraindications to antiplatelet or anticoagulant agents. The primary endpoint was recurrent stroke and death at 3 months, but patients were followed for 12 months. Secondary endpoints were ipsilateral TIA, stroke, death of any cause, major bleeding, or residual stenosis. The investigators enrolled 250 patients with ICAD and VAD between 2006 and 2013. The included patients presented with variable symptoms, such as stroke or TIA, and local symptoms, such as headache, neck pain, and Horner syndrome.

The CADISS data were published in early 2015 and the investigators found no difference in the efficacy of antiplatelet versus anticoagulant medications at preventing stroke and death in CeAD.[13] Overall, only 4 (2%) of 250 patients had stroke recurrence, 3 in the antiplatelet group and 1 in the anticoagulant group. One major bleed in the anticoagulant group occurred, with no deaths. The investigators note no major differences in the other secondary endpoints between the 2 treatment groups.[13] Therefore, similar to prior nonrandomized studies, the investigators concluded no difference in the efficacy of antiplatelet and anticoagulant medications at preventing stroke and death in patients with symptomatic ICAD and VAD.[13]

CADISS is a phase 2 feasibility study. The investigators planned a sample size of 250 to allow for an estimation of recurrent stroke and sample sizes for a phase 3 trial to be calculated. Essentially, CADISS is not powered enough to draw final conclusions between the use of antiplatelet and anticoagulant drugs.[99] The investigators note that up to 10,000 patients would be needed to detect a 1% difference in the occurrence of stroke or death or major bleeding between the 2 agents.[13] In addition, novel oral anticoagulants (NOACs) were not included in this trial, and given the popularity of these agents, it would be reasonable for future RCTs to include the NOACs. However, based on this clinical trial, either agent is reasonable to use in those patients with extracranial CeAD who do not require surgery or endovascular repair.

Surgical and Endovascular Repair

Although data on surgical therapy are limited, most investigators state that candidates for procedural therapy include those with recurrent ischemia despite medical treatment, patients with contraindications to anticoagulants or antiplatelet medications, patients with significantly compromised cerebral blood flow or with severe occlusion or luminal narrowing, and those with enlarging pseudoaneurysms.[3,48,80,81,84,86,100]

Recently, Moon and colleagues[100] followed 116 patients with extracranial CeAD treated with endovascular therapy for a mean of 41.6 months. Endovascular therapy included stent placement, coil occlusion of a parent artery, and stenting with contralateral vessel coil occlusion. Overall, the investigators found the patients with ICAD were more likely to have enlarging pseudoaneurysms, thromboembolic events, and failed medical therapy when compared with patients with VAD. Patients with ICAD were more likely to undergo stent placement. Importantly, the overall stroke rate was only 0.9% over 2825 patient years, and no patients worsened with regard to mRS after stent placement. The investigators conclude that endovascular intervention is effective and that it may be more relevant for those with failed medical therapy, pseudoaneurysms, and significant thrombotic events.[100]

The AHA/ASA recommends that angioplasty and stenting be considered when ischemic neurologic symptoms have not responded to medical therapy.[56] The AHA/ASA makes these recommendations only for ICAD and not VAD. They also do not mention exactly when medical therapy should be abandoned for surgical intervention. Nevertheless, several other studies have been conducted on endovascular repair of ICAD as well as VAD with successful results regarding safety and recurrent stroke[77,79,80,84,100–105] (**Box 2**).

PROGNOSIS

Overall, most patients with CeAD tend to do well. Most heal within 3 to 12 months, and based on the current literature available, short-term morbidity and mortality tend to be rare.[14,16,20,106] The risk of recurrent TIA or stroke in the first 3 to 6 months after dissection varies from 1.4% to 16.7%, but treatment regimens differ in the literature.[20,96,106] In a 2013 analysis of 970 patients with CeAD, 3-month follow-up was obtained, showing 2.3% recurrent TIA and 1.4% recurrent stroke.[20] Similarly, in the CADISS trial,

Box 2
Summary of treatment regimens

1. Thrombolysis for patients meeting thrombolytic criteria as in patients with nonthrombotic stroke.
2. Prevention of further stroke symptoms with an antiplatelet or anticoagulant medication.
3. Surgical or endovascular therapy for recurrent ischemia despite medical treatment, patients with contraindications to anticoagulants or antiplatelet medications, patients with severe occlusion or luminal narrowing, those with pseudoaneurysms, and patients with significantly compromised cerebral blood flow.

Data from Refs.[3,13,48,56,78,83,84,86]

only 2% of patients had recurrent stroke at 3 months, and all were in patients whose presenting symptoms were stroke.[13] Investigators also have observed relatively low mortality rates of both ICAD and VAD, ranging from 1.9% to 5.0%.[20,45,107]

Patients with CeAD who present with stroke have higher initial National Institutes of Health (NIH) scores, and have occlusive CeAD tend to do worse, while those with localized symptoms, such as headache, neck pain, tinnitus, and Horner syndrome, tend to have better overall outcomes, at least in the short term.[3,22,96] Most recently, a 2016 study followed 128 patients with CeAD over a period of 25 months and evaluated for favorable outcomes as defined by an mRS of 0 to 1. These patients were categorized by radiographic features including aneurysmal CeAD, stenotic CeAD, and occlusive CeAD. Accounting for NIH scores, types of therapy, and transcranial Doppler ultrasound results in the occlusive group, the aneurysmal and stenotic groups showed favorable outcomes, whereas the occlusive group was less favorable. Abnormal flow was on ultrasound was associated with stroke progression and overall poor outcomes, demonstrating that patients with occlusive CeAD with more severe flow abnormalities on ultrasound tend to do worse than the aneurysmal and stenotic subtypes of CeAD.[108]

SUMMARY

CeAD is a rare cause of stroke but should remain high on the differential in younger patients who present with strokelike symptoms. Patients may or may not report trauma, but CeAD can occur in patients who have sustained mild neck trauma. Imaging is key to diagnosis, and although various modalities can be used, MRI with MRA and CT-A are currently the recommended imaging studies. Strokelike symptoms are thought to be mostly due to thromboembolism, and anticoagulation or antiplatelet agents are the mainstay of treatment. Based on the current data, no differences have been seen between the 2 agents. Thrombolysis and surgical therapy are also options for treatment but will vary based on the patient. The NIH criteria should be applied as in non-CeAD stroke patients. Those with severe occlusion or pseudoaneurysm may require surgical therapy but will also be on a case-by-case basis. Overall prognosis tends to be good with rare exceptions. Patients who present with more severe stroke symptoms tend to fare worse, whereas those with localized symptoms have better overall outcomes.

REFERENCES

1. Kishi S, Kanaji K, Doi T, et al. A case of traumatic intracranial vertebral artery injury presenting with life threatening symptoms. Int Med Case Rep J 2012;5: 23–8.

2. Debette S, Grond-Ginsbach C, Bodenant M. Differential features of carotid and vertebral artery dissections. The CADISP study. Neurology 2011;77:1174–81.
3. Debette S, Leys D. Cervical-artery dissections: predisposing factors, diagnosis, and outcome. Lancet Neurol 2009;8:668–78.
4. Kristensen B, Malm J, Carlberg B, et al. Epidemiology and etiology of ischemic stroke in young adults aged 18 to 44 years in northern Sweden. Stroke 1997; 28(9):1702–9.
5. Schievink WI, Roiter V. Epidemiology of cervical artery dissection. Front Neurol Neurosci 2005;20:12–5.
6. Lichy C, Metso A, Pezzini A, et al. Predictors of delayed stroke in patients with cervical artery dissection. Int J Stroke 2015;10(3):360–3.
7. Grond-Ginsbach C, Metso TM, Metso AJ, et al. Cervical artery dissection goes frequently undiagnosed. Med Hypotheses 2013;80:787–90.
8. Leys D, Bandu L, Henon H, et al. Clinical outcome in 287 consecutive young adults (15 to 45 years) with ischemic stroke. Neurology 2002;59(1):26–33.
9. Engelter ST, Grond-Ginsbach C, Metso TM, et al. Cervical artery dissection: trauma and other potential mechanical trigger events. Neurology 2013;80: 1950–7.
10. Arauz A, Hoyos L, Espinoza C, et al. Dissection of cervical arteries: long-term follow-up study of 130 consecutive cases. Cerebrovasc Dis 2006;22(2–3): 150–4.
11. Debette S, Metso TM, Pezzini A, et al. CADISP genetics: an international project searching for genetic risk factors of cervical artery dissections. Int J Stroke 2009;4(3):224–30.
12. Cervical Artery Dissection in Stroke Study Trial Investigators. Antiplatelet therapy vs. anticoagulation in cervical artery dissection: rationale and design of the cervical artery dissection in stroke study (CADISS). Int J Stroke 2007;2(4): 292.
13. CADISS Trial Investigators. Antiplatelet treatment compared with anticoagulation treatment for cervical artery dissection (CADISS): a randomised trial. Lancet Neurol 2015;14(4):361–7.
14. Lee VH, Brown RD, Mandrekar JN, et al. Incidence and outcome of cervical artery dissection. A population-based study. Neurology 2006;67:1809–12.
15. Giroud M, Fayolle H, Andre N, et al. Incidence of internal carotid artery dissection in the community of Dijon. J Neurol Neurosurg Psychiatry 1994;57(11):1443.
16. Bejot Y, Daubail B, Debette S, et al. Incidence and outcome of cerebrovascular events related to cervical artery dissection: the Dijon stroke registry. Int J Stroke 2014;9:879–82.
17. Wilson L, Salmeen A, Field T, et al. Cervical artery dissections in the Vancouver General Hospital (VGH) stroke database: a common stroke mechanism? Neurology 2015;84(14 Suppl):P5–161.
18. Giossi A, Ritelli M, Costa P, et al. Connective tissue anomalies in patients with spontaneous cervical artery dissection. Neurology 2014;83:2032–7.
19. Metso TM, Debette S, Grond-Ginsbach C, et al. Age-dependent differences in cervical artery dissection. J Neurol 2012;259:2202–10.
20. VonBabo M, De Marchis GM, Sarikaya H, et al. Differences and similarities between spontaneous dissections of the internal carotid artery and the vertebral artery. Stroke 2013;44:1537–42.
21. Kim YK, Schulman S. Cervical artery dissection: pathology, epidemiology and management. Thromb Res 2009;123(6):810–21.

22. Lyrer PA, Brandt T, Metso TM, et al. Clinical import of Horner syndrome in internal carotid and vertebral artery dissection. Neurology 2014;82:1653–9.
23. Callaghan FM, Luechinger R, Kurtcuglu V, et al. Wall stress of the cervical carotid artery in patients with carotid dissection: a case-control study. Am J Physiol Heart Circ Physiol 2011;300(4):H1451–8.
24. Morel A, Naggara O, Touze E, et al. Mechanism of ischemic infarct in spontaneous cervical artery dissection. Stroke 2012;43:1354–61.
25. Volker W, Dittrich R, Nassenstein I, et al. The outer arterial wall layers are primarily affected in spontaneous cervical artery dissection. Neurology 2011;76:1463–71.
26. Debette S. Pathophysiology and risk factors of cervical artery dissection: what have we learnt from large hospital-based cohorts? Curr Opin Neurol 2014;27(1):20–8.
27. Saba L, Argiolas GM, Sumer S, et al. Association between internal carotid artery dissection and arterial tortuosity. Neuroradiology 2015;57:149–53.
28. Pelkonen O, Tikkakoski T, Leinonen S, et al. Extracranial internal carotid and vertebral artery dissections: angiographic spectrum, course and prognosis. Neuroradiology 2003;45(2):71–7.
29. Rist PM, Diener HC, Kurth T, et al. Migraine, migraine aura, and cervical artery dissection: a systematic review and meta-analysis. Cephalalgia 2011;31(8):886–96.
30. Mohammed I, Aaland M, Khan N, et al. A young pregnant woman with spontaneous carotid artery dissection-unknown mechanisms. BMJ Case Rep 2014;2014 [pii:bcr2013202541].
31. Mujtaba M, Kelsey MD, Saeed MA. Spontaneous carotid artery dissection: a rare cause of stroke in pregnancy and approach to diagnosis and management. Conn Med 2014;78(6):349–52.
32. Malek AM, Higashida RT, Halbach VV, et al. Patient presentation, angiographic features and treatment of strangulation-induced bilateral dissection of the cervical internal carotid artery. Report of three cases. J Neurosurg 2000;92(3):481–7.
33. Stapczynski JS. Strangulation injuries. Emerg Med Rep 2010;31(17):193–203.
34. Hauser V, Zangger P, Winter Y, et al. Late sequelae of whiplash injury with dissection of cervical arteries. Eur Neurol 2010;64:214–8.
35. Hwang DY, Pless ML. How can stretching maneuvers involving the neck cause vertebral artery dissection and transient ischemic attack? J Occup Environ Med 2010;52(7):764–5.
36. Arnolder C, Riss D, Wagenblast J. Tenth and twelfth nerve palsies in a patient with internal carotid artery dissection mistaken for cervical mass lesion. Skull Base 2010;20(4):301–4.
37. Fantaneanu T, Veinot JP, Torres C, et al. Cervical arterial dissections due to segmental mediolytic arteriopathy. Neurology 2011;77(3):295–7.
38. Headache Classification Committee of the International Headache Society (IHS). The international classification of headache disorders, 3rd edition (beta version). Cephalalgia 2013;33:629–808.
39. Amin FM, Larsen VA, Tfelt-Hansen P. Vertebral artery dissection associated with generalized convulsive seizures: a case report. Case Rep Neurol 2013;5(2):125–9.
40. Ryan P, Rehman S, Prince S. Acute tongue swelling, the only initial manifestation of carotid artery dissection: a case report with differentiation of clinical picture. Ann Vasc Surg 2015;29:365.e17-8.

41. Nguygen TTJ, Zhang H, Dziegielewski PT, et al. Vocal cord paralysis secondary to spontaneous internal carotid dissection: case report and systematic review of the literature. J Otolaryngol Head Neck Surg 2013;42:34.
42. Quinn C, Salameh J. Vertebral artery dissection causing an acute C5 radiculopathy. Neurology 2013;81(12):1101.
43. Silbert BI, Khangure M, Silbert PL. Vertebral artery dissection as a cause of cervical radiculopathy. Asian Spine J 2013;7(4):335–8.
44. Thomas LC, Rivett DA, Attia JR, et al. Risk factors and clinical features of craniocervical arterial dissection. Man Ther 2011;16:351–6.
45. Hassen WB, Machet A, Edjlali-Goujon M, et al. Imaging of cervical artery dissection. Diagn Interv Imaging 2014;95:1151–61.
46. Biousse V, D'Anglejan-Chatillion V, Touboul J, et al. Time course of symptoms in extracranial carotid artery dissections. A series of 80 patients. Stroke 1995; 26(2):235–9.
47. Jauch EC, Saver JL, Adams HP, et al. Guidelines for the early management of patients with acute ischemic stroke. A guideline for healthcare professionals from the American Heart Association/American Stroke Association. Stroke 2013;44:870–947.
48. Medel RM, Starke RM, Valle-Giler EP, et al. Diagnosis and treatment of arterial dissections. Curr Neurol Neurosci Rep 2014;14:419.
49. Cuvinciuc V, Viallon M, Momjian-Mayor I, et al. 3D fat-saturated T1 SPACE sequence for the diagnosis of cervical artery dissection. Neuroradiology 2013;55(5):595–602.
50. Vertinksy AT, Schwartz NE, Fischbein NJ, et al. Comparison of multidetector CT angiography and MR imaging of cervical artery dissection. AJNR Am J Neuroradiol 2008;29:1753–60.
51. Fusco MR, Harrigan MR. Cerebrovascular dissections—a review part I: spontaneous dissections. Neurosurgery 2011;68(1):242–57.
52. Teasdale E, Zampakis P, Santosh C, et al. Multidetector computed tomography angiography: application in vertebral artery dissection. Ann Indian Acad Neurol 2011;14:35–41.
53. Flis CM, Jager HR, Sidhu PS. Carotid and vertebral artery dissections: clinical aspects, imaging features and endovascular treatment. Eur Radiol 2007; 17(3):820–34.
54. Nazzal M, Herial NA, MacNealy MW. Diagnostic imaging in carotid artery dissection: a case report and review of current modalities. Ann Vasc Surg 2014;28:739.e5-9.
55. Steinke W, Rautenberg W, Schwartz A, et al. Noninvasive monitoring of internal carotid artery dissection. Stroke 1994;125(5):998–1005.
56. Brott TG, Halerin JL, Abbara S, et al. 2011 ASA/ACCF/AHA/AANN/AANS/ACR/ASNR/CNS/SAIP/SCAI/SIR/SNIS/SVM/SVS guideline on the management of patients with extracranial carotid and vertebral artery disease. Circulation 2011; 124:e54–130.
57. Arnold M, Baumgartner RW, Stapf C, et al. Ultrasound diagnosis of spontaneous carotid dissection with isolated Horner syndrome. Stroke 2008;39(1):82–6.
58. Benninger DH, Georgiadis D, Gandjour J, et al. Accuracy of color duplex ultrasound diagnosis of spontaneous carotid dissection causing ischemia. Stroke 2006;37(2):377–81.
59. Dittrich R, Nassenstein I, Bachmann R, et al. Polyarterial clustered recurrence of cervical artery dissection seems to be the rule. Neurology 2007;69(2):180–6.

60. Steinsiepe VK, Jung S, Goeggel-Simonetti B, et al. Spontaneous cervical artery dissections. Austin J Clin Neurol 2014;1(3):1012.
61. Goldberg HI, Grossman RI, Gomori JM, et al. Cervical internal carotid artery dissecting hemorrhage: diagnosis using MR. Radiology 1986;158(1):157–61.
62. Naggara O, Soares F, Touze E, et al. Is it possible to recognize cervical artery dissection on stroke brain MR imaging? A matched case-control study. AJNR Am J Neuroradiol 2011;32(5):869–73.
63. Zuber M, Meary E, Meder JF, et al. Magnetic resonance imaging and dynamic CT scan in cervical artery dissections. Stroke 1994;25:576–81.
64. Miller PR, Fabian TC, Croce MA, et al. Prospective screening for blunt cerebrovascular injuries: analysis of diagnostic modalities and outcomes. Ann Surg 2002;236:386–93.
65. Levy C, Laissy JP, Raveau V, et al. Carotid and vertebral artery dissections: three-dimensional time-of-flight MR angiography and MR imaging versus conventional angiography. Radiology 1994;190:97–103.
66. Stingaris K, Liberopoulos K, Giaka E, et al. Three-dimensional time-of-flight MR angiography and MR imaging versus conventional angiography in carotid artery dissections. Int Angiol 1996;1(1):20–5.
67. Auer A, Felber S, Schmidauer C, et al. Magnetic resonance angiography and clinical features of extracranial vertebral artery dissection. J Neurol Neurosurg Psychiatry 1998;64:474–81.
68. Mozayan M, Sexton C. Imaging of carotid artery dissection. J Community Hosp Intern Med Perspect 2012;2:18645.
69. Chen CJ, Tseng YC, Lee TH, et al. Multisection CT angiography compared with catheter angiography in diagnosing vertebral artery dissection. AJNR Am J Neuroradiol 2004;25:769–74.
70. Malhotra AK, Camacho M, Ivatury RR, et al. Computed tomographic angiography for the diagnosis of blunt carotid/vertebral artery injury: a note of caution. Ann Surg 2007;246:632–43.
71. Bub LD, Hollingworth W, Jarvik JG, et al. Screening for blunt cerebrovascular injury: evaluating the accuracy of multidetector computed tomographic angiography. J Trauma 2005;59:691–7.
72. Pugliese F, Crusco F, Cardaioli G, et al. CT angiography versus colour-Doppler US in acute dissection of the vertebral artery. Radiol Med 2007;112:435–43.
73. Fred HL. Drawbacks and limitations of computed tomography: views from a medical educator. Tex Heart Inst J 2004;31(4):345.
74. Arnold M, Fischer U, Bousser MG. Treatment issues in spontaneous cervicocephalic artery dissections. Int J Stroke 2011;6:213–8.
75. Zinkstock SM, Vergouwen MDI, Engelter ST, et al. Safety and functional outcome of thrombolysis in dissection-related ischemic stroke: a meta-analysis of individual patient data. Stroke 2011;42:2515–20.
76. Qureshi AI, Chaudhry SA, Hassan AE, et al. Thrombolytic treatment of patients with acute ischemic stroke related to underlying arterial dissection in the United States. Arch Neurol 2011;68(12):1536–42.
77. Asif KS, Lazzaro MA, Teleb MS, et al. Endovascular reconstruction for progressively worsening carotid artery dissection. J Neurointerv Surg 2015;7:32–9.
78. National Institute of Neurological Disorders and Stroke rt-PA Stroke Study Group. Tissue plasminogen activator for acute ischemic stroke. N Engl J Med 1995;333:1581–7.

79. Pham MH, Rahme RJ, Arnaout O, et al. Endovascular stenting of extracranial carotid and vertebral artery dissections: a systematic review of the literature. Neurosurgery 2011;68:856–66.
80. Alhelm F, Benz RM, Ulmer S, et al. Endovascular treatment of cervical artery dissection: ten case reports and review of the literature. Interv Neurol 2012;1: 143–50.
81. Biffl WL, Moore EE, Offner PJ, et al. Blunt carotid arterial injuries: implications of a new grading scale. J Trauma 1999;47(5):845–53.
82. Engelter ST, Rutgers MP, Hatz F, et al. Intravenous thrombolysis in stroke attributable to cervical artery dissection. Stroke 2009;40:3772–6.
83. Hacke W, Kaste M, Bluhmki E, et al. Thrombolysis with alteplase 3 to 4.5 hours after acute ischemic stroke. N Engl J Med 2008;359:1317–29.
84. Xianjun H, Zhiming Z. A systematic review of endovascular management of internal carotid artery dissections. Interv Neurol 2012;1:164–70.
85. Tsivgoulis G, Safouris A, Alexandrov AV. Safety of intravenous thrombolysis for acute ischemic stroke in specific conditions. Expert Opin Drug Saf 2015; 14(6):845–64.
86. Georgiadis D, Caso V, Baumgartner RW. Acute therapy and prevention of stroke in spontaneous carotid dissection. Clin Exp Hypertens 2006;28:365–70.
87. Jensen J, Salottolo K, Frei D, et al. Comprehensive analysis of intra-arterial treatment for acute ischemic stroke due to cervical artery dissection. J Neurointerv Surg 2017;9(7):654–8.
88. Fuentes B, Masjuan J, de Lecin MA, et al. Benefits of intravenous thrombolysis in acute ischemic stroke related to extracranial internal carotid dissection. Dream or reality? Int J Stroke 2012;7:7–13.
89. Cohen JE, Gomori JM, Grigoriadis S, et al. Intra-arterial thrombolysis and stent placement for traumatic carotid dissection with subsequent stroke: a combined, simultaneous endovascular approach. J Neurol Sci 2008;269:172–5.
90. Lavalee PC, Mazighi M, Stain-Maurice JP, et al. Stent-assisted endovascular thrombolysis versus intravenous thrombolysis in internal carotid artery dissection with tandem internal carotid and middle cerebral artery occlusion. Stroke 2007;38:2270–4.
91. Cerratto P, Berardino M, Bottachhi E, et al. Vertebral artery dissection complicated by basilar artery occlusion successfully treated with intra-arterial thrombolysis: three case reports. Neurol Sci 2008;29:51–5.
92. Lin J, Sun Y, Zhao S, et al. Safety and efficacy of thrombolysis in cervical artery dissection-related ischemic stroke: a meta-analysis of observational studies. Cerebrovasc Dis 2016;42(3–4):272–9.
93. Tsivgoulis G, Zand R, Katsanos AH, et al. Safety and outcomes of intravenous thrombolysis in dissection-related ischemic stroke: an international multicenter study and comprehensive meta-analysis of reported case series. J Neurol 2015;262(9):2135–43.
94. Engelter ST, Dallongeville J, Kloss M, et al. Thrombolysis in cervical artery dissection–data from the cervical artery dissection and ischaemic stroke patients (CADISP) database. Eur J Neurol 2012;19:1199–206.
95. Menon R, Kerry S, Norris JW, et al. Treatment of cervical artery dissection: a systematic review and meta-analysis. J Neurol Neurosurg Psychiatry 2008;79: 1122–7.
96. Yaghi S, Maalouf N, Keyrouz SG. Cervical artery dissection: risk factors, treatment, and outcome; a 5 year experience from a tertiary care center. Int J Neurosci 2012;122:40–4.

97. Georgiadis D, Arnold M, vonBuedingen HC, et al. Aspirin vs anticoagulation in carotid artery dissection. A study of 298 patients. Neurology 2009;72:1810–5.
98. Arauz A, Ruiz A, Pacheco G, et al. Aspirin versus anticoagulation in intra- and extracranial vertebral artery dissection. Eur J Neurol 2013;20:167–72.
99. Conforto AB. Challenges in diagnosis and treatment of cervico-cephalic arterial dissections. Arq Neuropsiquiatr 2016;74(4):273–4.
100. Moon K, Albuquerque F, Cole TS, et al. 355 Endovascular management of cervical carotid and vertebral artery dissection: indications, techniques, and outcomes from a 20-year experience. Neurosurgery 2016;63:205.
101. Kashiwazaki D, Ushikoshi S, Asano T, et al. Long-term clinical and radiological results of endovascular internal trapping in vertebral artery dissection. Neuroradiology 2013;55(2):201–6.
102. Hernandez-Duran S, Ogilvy CS. Clinical outcomes of patients with vertebral artery dissection treated endovascularly: a meta-analysis. Neurosurg Rev 2014; 37:569–77.
103. Ohta H, Natarajan SK, Hauck EF, et al. Endovascular stent therapy for extracranial and intracranial carotid artery dissection: single-center experience. J Neurosurg 2011;115:91–100.
104. Sadato A, Maeda S, Hayakawa M, et al. Endovascular treatment of vertebral artery dissection using stents and coils: its pitfall and technical considerations. Minim Invasive Neurosurg 2010;53:243–9.
105. Stella N, Palombo G, Filippi F, et al. Endovascular treatment of common carotid artery dissection via the superficial temporal artery. J Endovasc Ther 2010;17: 569–73.
106. Weimar C, Kraywinkel K, Hagemeister C, et al. Recurrent stroke after cervical artery dissection. J Neurol Neurosurg Psychiatry 2010;81:869–73.
107. Dziwas R, Konrad C, Drager B, et al. Cervical artery dissection—clinical features, risk factors, therapy and outcome in 126 patients. J Neurol 2003;250: 1179–84.
108. Lee WJ, Jung KH, Moon J, et al. Prognosis of spontaneous cervical artery dissection and transcranial Doppler findings associated with clinical outcomes. Eur Radiol 2016;26(5):1284–91.

Deep Venous Thrombosis

Mark Olaf, DO[a,*], Robert Cooney, MD, MSMedEd, RDMS[b]

KEYWORDS

- Deep venous thrombosis • Venous thromboembolism • Anticoagulation
- Novel oral anticoagulant • Vitamin K antagonist

KEY POINTS

- Deep venous thrombosis (DVT) is part of the venous thromboembolic spectrum and is a relatively common condition.
- Evaluation and diagnosis are performed by risk stratification utilizing the Wells score, d-dimer testing, and duplex ultrasound.
- Treatment depends on individual conditions, but usually consists of anticoagulation for a finite or infinite period of time, depending on the suspected etiology of the thrombosis.
- Adjunctive therapies such as caval filters, thrombolysis, and clot extraction play specific and limited roles.
- Risks and benefits of anticoagulation or other modalities should be discussed with and individualized for patients.
- An adjunctive search for causes of venous thromboembolism (VTE) should be investigated, beginning by looking for causes of provoked DVT, considering malignancy in the appropriate population, and finally assessing personal and family history in consideration of risks for thrombophilia.
- Upper Extremity DVT is a rare condition that is usually associated with catheters, implantable devices, malignancy, or thrombophilia and is primarily treated with anticoagulation.

INTRODUCTION

Deep venous thrombosis (DVT) is part of a spectrum of venous thromboembolic disorders that includes superficial thrombophlebitis and pulmonary embolism.[1] DVT may be defined as "the formation of a blood clot within a deep vein.[2]" Although DVT most commonly occurs in the deep veins of the lower leg and thigh, it may also occur within the upper limb deep veins, visceral veins, and even the vena cava.[2]

Disclosures: The authors attest that they have no commercial or financial conflicts of interest relevant to the material presented.
[a] Department of Emergency Medicine, Geisinger Medical Center, 100 North Academy Avenue, Danville, PA 17822-2005, USA; [b] Emergency Medicine Residency Program, Geisinger Medical Center, 100 North Academy Avenue, Danville, PA 17822-2005, USA
* Corresponding author.
E-mail address: mfolaf@geisinger.edu

Emerg Med Clin N Am 35 (2017) 743–770
http://dx.doi.org/10.1016/j.emc.2017.06.003

EPIDEMIOLOGY

The true incidence of DVT is unknown. The estimated risk for first time venous thromboembolism (VTE) is 100 cases per 100,000 persons per year, yielding an annual incidence of 0.1%[3] and generating an annual US incidence of over 1 million patients per year. The incidence of DVT appears to be equal between the sexes,[4] although women present 1.6 times more often for evaluation of suspected DVT.[5] DVT occurs more commonly as people age, with the rate in persons aged 60 years and older rising to nearly 1%.[6] VTE remains a disease with high morbidity and mortality. The case fatality rate for VTE has been reported to be 10.6% at 30 days and 23% at 1 year.[7] With prompt diagnosis and treatment, mortality declines dramatically. The 10-year recurrence rate after diagnosis of first-time DVT is approximately 25%. This peaks at 6 months and gradually declines to 2% per patient per year after 3 years, but is dependent on the etiology of the thrombosis.[8] The estimated overall mortality from VTE in the United States ranges from 60,000 to 100,000 deaths per year.[9] A subset of DVT is upper extremity DVT (UEDVT), which is far less common than lower extremity DVT (LEDVT). The prevalence of UEDVT is 0.15%, which constitutes about 1% to 4% of all DVTs.[10] Survival rates of patients with UEDVT are also lower than those with LEDVT.[10]

PATHOPHYSIOLOGY

Virchow's triad of alterations in blood flow, endothelial vascular injury, and derangements in the constitution of blood remain relevant over 150 years after they were first described.[11] Stasis, whether caused by obstruction or immobilization, is thought to prevent the clearance and dilution of activated clotting factors.[12] Injury to the vascular endothelium prevents the inhibition of coagulation and activates the clotting cascade. A propensity toward clotting secondary to hypercoagulability may be inherited or acquired.[12]

DVT commonly begins in the calf, and, less commonly, the proximal veins of the lower extremity. Obstruction of venous outflow leads to swelling and pain with the subsequent activation of the inflammatory cascade.[12] Many DVTs isolated within the calf veins will spontaneously resolve and are unlikely to embolize and cause pulmonary embolism (PE).[13] Twenty-five percent of isolated calf vein DVTs will subsequently extend into more proximal deep veins.[14] It is estimated that 50% of these may embolize, resulting in PE.[15] DVT occasionally compromises vascular flow within the extremity, resulting in phlegmasia cerulea dolens, a painful and limb-threatening vascular disorder.[12]

There are many risk factors for the development of DVT (**Table 1**). Pregnancy increases the risk secondary to mechanical obstruction of the inferior vena cava, relative immobility, and hormonal influence. The increase in risk is approximately 0.13% and begins in the first trimester.[2] Oral contraceptive (OCP) use roughly doubles the risk of VTE in patients, but the overall risk remains low because of the use of OCPs in generally healthy and young patients.[2] Malignancies may double the risk of developing a DVT, although this risk is highly dependent upon the type of cancer, the use of chemotherapy or surgical treatment options, and immobility.[2] **Table 1** shows estimated relative risks for multiple conditions.[12]

In hospitalized surgical patients of all types, older data[2] suggest that up to 25% of postoperative patients suffer VTE when not given prophylaxis, with higher rates (40%–60%) noted in postoperative orthopedic patients. Newer data suggest that with appropriate prophylaxis, this rate worldwide has dropped to 1%, and is perhaps 2% to 3% in the United States.[2] Medical patients admitted to the hospital also have about a 25%

Table 1
Selected conditions and associated relative risks for venous thromboembolism

Condition	Approximate Relative Risk
Antithrombin deficiency	25
Protein C or S deficiency	10
Factor V Leiden mutation	Heterozygous: 5; homozygous: 50
Prothrombin gene mutation	2.5
Major surgery or trauma	5–200
History of VTE	50
Antiphospholipid antibodies	2–10
Cancer	5
Medical illness with hospitalization	5
Age >50	5
Age >70	10
Pregnancy	7
Estrogen	OCPs: 5; hormone replacement: 2
Estrogen chemotherapy	Tamoxifen: 5; raloxifene: 3
Obesity	1–3
Hyperhomocysteinemia	3
Elevated factors VIII, IX or X (>90th percentile)	2.2–3

Data from Bates SM, Ginsberg JS. Clinical practice. Treatment of deep-vein thrombosis. N Engl J Med 2004;351(3):268–77.

risk of VTE without DVT prophylaxis.[2] Among these patients, stroke patients carry the highest risk, up to 50%. Acute coronary syndrome patients have VTE rates of about 20% without prophylactic measures.[2] Obesity is associated with increased risk of VTE. A body mass index (BMI) over 30 is estimated to roughly double the risk of VTE through a mechanism of venous stasis related to decreased lower extremity muscle contraction and venous pump.[2] Individuals with a personal history of VTE are at increased risk for subsequent VTE 5 times above the normal population.[2] Although often suspected by patients and some clinicians, there is no evidence to suggest uncomplicated varicose veins increase risk of VTE.[2]

Long-haul flights are often assumed to be an independent risk for VTE, although the medical literature fails to adequately describe the associated risk. The proposed pathogenesis of VTE during air travel is related to relative hypoxia in airplane cabins, venous stasis from prolonged sitting, and dehydration.[16] The rate of VTE (PE or DVT) on long-haul flights has been estimated to lie between 1.1 case per million person-days (roughly the rate of VTE in the healthy population) to 2000 times that (3%–12% of travelers).[16] One analysis postulates flights of 8 hours or more may pose an increased risk of VTE if additional risk factors are present.[17] In a separate outcome study in which 545 patients (6.9%) had VTE, risks of VTE were substantially increased by the presence of limb, whole-body, or neurologic immobility, but not by travel greater than 8 hours.[18] There is general consensus in the literature that many underlying prothrombotic conditions (age >40, obesity, OCP use, genetic thrombophilia) enhance the risk of developing VTE during long travel, whether by airplane, train, or car.[16]

Superficial thrombophlebitis (ST) is a distinct disease entity from DVT but has similar causal mechanisms, with an associated risk of DVT of 6.8% to 40%.[19] The high range of associated DVT is thought to be caused by variation in study design; therefore ST is not thought to be an independent risk for DVT. However, it is considered prudent to perform a duplex ultrasound of the affected limb to evaluate for ST and concomitant DVT.[19] Complete assessment and treatment of ST are beyond the scope of this article, but when DVT is diagnosed in the setting of nonsuppurative ST, the treatment of DVT is unchanged.

Underlying thrombophilia is an independent risk for VTE, above and beyond the aforementioned risks. Approximately 50% of individuals with VTE are found to have inherited thrombophilia disorders.[2] Thrombophilic testing identifies an etiology in about one-third of patients but has not been shown to alter outcome or duration of therapy in the past.[12] **Table 2** demonstrates the quantified risks of recurrent VTE from specific thrombophilic disorders.

Thrombophilia is broadly classified into loss-of-function (protein C, protein S, antithrombin III) or gain-of-function (factor V Leiden and prothrombin 20210A gene mutation) protein disorders that fail to provide homeostasis between clot formation and dissolution. Factor V Leiden is present in about 5% of the population, with heterozygotes at 3 times increased risk of VTE compared with the normal population, and homozygotes 50 to 80 times the normal population.[2] Prothrombin 20210A is a noncoding gene mutation that leads to elevated plasma prothrombin levels. Hyperhomocysteinemia and elevated levels of coagulation factors VIII, IX, and XI are suggested to have an additive, but not independent, effect in generating VTE.[2]

In cases of UEDVT, the subclavian (74%) and axillary (38%) veins are most commonly affected.[10] Risk factors for UEDVT are cancer, central venous catheters, and thrombophilia. Central venous catheters (CVCs) are the largest independent risk for the development of UEDVT, but only 3% of those with these devices develop a clot. Cancer appears to be an important risk factor in UEDVT in those DVTs that are not related to CVCs.[10] Implantable pacemakers have a rate of UEDVT of about 5%. UEDVT is thought to be less common than LEDVT because of higher rates of flow, increased mobility, and use of the upper extremity compared with the lower extremities and less stasis from gravity.[10]

PRESENTATION

The presentation of DVT can range from completely asymptomatic to pain, heaviness, or a cramping sensation in the affected extremity. Local swelling or discoloration of the

Table 2
Selected inherited conditions and estimated risks of recurrent venous thromboembolism after cessation of anticoagulant therapy

Risk Factor	Estimated Relative Risk of Recurrent Venous Thromboembolism
Antithrombin deficiency	1.5–3
Protein C or S deficiency	1.5–3
Factor V Leiden mutation	1–4
Prothrombin gene mutation	1–5
Antiphospholipid antibodies	2–4
Elevated factor VIII or IX levels	1–7
Hyperhomocysteinemia	1–3

Data from Bates SM, Ginsberg JS. Clinical practice. Treatment of deep-vein thrombosis. N Engl J Med 2004;351(3):268–77.

affected limb may accompany these complaints.[5] Multiple eponymous signs and tests (Michaelli sign, Mahler sign, Homan test, Loewenberg test) attempt to quantify or qualify the history and examination findings.[5] Despite the focus on calf tenderness, the signs and tests have failed to consistently or adequately diagnose DVT and have diagnostic accuracies around 50%.[20,21] Thus, these subjective and objective findings lack the sensitivity and specificity to diagnose DVT.[22]

The differential diagnosis for LEDVT is broad. In one study, DVT was found in 21% of patients, while alternative diagnoses were found 8% of the time or less and included Baker cyst (3%), general edema (8%), calf hematoma (4%), superficial vein thrombosis (5%), muscle vein thrombosis (4%), cellulitis and erysipelas (4%), and varicose veins (3%).[5] Also included in the differential are Achilles tendonitis, trauma, abscess, torn gastrocnemius muscle, acute arterial ischemia, venous or lymphatic obstruction, femur fracture, hemarthrosis of the knee, torn meniscus, congestive heart failure, nephrotic syndrome, liver failure, soft tissue tumor, and others.[5]

UEDVT is most commonly found after a patient develops swelling of the upper extremity. Few are associated with erythema (6% in one study), although pain (40%) was the most common associated complaint.[10] CVC-related UEDVT is less commonly associated with pain or symptoms because of slower clot growth. These CVC-associated clots are often more subtle and suggested by transient hand edema after dialysis, high dialysis pressures, or difficulty drawing blood from the catheter.[10]

DIAGNOSING DEEP VENOUS THROMBOSIS

As already indicated, physical examination and elements of a patient's history are poor independent predictors of VTE and are therefore not sufficient for the diagnosis of DVT. Comprehensive evaluation for VTE should always begin with risk stratification, followed by adjunctive testing based upon an identified level of risk. Adjunctive testing for DVT usually includes d-dimer or duplex ultrasound testing, and in very limited cases may include venography.

Risk Stratification

To improve upon the poor sensitivity and specificity of clinical examination findings, several scoring systems have been developed. Despite these objective analysis tools, 1 meta-analysis demonstrated that nonformal physician judgment was comparable to the validated scoring systems.[23]

The Wells Scoring System

Developed in 1995, the Wells score (**Table 3**) is the most widely used clinical decision instrument (CDI) for the diagnosis of DVT.[5] The CDI risk stratifies patients into low, intermediate, or high risk for DVT based upon a point system that identifies risk factors and has been further developed to dichotomize patients into high and low probability categories.[24] The interobserver reliability of the Wells score is excellent (kappa 0.85), with the most variability seen in the element of the score that considers the likelihood of an alternative diagnosis.[24] Currently, the Wells score is recommended for use in practice in order to dichotomize or trichotomize patients into risk categories, and both methods have been independently validated.[25,26]

In the original, 3-part risk stratification assessment, a Wells score (see **Table 3**) indicates levels of risk and includes low (Wells score 0 or less), moderate (Wells score 1–2), and high pretest probability (Wells score 3 or more) categories.[26]

Table 3
The Wells scoring system for deep venous thrombosis

Findings on History and Examination	Point Value
Active cancer Treatment or palliation within 6 mo	1
Bedridden recently ≥3 d or major surgery within 12 wk	1
Calf swelling >3 cm compared with the other leg Measured 10 cm below tibial tuberosity	1
Collateral (nonvaricose) superficial veins present	1
Entire leg swollen	1
Localized tenderness along the deep venous system	1
Pitting edema, confined to symptomatic leg	1
Paralysis, paresis, or recent plaster immobilization of the lower extremity	1
Previously documented DVT	1
Alternative diagnosis to DVT at least as likely	−2

A 2-level risk assessment is also valid and combines the moderate- and higher-risk patients into one category. Low-risk (<2 points) and combined intermediate/high-risk (2 or more points) categories are thus created.[26]

Both the 2-level and 3-level risk stratification techniques are used in clinical practice with adjunctive d-dimer and duplex ultrasound scanning to evaluate for DVT. A 2003 clinical policy recommendation from the American College of Emergency Physicians supports the use of DVT risk stratification using the Wells criteria along with d-dimer testing to safely exclude DVT (Level B recommendation).[27]

D-dimer

D-dimer is a molecular marker that results from the dissolution of cross-linked fibrin. It is often elevated in thrombotic conditions; however, it may also be elevated in nonthrombotic conditions including pregnancy, malignancy, trauma, infection, and inflammatory conditions and is therefore not a specific marker for DVT.[2,28] Multiple assays are available, with the enzyme linked immunosorbent assay (ELISA) possessing the highest sensitivity (94%).[2,28] The current recommended testing strategy for first-time DVT includes assessment of pretest probability combined with high sensitivity d-dimer testing and compression ultrasound assessment.[25]

In the dichotomized risk stratification approach, patients in the low category can safely undergo d-dimer testing, and if negative, the diagnosis of DVT can be reasonably excluded. If the d-dimer level is elevated, or if the pretest probability of DVT is intermediate or high based on the CDI, a duplex of the lower extremity should be performed.[26,27]

In the trichotomized version, low-probability patients (Wells score 0 or less), should be offered the use of d-dimer, or proximal vein ultrasound. In moderate-probability patients (Wells score 1–2), highly sensitive d-dimer, proximal-vein ultrasound, or whole-leg ultrasound is favored over other modalities. In low- and moderate-risk patients, if d-dimer is negative, no further testing is warranted, while a positive d-dimer testing prompts compression ultrasound, but does not necessitate treatment.[25] In high pretest probability patients, d-dimer testing should not be utilized, and one should proceed with duplex ultrasound of the extremity to evaluate for DVT.[25] In addition, in a patient with a moderate or high pretest probability, if compression ultrasound is utilized and is initially negative, repeat testing with compression ultrasound or a moderate or high sensitivity d-dimer is recommended at 1 week follow-up.[25] In cases where a patient has high pretest probability and there is no immediate access to utrasound, a single dose of low molecular weight heparin and a return visit within 12 hours for planned ultrasound are reasonable.

Testing for recurrent DVT is controversial, but recommendations favor the same modalities as for primary DVT assessment. Repeat duplex testing is warranted if d-dimer is positive but initial duplex is negative.[26]

Age-Adjusted D-dimer

Increased age has the propensity to increase d-dimer values and may therefore decrease the diagnostic accuracy and specificity of the d-dimer. A 2014 systematic review found that age-adjusted (age $\times$ 10 μg per liter as the upper limit of normal) d-dimer values in older, nonhigh-risk patients increased the specificity and did not significantly decrease the sensitivity of the study.[29] It is important to note that this was a derivation study, not a validation study, and to date the results have not undergone validation. Although not specifically evaluating the age-adjusted D-dimer on DVT, the ADJUST-PE trial did validate age-adjusted D-dimer for use in the evaluation of acute PE.[30]

Pregnancy Adjusted D-dimer

Data have shown a consistent elevation in d-dimer levels as pregnancy progresses.[31,32] This would serve to reduce the specificity of the d-dimer test, prompting unnecessary further evaluation. In 1 small study of asymptomatic women, none of the women had a d-dimer value less than the traditional cutoff value of 0.50 mg/L in the third trimester. The authors advocate for a prospective validation of cutoff values at 0.750, 1.0, and 1.5 mg/L for the first, second, and third trimesters, respectively. A small trial prospectively validated 3 d-dimer cutoff values at 286, 457, and 644 ng/mL in the first, second, and third trimesters, respectively and found 100% sensitivity for the adjusted values. The authors note their trial should be viewed as a pilot study and advocate for additional, larger studies.[32]

Ultrasound

Duplex ultrasound imaging, which includes B-mode imaging of veins as well as pulsed Doppler flow assessment, can evaluate for DVT in the proximal veins with specificity of 94% and sensitivity of 90%.[28] A meta-analysis pooled 7 studies and demonstrated a 0.57% 3-month rate of VTE after single negative LE compression ultrasound.[33] Duplex imaging modalities may include proximal-vein-only methods or whole leg scanning. Positive compression ultrasound of the lower extremity is sufficient to warrant treatment, and venography is not recommended for confirmation.[25] Although venography remains an option, it may be associated with decreased availability, increased discomfort, and more complications, but it has a lower false-positive rate.[25] A 2003 clinical policy recommendation from ACEP supports (level B evidence) the use of venous ultrasonography to safely exclude all proximal and symptomatic distal DVT.[27] Serial ultrasounds are recommended for high-probability cases with negative initial imaging.[27]

Ultrasound Sites

A 2014 study identified 362 individuals with DVT on compression ultrasound, of whom 6.3% had findings of isolated thrombi in proximal veins. The study authors used the data to support the recommendation of the addition of femoral and deep femoral vein evaluation to standard compression ultrasound of the common femoral and popliteal veins.[34] In agreement with this are the 2015 guidelines from the American Institute of Ultrasound in Medicine (AIUM), which recommend[35]:

"The fullest visualized extent of the common femoral, femoral, and popliteal veins must be imaged using an optimal gray scale compression technique. The popliteal vein is examined distally to the tibioperoneal trunk. The proximal deep femoral and proximal great saphenous veins should also be examined. Venous compression is applied every 2 cm or less in the transverse (short axis) plane with adequate pressure on the skin to completely obliterate the normal vein lumen."

In addition, focal symptoms require individualized assessment.[35]

For a normal examination, the minimum assessment and imaging documentation should include gray scale images with and without compression of the[35]

- Common femoral vein
- Junction of the common femoral vein with the great saphenous vein
- Proximal deep femoral vein separately or along with the proximal femoral vein
- Proximal femoral vein
- Distal femoral vein
- Popliteal vein

In addition, color spectral Doppler waveforms from the long axis should be recorded at these levels[35]:

- Right common femoral or external iliac vein
- Left common femoral or external iliac vein
- Popliteal vein on symptomatic side or on both sides if the examination is bilateral

Abnormal examination findings require documentation and imaging of the abnormal finding.[35]

For upper extremity assessment, the 2015 AIUM guidelines recommend that gray scale images or cine loops should be recorded without and with compression at each of the following levels[35]:

- Internal jugular vein
- Peripheral subclavian vein
- Axillary vein
- Brachial vein in the upper arm
- Cephalic vein in the upper arm
- Basilic vein in the upper arm
- Focal symptomatic areas, if present

Color and spectral Doppler images are recorded at each of the following levels using the appropriate color technique to show filling of the normal venous lumen:

- Internal jugular vein
- Subclavian vein
- Axillary vein

If seen, the innominate vein should be recorded with color Doppler imaging.

At a minimum, both the right and left subclavian venous spectral Doppler waveforms should be recorded to evaluate for asymmetry or loss of cardiovascular pulsatility and respiratory phasicity.[35]

Emergency Department Physician-Performed Imaging

A 2013 meta-analysis of 16 studies that assessed the diagnostic accuracy of emergency department physician lower extremity ultrasound for DVT demonstrated a kappa value of 0.83 between investigators, with a mean sensitivity of 96.5%.[36] In the studies analyzed, there was high variability in training among emergency department physicians and variable study type (whole leg, 2 point, 3 point). Additional studies regarding emergency department physician DVT diagnoses have been conducted and have demonstrated highly variable results (sensitivity from 66% to 100%) but were subject to poor study methods.[37] Overall, the studies seem to demonstrate that bedside performance of ultrasound for the evaluation of LEDVT by emergency department physicians is reasonable, but perhaps dependent upon experience and level of training.

Upper Extremity Deep Venous Thrombosis

Only about 50% of clinical investigations identify DVT in patients with suspected UEDVT. Contrast venography is the gold standard but invasive and requires contrast use. Ultrasound is 82% to 97% sensitive and 82% to 96% specific, and benefits from portability and lack of radiation use.[10] Recommendations for the evaluation of UEDVT begin with risk stratification of patients into high or low probability. Both groups should begin their evaluation with color flow duplex ultrasonography. If UEDVT is found on ultrasound, treatment should be initiated. In low-risk patients in whom ultrasound is negative, serial ultrasound can be considered, or the evaluation can be stopped. In high-risk patients, contrast venography is recommended for further evaluation.[10]

The approach to evaluation for LEDVT is summarized in **Fig. 1**.

MANAGEMENT

The management of DVT depends upon individual patient factors including the underlying etiology of the DVT, risks for bleeding, symptom severity, and patient preference.

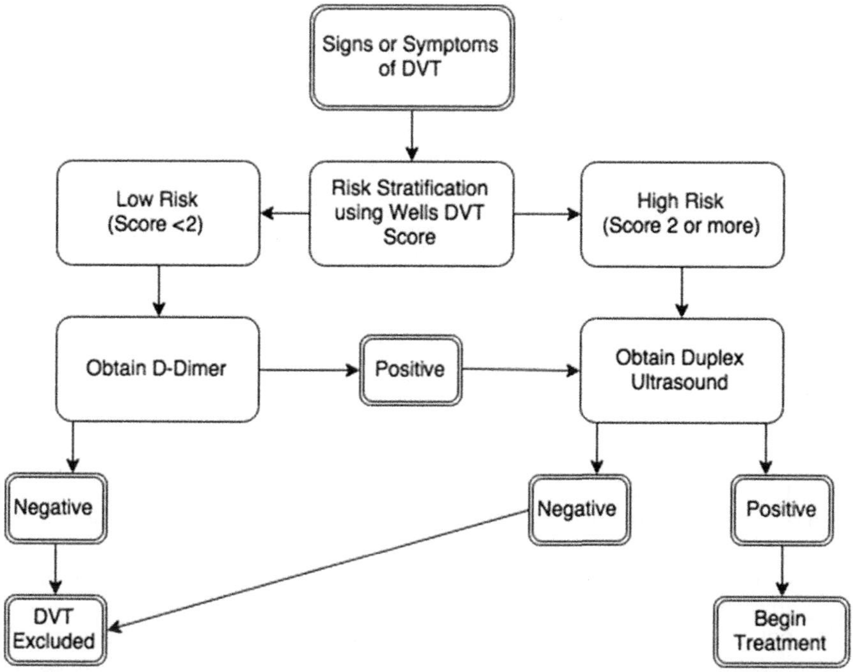

Fig. 1. The two-tiered algorithmic approach to diagnosing DVT.

Given the multitude of combinations and possibilities, The American College of Chest Physicians has published guidelines for evaluation and management of VTE. These consensus guidelines are evidence based and updated every few years, referred to as the CHEST guidelines.[38,39]

Isolated Distal Calf Deep Venous Thrombosis

Isolated distal calf VTE is special, as these cases may not progress to proximal DVT or PE. Authors suggest that all proximal LEDVT be treated and that calf vein DVT should either be treated empirically or followed with serial ultrasound to devaluate for proximal progression.[26] Some authors recommend acute isolated DVT without severe symptoms or risks for progression be followed with serial ultrasound rather than anticoagulation, while those patients with severe symptoms or high risk for progression be treated with anticoagulation.[39] Shared decision-making plays a large role in the decision to treat or perform serial imaging in isolated distal DVT, as patient preference may affect adherence to the treatment plan.[26]

The remaining discussion of therapies reflects the treatment of proximal LEDVT.

Compression Stockings

Graded compression elastic stockings utilized for 2 years have demonstrated no decreased risk of recurrence of DVT, but did reduce the risk of post-thrombotic syndrome (PTS) at 5 years.[40] In patients with acute DVT of the leg, the CHEST guidelines suggest not using compression stockings routinely to prevent PTS.[38] This recommendation focuses on prevention of the chronic complication of PTS and not on the treatment of symptoms. For patients with acute or chronic symptoms, a trial of graduated compression stockings is often justified.[38] No specific compression value is mentioned by the authors, and reference is only made to graded compression stockings.[38]

Inferior Vena Cava Filters

In patients with acute DVT or PE who are treated with anticoagulants, the routine use of inferior vena cava (IVC) filters is not recommended.[25] Although early embolism was reduced by filter placement in one study, the effect was transient, and data at 2 years indicated no significant reduction in mortality or recurrent symptomatic PE.[41] In fact, another study showed increased risk of subsequent DVT at 2-year follow-up after IVC filter placement.[41] IVC filters might be considered in patients who have acute DVT and suffer complications necessitating cessation of anticoagulation, and in those who have failed multiple forms of anticoagulation, including vitamin K antagonists (VKAs) at both the traditional international normalized ratio (INR) of 2.0 to 3.0, as well as an elevated INR of 3.0 to 4.0, and other therapies including low molecular weight heparin (LMWH) or novel oral anticoagulants (NOACs).[2]

Aspirin

Aspirin therapy is not considered an adequate alternative to anticoagulation for treatment of DVT or PE.[39] However, after completion of traditional therapy, aspirin may be an effective measure to prevent recurrence. The WARFASA and ASPIRE studies both evaluated ASA versus placebo in patients with unprovoked (noncancer- and nonimmobility-related VTE) after completion of traditional treatment for VTE. Both studies demonstrated reduced rates of VTE in the aspirin groups.[42,43] Multiple studies of varying design, including 2 meta-analyses, have demonstrated reductions in VTE among patients on ASA or placebo for cardiovascular risk control (primary prevention).[44–46] Pitfalls of studies related to the primary prevention of VTE with aspirin are largely related to VTE prevention being a secondary outcome or the result of post-hoc analysis. In none of these studies was prevention of PE by ASA a primary end point. Other large, population-based observational studies have failed to demonstrate an effect on VTE prevention by ASA.[47,48]

Given the previously mentioned data, the risks and benefits of aspirin for prevention of recurrent DVT should be considered upon cessation of traditional anticoagulation. Although the data are not conclusive, aspirin therapy for secondary prevention of DVT seems a reasonable and probably effective measure, and should be considered and weighed against the risk of bleeding in the appropriate patient. In those patients with unprovoked DVT and low risk of bleeding, and in whom cessation of therapy is planned, the CHEST guidelines recommend aspirin therapy, as long as there is no contraindication to such therapy.[39] Additionally, the use of aspirin for other primary or secondary prevention purposes (eg, stroke) should be assessed.[49]

Aspirin has also been studied for primary prevention of VTE after orthopedic surgery, with conflicting results. The American Academy of Orthopedic Surgeons, in a 2009 statement, recommended primary prevention of VTE with ASA, based on the Pulmonary Embolism Prevention Study.[44,50] CHEST recommendations now recommend ASA therapy as an alternative therapy to heparin or LMWH. A study published in 2013 was halted prematurely because of poor patient recruitment, but has been cited as evidence of aspirin noninferiority compared with dalteparin treatment.[44,51]

Anticoagulation

A seminal work by Barritt and Jordan was a small and technically poor study that seemingly demonstrated the efficacy of anticoagulation for the prevention of progression of VTE following initial diagnosis.[52] Although their methods were flawed, several more rigorous subsequent studies have proven the benefit of anticoagulation on morbidity and mortality.[40]

Current options for anticoagulation in VTE include

1. Anticoagulation with heparin or a LMWH, with transition to a VKA until the INR is greater than 2 on 2 consecutive days
2. Oral dabigatran or edoxaban after 5 days of heparin or LMWH
3. Oral apixaban or rivaroxaban only, with loading doses
4. LMWH treatment only for those patients with active cancer[53]

Treatment options regarding anticoagulation are categorized by the mechanism or class of drug when studied or described in the literature.

Unfractionated heparin

Unfractionated heparin (UFH) is an anticoagulant that complexes with antithrombin III (ATIII), producing a conformational change and converting the ATIII molecule into a potent inhibitor of thrombin. ATIII exerts its anticoagulant effect through inhibition of thrombin and factor Xa.[54]

UFH is delivered intravenously and requires partial thromboplastin time (PTT) monitoring.[12] The range of PTT depends on reagent and desired coagulation parameters. A fixed ratio of 1.5 to 2.5 times the control value is suggested but often results in variable and subtherapeutic degrees of anticoagulation.[12] More ideal is the correlation of PTT values with ex vivo values of antifactor Xa between 0.3 and 0.7 u/mL.[12] Weight-based nomograms are often used to estimate the amount of heparin required for anticoagulation.[12] Adverse effects include hemorrhage in up to 7% of patients and osteoporosis in patients with prolonged (longer than one month) use.[12] The risk of hemorrhage is affected by age and concomitant use of thrombolytic or antiplatelet agents.[12] Heparin-induced thrombocytopenia (HIT) is an immune-mediated phenomenon defined by the presence of heparin-dependent immunoglobulin G (IgG) antibodies, which appear to activate platelets in a complex of heparin, platelet, and platelet factor 4, occurring in up to 2.7% of patients receiving heparin.[55] The thrombocytopenia can be complicated by thrombotic events, likely through platelet activation, and usually occurs on or after day 5 of heparin therapy. Patients with a history of HIT should receive heparin alternatives to anticoagulation.[12]

Low Molecular Weight Heparins

LMWHs differ from unfractionated heparins in their pharmacokinetic and biologic properties, namely decreased plasma protein binding and increased serum bioavailability when delivered via a subcutaneous route. LMWH drugs can thus be administered subcutaneously, do not require frequent laboratory monitoring, and exhibit fewer biologic phenomena than unfractionated heparin.[54]

A 1999 meta-analysis found the use of LMWH decreased mortality in the treatment of DVT when compared with UFH. In addition, the LMWH products demonstrated similar safety profiles with respect to bleeding and were as effective as UFH in preventing recurrent DVT.[56] Most patients can be treated safely and effectively with LMWH, with appropriate infrastructure in place.[12] Outpatient treatment with LMWH is reasonable in many patients, provided a high risk of bleeding (very advanced age, recent surgery, history of renal of liver disease), serious coexisting illness, and massive thrombosis are absent. Direct comparisons of LMWH and UFH have shown lower VTE recurrence rates, less major bleeding, and lower mortality rates with treatment using LMWH.[57]

In patients who have recurrent VTE on long-term LMWH (and are believed to be compliant), increasing the dose of LMWH by one-quarter to one-third is recommended.[39] Recurrent VTE while on therapeutic-dose anticoagulant therapy is unusual and should prompt evaluation for underlying malignancy, antiphospholipid syndrome, evaluation of compliance with anticoagulation, and whether the perceived recurrent VTE is an acute finding or a chronic VTE.[39]

In patients who have recurrent VTE on VKA therapy (in the therapeutic range) or NOACs and are believed to be compliant, the CHEST guidelines recommend switching to treatment with LMWH, at least temporarily.[39]

Specific adverse events associated with LMWH include the HIT phenomena, as well as bleeding. LMWH can cross-react with the antibodies that cause HIT and should thus be avoided in patients with a history of HIT.[12] Use of LMHW (dalteparin) in women during pregnancy demonstrated less decline in bone mineral density compared with UFH during and no significant difference in osteoporosis 3 years after delivery, compared with healthy women who did not require anticoagulation.[58]

Warfarin and Vitamin K Antagonists

VKAs include warfarin, acenocoumarol, phenprocoumon, and others, which inhibit gamma carboxylation of factors II, VII, IX, X, C, and S. Drug absorption is rapid and complete, but therapeutic levels take 4 to 5 days to obtain, owing to the mechanism of action of the drugs.[53]

VKA therapy is traditionally started on the same days as parenteral anticoagulation with heparin or LMWH and titrated to an INR of 2 to 3.[12] A small randomized controlled trial demonstrated a significant reduction (20% vs 6.7%) in VTE recurrence in those patients treated with intravenous unfractionated heparin and transitioned to a vitamin K antagonist versus a vitamin K antagonist alone, respectively.[53] Utilized at an INR of 2.0 to 3.0, VKAs have been shown to reduce the risk of recurrent thromboembolism.[12] INRs higher than 3 have demonstrated increased risks of bleeding without benefit of reduced recurrence of DVT. Although INRs higher than 3 were recommended for the management of DVT in patients with antiphospholipid syndrome, 2 trials failed to demonstrate superiority compared with standard (INR 2–3) recommendations.[59,60]

In trials comparing VKA therapy to novel (or direct) oral anticoagulant therapy, VTE recurrence rates for LMWH/VKA therapy were 2.2% to 3.5% in patients treated for 3 to 12 months, with a risk of major bleeding 8.5% to 10.3%.[53] A large VTE registry found VTE recurrence rates of 2.5%, similar to recent trials, but increased risk of major bleeding, about 2.5% beyond that seen in the same trials.[53]

In addition to bleeding risks, adverse effects of warfarin therapy include vascular purpura and consequent skin necrosis in the first few weeks of therapy, which has been associated with protein C deficiency and malignancy. Coumarin derivatives are known teratogens and should be avoided in pregnancy.[61] The rate of recurrent DVT while on well-coordinated VKA is about 2%.[38] The risk of bleeding at 90 days is about 2.2%.[62] Long-term therapy with VKAs has demonstrated decreased risks of recurrent VTE compared with short-term (3 months) therapy (relative risk 0.20), but was associated with increased risks of bleeding (relative risk 3.44) and no significant difference in mortality.[63]

Novel (Direct) Oral Anticoagulant Therapy

The direct or novel oral anticoagulant therapies differ from VKAs in mechanism, from UFH and LMWH at their sites of action, and from argatroban, in that these novel medications are orally bioavailable. Dabigatran, like argatroban, is a univalent direct thrombin inhibitor, inhibiting thrombin (factor IIa) at its active site. Rivaroxaban, apixaban, and edoxaban are factor Xa inhibitors. Collectively, the NOAC drugs exhibit relatively rapid onsets of action, with peak levels being achieved 1 to 4 hours after oral dosing. The half-lives approximate 12 hours.[64] Advantages of these therapies include ease of dosing, lack of need for monitoring, and improved management for anticoagulation for procedures that might cause bleeding.[49] In support of this is the fact that antifactor IIa and antifactor Xa activities are directly proportional to drug levels.[53] Renal function plays a large role in the elimination of these drugs, and compromised renal function may lead to accumulation, supratherapeutic drug levels, and consequential bleeding. Apixaban and Rivaroxaban have the advantages of not requiring heparin bridging to attain therapeutic levels. In addition, the NOACs have far fewer drug-drug interactions when compared with warfarin, allowing for more stable levels and drug effects.[65] It is important to note that potent inhibitors or inducers of CYP3A4 or p-glycoproteins can affect NOAC drug levels.[65]

All of the trials for the NOACs were designed as noninferiority trials when compared with LMWH or VKAs, although different criteria for noninferiority were utilized across studies. The details of individual trials are discussed, but in general, consistent findings of noninferiority of the NOACs were present throughout.[65] Recurrence rates for VTE in these trials was about 2% for DOACs compared with 2.2% for VKAs; however, study parameters for duration of treatment differed among the trials.[53] Recent meta-analyses showed similar rates of recurrent DVTs between the NOACs and traditional therapies but reduced rates of major and fatal bleeding, as well as all-cause mortality with the NOACs.[66,67] A significant reduction in bleeding among the NOACs was noted, with a number needed to treat (with NOAC as opposed to VKAs) between 19 and 167.[65] There are limited real-world data to determine the outcomes for patients outside of the selected study groups for the phase III trials for these drugs.[53]

Direct Thrombin Inhibitors

Dabigatran etexilate

RE-COVER and RE-COVER II were double-blinded trials that compared the treatment of VTE with warfarin. Both demonstrated noninferiority for recurrent VTE or VTE-related death and reduction in bleeding.[68,69] The RE-MEDY study was a randomized study that demonstrated the noninferiority of dabigatran to warfarin for extended therapy for VTE, with a nonstatistically significant reduction in bleeding.[69] RE-SONATE was a placebo-controlled, double-blinded study with dabigatran versus placebo for extended therapy after initial completion of VTE treatment for first VTE. Dabigatran significantly reduced recurrent VTE in the study population.[69]

When dabigatran was compared with VKAs for long-term treatment of VTE, the data showed an anticipated absolute risk difference of 5 fewer (per 1000) episodes (95% confidence interval [CI]: 2–10) of major bleeding.[38] Specifically, in the RE-LY trial, major gastrointestinal (GI) bleeding compared with warfarin was significantly increased in the twice-daily 150 mg dose, but comparable at the 110 mg twice-daily dose. Bleeding in the 75 mg twice-daily dose was not assessed.[70] Dabigatran at both the 150 mg and 110 mg dosing was associated with significantly less intracranial hemorrhage compared with warfarin.[71] The RE-COVER trial showed lower rates of intracranial hemorrhage in the dabigatran group as well.[71]

Factor Xa Inhibitors

Rivaroxaban

The EINSTEIN study assessed rivaroxaban against placebo for extended VTE prevention after initial traditional anticoagulation for first VTE and demonstrated superior efficacy compared with placebo.[72] EINSTEIN-DVT and EINSTEIN-PE were open-label trials that demonstrated noninferiority of rivaroxaban compared with warfarin in the treatment of DVT and PE, respectively. Similar bleeding rates were noted between rivaroxaban and vitamin K antagonists.[72,73]

When rivaroxaban was compared with LMWH and VKAs in 2 studies that assessed the acute and the long-term treatment of VTE, the anticipated absolute risk difference in major bleeding was 8 fewer (per 1000) episodes (95% CI: 3–11).[38] In the ROCKET-AF trial, rivaroxaban 20 mg daily demonstrated an increased risk of major GI bleeding when compared with warfarin (hazard ratio 1.61).[70] A post hoc analysis of data showed similar rates of life-threatening bleeding (4 or more units of packed red blood cells transfused) between the 2 groups and fewer (1 vs 5) fatal events with rivaroxaban. The ROCKET-AF trial also demonstrated rivaroxaban to have significantly less acute intracranial hemorrhage when compared with warfarin, with lower rates of both intracerebral hemorrhage and subdural hemorrhage.[71] In the EINSTEIN-DVT trial, intracranial hemorrhage rates were not reported separately, but bleeding in a critical location was similar between the rivaroxaban and warfarin groups.[71] In EINSTEIN-PE, lower rates of intracranial hemorrhage were observed in the rivaroxaban group.[71]

Apixaban

The AMPLIFY study evaluated patients treated for first VTE and randomized patients to 3 groups: 2.5 mg apixaban, 5 mg apixaban, or placebo for 12 months. Both doses of apixaban demonstrated superior efficacy at preventing death compared with placebo and equivalent rates of bleeding.[74]

In a comparison of apixaban to LMWH and VKAs for the acute and long-term treatment of VTE, the absolute anticipated risk of major bleeding was 13 fewer episodes (per 1000) (95% CI: 2 more to 10 fewer).[39] The ARISTOTLE trial showed no significant differences in major GI bleeding between apixaban and warfarin and demonstrated lower rates of intracranial hemorrhage in favor of apixaban.[70]

Edoxaban

A randomized, double-blinded, 12-month noninferiority trial demonstrated that in VTE treated first with LMWH or heparin, edoxaban showed no significant difference in recurrent VTE (3.2% vs 3.5% respectively), compared with warfarin. Additionally, a significantly lower rate of major or clinically relevant nonmajor bleeding (8.5% vs 10.3% respectively) was observed.[75] Another randomized, double-blind trial (ENGAGE AF-TIMI 48) evaluated over 21,000 patients with atrial fibrillation and increased risk of stroke. Significant reductions in rates of major bleeding (2.75% vs 3.43%), intracranial bleeding (0.39% vs 0.85%), and cardiovascular death (2.74%vs 3.17%) were observed with edoxaban.[76] Edoxaban compared with VKA for long-term treatment of VTE showed an anticipated absolute risk difference of 2 fewer episodes (per 1000) (95% CI: 3 more to 6 fewer) for major bleeding.[25]

Direct comparisons of GI bleeding, intracranial bleeding, or other types of bleeding among the NOACs are not yet available but should be performed in the future to more thoroughly assess the associated risks with each agent.

The safety of NOACs in pregnancy and children has not yet been sufficiently evaluated, and therefore specific recommendations cannot be made for the NOACs in the treatment of DVTs in these populations. Studies in pregnancy have not yet been conducted, and studies in children are underway currently.

Thrombolysis for deep venous thrombosis

Because of the risk of bleeding, thrombolysis of DVT is usually reserved for patients with a low risk of bleeding and limb-threatening thrombosis.[12,27] A Cochrane database review of 17 studies suggested that any type of thrombolysis improved clot resolution and reduced the risk of post-thrombotic syndrome, with an expected increase in bleeding complications.[77] UK guidelines recommend considering thrombolysis in specific patients with low risk of bleeding, good functional status, and iliofemoral DVT.[28]

Catheter-directed thrombolysis

In patients with acute proximal DVT of the leg, anticoagulant therapy alone over catheter-directed thrombolysis (CDT) is recommended.[25] A retrospective observational study of over 90,000 patients with lower extremity proximal DVT demonstrated no difference in mortality between CDT plus anticoagulation versus anticoagulation only, but did find an increased incidence of adverse events in the thrombolysis group.[78] However, a subset of patients with acute (within 14 days) iliofemoral DVT, good functional status, and a life expectancy of at least a year with a low risk of bleeding might be the most optimal candidates for the therapy, in cases where it is offered.[28]

Recommendations by type of anticoagulant therapy

Choosing the type anticoagulant can be daunting. One can begin to narrow the options by basing the decision on the patient's presumed underlying DVT etiology, individual risks, and clinical condition. Heparin is a reasonable choice for those individuals with extensive or massive DVT or PE or high risk of bleeding, so that levels may be monitored and doses properly titrated. This requires hospitalization. NOACs may not be appropriate for these patients, as they have not been evaluated in these respects. In cases of DVT in pregnancy or in the setting of active malignancy, LMWH appears to be the best option. NOACs play a specific role at this time and require that a particular set of conditions be met. In cases in which NOACs are available; consistent oral dosing is obtainable; patient preference is for no need for monitoring; and in patients with normal renal function (Cr clearance >30 mL/min), the NOACs rivaroxaban, apixaban, and edoxaban seem to be the best option. Anticoagulation parameters are not required on a regular basis. However, in cases in which NOACs are prohibited by cost, or the previously mentioned conditions are not met, LMWH with transition to warfarin is the best option. In more specific cases, patients with dyspepsia or recent acute coronary syndrome should avoid dabigatran. Patients with recent upper GI bleeding had less recurrent bleeds while on apixaban (compared with other NOACs) and should be offered this therapy as a first choice.[65]

Upper extremity deep venous thrombosis management

Treatment options for UEDVT are as varied as those for LEDVT. Treatment of UEDVT is related to risks of developing PE (which is lower in UEDVT than LEDVT), symptom management, the development of recurrent DVT or PE, and management of patient symptoms. Anticoagulation is the preferred management of UEDVT, and recommendations largely mimic those for the treatment of LEDVT.[10,39] Initial treatment recommendations are for 3 months. The decision concerning removing a CVC related to UEDVT is an individualized decision that is influenced by the symptoms of the DVT as well as the necessity of the device. Although anticoagulation is routinely preferred over thrombolysis, individualized treatment plans for thrombolysis can be made in specific situations to help manage severe or refractory symptoms.[10]

COMPLICATIONS OF DEEP VENOUS THROMBOSIS

After diagnosis and treatment of VTE, monitoring of complications, evaluation of potential causes, and duration of treatment should be investigated. Among complications of VTE, post-thrombotic syndrome (PTS) occurs in about 20% to 50% of patients after DVT.[39] PTS is a constellation of chronic clinical findings that are induced by DVT. Symptoms may include leg heaviness, pain, cramps, pruritis, and paresthesias. Objective signs may include pretibial edema, skin induration, hyperpigmentation, ectatic veins, ulcers, and painful calf compression. The highest risks for developing PTS are extensive proximal DVT, ipsilateral recurrent DVT, and ineffective or absent anticoagulation therapy.[79] Phlegmasia cerulea dolens (PCD) and phlegmasia alba dolens (PAD) are uncommon but catastrophic complications of DVT. Both conditions describe fulminant DVT of the extremity, with PCD including obstructed arterial flow caused by increased compartmental pressures.[80] Significant morbidity and mortality are seen with PCD, with 12% to 15% of survivors requiring amputation and a mortality rate of 25%.[81] Although the exact incidence of the disease is poorly reported, in 1 study of PCD, the observed rate was just 7 times over 4.5 years.[82] As noted previously, about 25% of DVTs will demonstrate proximal progression, and 50% of these with result in PE.[14,15] Aside from these inherent complications from DVT, the remainder of complications stem from bleeding related to treatment of DVT.

Even with treatment, VTE carries a high risk of death, but rates vary widely in the literature.[83] Short-term survival estimates from DVT range from 95% to 97%, while long-term survival estimates range between 61% to 75%.[83] In 1 study, estimates of 30-day mortality after diagnosis of DVT and PE were 6% and 12%, respectively.[65] In another study, rates of survival for DVT were 96.2% at 7 days, 94.5% at 30 days, and 94.5% at 1 year. These values were significantly different from the rates of PE, which were 59.1%, 55.6%, and 47.7%, respectively.[83]

FURTHER EVALUATION

In those patients with unprovoked DVT, undiagnosed malignancy is an additional concern. Recommendations from the United Kingdom suggest that all patients with unprovoked DVT undergo a full physical examination, chest radiograph, and laboratory testing including complete blood count, serum calcium, liver function testing, and urinalysis. In patients over 40 years of age with unprovoked DVT and without abnormal findings on the initial screening tests, abdominal-pelvic computed tomography (CT) scanning is recommended to search for malignancy.[28]

Thrombophilia evaluation should be pursued in patients only after the cessation of anticoagulation in the setting of unprovoked DVT.[2] A review of available literature found no North American guidelines for thrombophilia testing after unprovoked DVT. UK guidelines (which were created with consideration of both economic and disease-related factors) recommend no additional thrombotic workup for patients who will continue anticoagulation.[28] For those patients with unprovoked DVT who will stop anticoagulation, antiphospholipid antibody screening is recommended. For those patients with a first-degree relative with a history of VTE, additional thrombophilia testing is warranted.[28]

TREATMENT DURATION

Although it is often beyond the scope of care in the emergency department for the acute VTE patient, the duration of treatment for VTE is a concern to many patients, and it is reasonable for the emergency physician to be familiar with recommendations for duration of treatment to provide general counseling at the time of diagnosis. Transient and nontransient risk factors can be identified, and risk of bleeding related to age and history of bleeding can be evaluated. A great deal of the decision for duration focuses on risk of recurrence, comorbidities, and bleeding risk, and this review will focus on these aspects.

Risk and Rates of Recurrence

Rates of recurrence are correlated to duration of treatment; as risk of recurrent DVT increases, duration of therapy is theoretically prolonged. Therefore, to understand duration of treatment, one must understand rates and risk of recurrence.

One manner of analyzing risk of recurrence is through the associated cause. The rate of recurrence of VTE after trauma or surgery is about 3% per year.[84–86] Cancer-associated recurrent VTE occurs at a rate of 10% per year.[84–86] Unprovoked VTE has a risk of recurrence of about 15% over the first 2 years. Rates of recurrence also vary by time and are influenced by provocative factors.[40,87] **Table 4** categorizes recurrence rates by risk factor and time period.

Table 4
Rates of recurrence of venous thromboembolism can also be categorized by time

Time	Transient Risk Factor Rate	Nontransient Risk Factor Rate
6 wk to 3 mo	2.5% per year	5% per year
3 mo to 6 mo	2.5% per year	5% per year
6 mo to 2 y	5% per year	10% per year
Beyond 2 y	2% per year	4% per year

From Prins MH, Hutten BA, Koopman MM, et al. Long-term treatment of venous thromboembolic disease. Thromb Haemost 1999;82(2):892–8.

Bleeding Risk

The associated risk of recurrence must be weighed against the risk of bleeding. Many factors influence the risk of bleeding, and advancing age is well known to increase the risk of bleeding (from VKAs) as follows[40]:

- Less than 40 years: 0.6% per year
- 40 to 49 years: 1.0% per year
- 50 to 59 years: 1.5% per year
- 60 to 69 years: 2.2% per year
- 70 years and beyond: 3.2% per year

In addition to advancing age, the following risk factors have been identified as independent and cumulative risks for bleeding:

- Previous bleeding
- Cancer
- Metastatic Cancer
- Renal failure
- Liver failure
- Thrombocytopenia
- Previous stroke
- Diabetes
- Anemia
- Antiplatelet therapy
- Poor anticoagulant control
- Comorbidity and reduced functional capacity
- Recent surgery
- Alcohol abuse
- Nonsteroidal anti-inflammatory drugs

With none of the previously mentioned risk factors present, the baseline risk for bleeding is estimated at 0.6%. Adding anticoagulant therapy increases the risk to 1.6%. If 1 risk factor is present, the baseline risk is 1.2%, and adding anticoagulation increases the risk of bleeding to 3.2%. If 2 or more risk factors are present, the baseline risk of bleeding is 4.8%, and adding anticoagulation increases this risk to 12.8%.[39] These data are based on aggregate data and largely on VKA therapy. The authors note that variability will exist from patient to patient, and that although the increased risk of bleeding has not been validated in the manner described previously, the risk of bleeding is cumulative from multiple risk factors.[39]

Multiple clinical tools and predictors have been created to assess risk of bleeding in an objective and individualized manner for each specific patient. Unfortunately, a calculator or prediction tool specific to VTE is unavailable.

The HAS-BLED score is used to estimate risk of bleeding for patients using anticoagulation for the prevention of stroke due to atrial fibrillation.[88] The tool identifies the following risks: hypertension, abnormal renal/liver function, history of stroke, bleeding history or predisposition, labile INR, elderly, and the use of drugs/alcohol concomitantly. The score has been validated in comparison to other scores, and the data set utilized a direct thrombin inhibitor (ximelagatran) in comparison to warfarin.[88] It is important to note that the validation study also identified concurrent aspirin use, diabetes, and heart failure or left ventricular dysfunction as significant risks for bleeding while on anticoagulation.[88]

Another validated tool is the Outpatient Bleeding Risk Index, which was validated on a data set of patients diagnosed with DVT or PE and undergoing standard LMWH/VKA therapy.[89] The data set suffered from not having many high-risk bleeding patients, but did have adequate numbers to discriminate between low and moderate risks of bleeding, making it uniquely appropriate for risk assessment in lower-risk patients. In the study, rates of major hemorrhage were zero per hundred person-years (0%–2.8% 95% CI) and 4.3% (1.1%–11.1% 95% CI) for the low-risk and moderate-risk groups, respectively.[89]

Treatment Duration

The efficacy of treatment and the associated reduction in morbidity and mortality should be weighed against the probability of bleeding. It would be reasonable, for example, to treat a younger individual for a more prolonged period (eg, 2 years), in the setting of unprovoked DVT, and just as reasonable to treat an elderly individual (eg, 70 years) for only 6 months, given the relative risks of recurrence, case fatality, and bleeding.

The efficacy of prevention of recurrence can be expressed in terms of a reduction of risk associated with a unit of time (eg, months of treatment needed to prevent an additional event).[40] Multiple studies have demonstrated that short-term anticoagulation (6 weeks to 6 months) demonstrates more robust efficacy in terms of prevented DVT per month, as compared with extended anticoagulation. Authors have suggested alterable risk factors (eg, immobilization, recent surgery) that might cause of VTE may suggest a need for a shorter period of anticoagulation.[40]

Novel Oral Anticoagulant Efficacy and Risk for Extended (More than 3 Months) Therapy

In cases in which extended therapy is pursued due to an estimated high risk of recurrence and low risk of bleeding, some NOACs offer advantages. The agents dabigatran, apixaban, and rivaroxaban were all superior to placebo, with low major rates of bleeding. In addition, a prophylactic dose (2.5 mg as opposed the therapeutic dose of 5 mg) of apixaban significantly reduced VTE recurrence and had a trend toward even lower rates of bleeding. Although no trial has been conducted, the data would suggest that an investigation into extended therapy at lower doses would be warranted. Similar trials with lower INR goals with warfarin did not prove beneficial in preventing recurrent DVT.[65] As mentioned previously, aspirin therapy as opposed to no therapy after cessation of anticoagulant use remains a viable option and should be based on risk of bleeding.

Specific Recommendations

Weighing individual risks and benefits for each patient is ideal. Identifying risk thresholds for starting and stopping anticoagulation on an individual basis is best, but may be difficult to calculate and translate. Therefore, the authors recommend the previously discussed CHEST guidelines to assist in the management cases, while still contextualizing and individualizing therapy for the patient. A recommended treatment algorithm, based on these guidelines, is provided in **Fig. 2**. Treatment guidelines and algorithm serve to broadly contextualize treatment, but each patient requires individualized therapy for his or her specific situation.

Provoked Deep Venous Thrombosis

Transient and alterable risks

For individuals with proximal lower extremity DVT whose risk for VTE can be altered (eg, provoked DVT related to surgery, immobilization, or exogenous estrogen use), 3 months of therapy are often adequate and recommended when compared with no therapy at all or when compared with longer or shorter-term therapy.[39] In these cases, dabigatran,

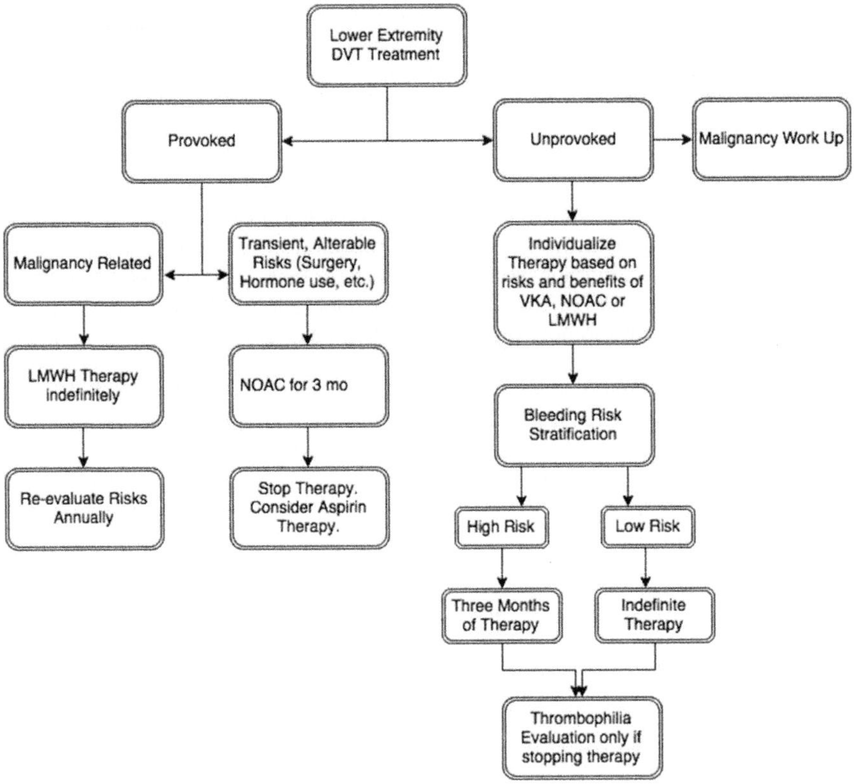

Fig. 2. Recommended treatment algorithm based on the 2016 CHEST guidelines. (*Data from* Kearon C, Akl EA, Ornelas J, et al. Antithrombotic therapy for VTE disease: CHEST guideline and expert panel report. Chest 2016;149(2):315–52.)

rivaroxaban, apixaban, and edoxaban are recommended over VKA therapy.[39] In patients with a proximal DVT of the leg or PE provoked by a nonsurgical but transient risk factor, treatment is recommended for 3 months regardless of bleeding risk.[39]

Malignancy-associated deep venous thrombosis

For individuals with cancer-associated VTE, LMWH is the preferred and recommended initial therapy over VKA therapy. Patients taking only LMWH versus those bridged to VKAs have about half the rate of recurrent events.[39,90]

In patients with DVT of the leg or PE and active cancer (cancer-associated thrombosis), regardless of bleeding risk, extended anticoagulant therapy (no scheduled stop date) is recommended over 3 months of therapy. It is recommended to reassess the necessity of anticoagulation and anticipated duration on an annual basis.[39] For those patients who require continuation of therapy beyond 3 months, there is no need to change the choice of anticoagulant after the first 3 months.[39]

Unprovoked Deep Venous Thrombosis

In patients with an unprovoked DVT of the leg, treatment with anticoagulation is recommended for at least 3 months over treatment of a shorter or longer duration.[39] D-dimer and patient sex may be considered in the decision to extend anticoagulant therapy 1 month after cessation.[39]

In patients with a first DVT (ie, an unprovoked proximal DVT of the leg) and a low or moderate bleeding risk, extended anticoagulant therapy (at least 3 months, no scheduled stop date) is preferred. However, in those patients with unprovoked DVT and high bleeding risk, 3 months of anticoagulant therapy are suggested.

In the case in which a second unprovoked VTE occurs after cessation of therapy in a patient who has a low or moderate bleeding risk, extended anticoagulant therapy (no scheduled stop date) is recommended. In patients with high bleeding risk and recurrent unprovoked VTE, 3 months of anticoagulant therapy are recommended.[39]

Regardless of the etiology, the CHEST guidelines on duration of therapy serve as a reminder to reassess the need for anticoagulation annually.

Isolated Distal Deep Venous Thrombosis

In patients with acute isolated distal DVT of the leg without severe symptoms or risk factors for extension, serial imaging of the deep veins for 2 weeks is recommended over initial anticoagulation.[39] Consideration should be given to risk of bleeding, and in those patients with a high bleeding risk, serial imaging is likely the preferred strategy.

If the thrombus demonstrates no extension in those patients with acute isolated distal DVT of the leg who are managed with serial imaging, no anticoagulation is recommended, unless severe symptoms are present. If the thrombus extends, anticoagulation is recommended.[39]

In the case in which acute isolated distal DVT of the leg manifests with severe symptoms or high risk of extension, empiric anticoagulation is recommended.[39] In patients with acute isolated distal DVT of the leg who are managed with anticoagulation, the same recommendations for proximal lower extremity DVT treatment should be followed.[39]

CONTROVERSIES

The advent of the NOACs has been met with appropriate skepticism regarding the efficacy and adverse effects of these novel drugs. Recent literature has demonstrated the noninferiority of dabigatran, rivaroxaban, apixaban, and edoxaban when compared with traditional VKAs in the treatment of VTE.[65,72,91–93]

Despite the estimated lower risks of bleeding demonstrated in the phase 3 trials for the NOACs (as well as data from a meta-analysis of 102,607 patients),[94] 1 concern among many practitioners has been the lack of a reversal agent when unanticipated or catastrophic bleeding occurs. Reversal of anticoagulation for anticipated procedures (minor or major surgeries) is a justified but smaller concern, as the drugs all have relatively short half-lives, and cessation of the drug alone is enough to adequately reverse anticoagulation in 24 to 72 hours depending on the half-life of the specific drug used and renal clearance of the patient. Risk of bleeding from surgery is also a consideration, as is the reason for anticoagulation, when stopping anticoagulation for anticipated procedures.

In cases of catastrophic bleeding in which emergent reversal of anticoagulation is needed, in contrast to the traditionally used VKAs, heparin, or LMWH, the NOACs initially did not have US Food and Drug Administration (FDA)-approved specific agents for reversal. It is well known that warfarin and the VKAs can be reversed with vitamin K, prothrombin complex concentrates (PCCs), and fresh-frozen plasma (FFP). Heparin (and to some extent LMWH) can be reversed with protamine sulfate. To add to the problem, standardized anticoagulation parameters such as the PT, activated partial thromboplastin time (aPTT), and INR are not informative in assessing the degree of anticoagulation with the NOACs.[65]

Consideration for reversal of anticoagulation with NOACs begins with risk assessment. Vital signs and rate of blood loss should be first assessed to determine any emergent need for reversal. The location of bleeding and whether pressure can be applied to a bleeding site should also be considered. In sources of occult bleeding or that which cannot be visualized directly (eg, GI tract bleeding), serial blood counts may prove beneficial. One should also consider alternative etiologies of bleeding, including thrombocytopenia or qualitative platelet dysfunction. Few data exist regarding effective drug therapies for reversal of NOAC-associated bleeding. Options that have been described in the literature include[95]

- Alteration of pharmacokinetics (decrease absorption from GI tract, remove from circulation with hemodialysis)
  - Of the agents available, dabigatran is the only drug with which hemodialysis is expected to be of benefit
  - Activated charcoal is expected to decrease absorption of dabigatran and apixaban, with unknown efficacy in the other NOACs
- Antifibrinolytic therapies (eg, aminocaproic acid, tranexamic acid)
- Plasma factor therapy: FFP, PCCs, cryoprecipitate
  - These therapies collectively have limited data for efficacy
  - Studies that have been performed have only investigated surrogate markers for clinical outcome (eg, reversal of INR and bleeding time) and have demonstrated no data on actual patient outcomes[95]
- Specific antidotes[95] bind the drug or inhibit a drug or class of drugs at the active site, rendering the NOACs ineffective
  - Ciraparantag, which reverses the effects of direct thrombin inhibitors, factor Xa inhibitors, and heparins
  - Andexanet alfa, which reverses the effect of factor Xa inhibitors
  - Idarucizumab, a humanized mouse monoclonal antibody fragment that reverses the effects of dabigatran and was FDA approved in October, 2015
  - Investigations into the efficacy and safety of these drugs are all being performed. Considerations for procoagulant effects are among the highest concern and have been demonstrated in 5 of 90 patients analyzed at a phase III interim analysis. The true procoagulant effect cannot be analyzed based on these data, as there was no placebo group for comparison[95]

One important consideration when evaluating the efficacy of anticoagulation reversal with the NOACs is a comparison to the efficacy of reversal of more commonly used agents, including VKAs. Although analysis of coagulation parameters seems helpful, patient based outcomes are far more important. For example, improvement of an INR, PT, or PTT value is meaningless if a patient suffers a catastrophic intracranial hemorrhage that is not prevented or treated by use of the reversal agent. The availability of FFPs, PCCs, and Vitamin K for reversal of an INR does not necessarily translate into efficacy in terms of patient outcome. Even the most recent trials utilizing 4-factor PCCs have focused on INR reduction or surrogate markers of bleeding as opposed to patient outcomes.[96,97] As the NOACs are more commonly used and specific antidotes are developed, trials assessing patient outcomes should be conducted in order to assess the efficacy of reversal of the NOACs in comparison to traditional reversal of VKAs.

SUMMARY

VTE ranges from an isolated and self-limited disease, in the case of distal calf vein thrombosis, to catastrophic disease in the setting of large DVTs that cause localized swelling and pain and place patients at high risk of pulmonary embolism that could ultimately prove fatal. Assessment for DVT begins with risk factors and utilizes adjunctive testing based on the perceived level of risk. Most DVTs are managed with anticoagulant therapy, the type and duration of which varies with the patient's own history of VTE, cancer, or other risk factors. Adjunctive therapies to anticoagulation play a limited role in the management of DVT. Recent advances in anticoagulant therapies have allowed for more regular dosing, less need for monitoring, and decreased risks of bleeding, which ultimately may prove more satisfactory for patients, in addition to the obvious safety benefits. In the future, additional studies should continue to evaluate the efficacy of novel anticoagulants in comparison to traditional agents, refine the role of these agents based on individual risk factors, and compare the efficacy of reversal agents in circumstances of catastrophic bleeding in terms of patient outcomes.

REFERENCES

1. Fields JM, Goyal M. Venothromboembolism. Emerg Med Clin North Am 2008; 26(3):649–83, viii.
2. Bevis PM, Smith FCT. Deep vein thrombosis. Surgery (Oxford) 2016;34(4): 159–64.
3. Nordström M, Lindblad B, Bergqvist D, et al. A prospective study of the incidence of deep-vein thrombosis within a defined urban population. J Intern Med 1992; 232(2):155–60.
4. Bauersachs RM, Riess H, Hach-Wunderle V, et al. Impact of gender on the clinical presentation and diagnosis of deep-vein thrombosis. Thromb Haemost 2010; 103(4):710–7.
5. Bauersachs RM. Clinical presentation of deep vein thrombosis and pulmonary embolism. Best Pract Res Clin Haematol 2012;25(3):243–51.
6. Silverstein MD, Heit JA, Mohr DN, et al. Trends in the incidence of deep vein thrombosis and pulmonary embolism: a 25-year population-based study. Arch Intern Med 1998;158(6):585–93.
7. Tagalakis V, Patenaude V, Kahn SR, et al. Incidence of and mortality from venous thromboembolism in a real-world population: the Q-VTE Study Cohort. Am J Med 2013;126(9):832.e13-21.
8. Martinez C, Cohen AT, Bamber L, et al. Epidemiology of first and recurrent venous thromboembolism: a population-based cohort study in patients without active cancer. Thromb Haemost 2014;112(2):255–63.
9. Beckman MG, Hooper WC, Critchley SE, et al. Venous thromboembolism: a public health concern. Am J Prev Med 2010;38(4 Suppl):S495–501.
10. Marshall PS, Cain H. Upper extremity deep vein thrombosis. Clin Chest Med 2010;31(4):783–97.
11. Dickson BC. Venous thrombosis: on the history of Virchow's triad. Univ Toronto Med J 2004;81(3):166–71.
12. Bates SM, Ginsberg JS. Clinical practice. Treatment of deep-vein thrombosis. N Engl J Med 2004;351(3):268–77.
13. Negus D, Pinto DJ. Natural history of postoperative deep-vein thrombosis. Lancet 1969;2(7621):645.
14. Lagerstedt CI, Olsson CG, Fagher BO, et al. Need for long-term anticoagulant treatment in symptomatic calf-vein thrombosis. Lancet 1985;2(8454):515–8.
15. Moser KM, Fedullo PF, LitteJohn JK, et al. Frequent asymptomatic pulmonary embolism in patients with deep venous thrombosis. JAMA 1994;271(3):223–5.

16. Gavish I, Brenner B. Air travel and the risk of thromboembolism. Intern Emerg Med 2011;6(2):113–6.
17. Adi Y, Bayliss S, Rouse A, et al. The association between air travel and deep vein thrombosis: systematic review & meta-analysis. BMC Cardiovasc Disord 2004;4:7.
18. Beam DM, Courtney DM, Kabrhel C, et al. Risk of thromboembolism varies, depending on category of immobility in outpatients. Ann Emerg Med 2009;54(2):147–52.
19. Litzendorf ME, Satiani B. Superficial venous thrombosis: disease progression and evolving treatment approaches. Vasc Health Risk Manag 2011;7:569–75.
20. Flanc C, Kakkar VV, Clarke MB. The detection of venous thrombosis of the legs using 125-I-labelled fibrinogen. Br J Surg 1968;55(10):742–7.
21. Haeger K. Problems of acute deep venous thrombosis. I. The interpretation of signs and symptoms. Angiology 1969;20(4):219–23.
22. Anand SS, Wells PS, Hunt D, et al. Does this patient have deep vein thrombosis? JAMA 1998;279(14):1094–9.
23. Goodacre S, Sutton AJ, Sampson FC. Meta-analysis: the value of clinical assessment in the diagnosis of deep venous thrombosis. Ann Intern Med 2005;143(2):129–39.
24. Wells PS, Hirsh J, Anderson DR, et al. Accuracy of clinical assessment of deep-vein thrombosis. Lancet 1995;345(8961):1326–30.
25. Bates SM, Jaeschke R, Stevens SM, et al. Diagnosis of DVT: antithrombotic therapy and prevention of thrombosis, 9th ed: American College of Chest Physicians evidence-based clinical practice guidelines. chest 2012;141(2 Suppl):e351s–418.
26. Dupras D, Bluhm J, Felty C, et al. Venous thromboembolism diagnosis and treatment. Institute for Clinical Systems Improvement; 2013. Available at: http://bit.ly/VTE0113.
27. American College of Emergency Physicians (ACEP) Clinical Policies Committee, ACEP Clinical Policies Subcommittee on Suspected Lower-Extremity Deep Venous Thrombosis. Clinical policy: critical issues in the evaluation and management of adult patients presenting with suspected lower-extremity deep venous thrombosis. Ann Emerg Med 2003;42(1):124–35.
28. National Clinical Guideline Centre (UK). Venous thromboembolic diseases: the management of venous thromboembolic diseases and the role of thrombophilia testing [Internet]. London: Royal College of Physicians (UK); 2012. Available at: https://www.ncbi.nlm.nih.gov/books/NBK132796/. Accessed July 28, 2017.
29. Adams D, Welch JL, Kline JA. Clinical utility of an age-adjusted D-dimer in the diagnosis of venous thromboembolism. Ann Emerg Med 2014;64(3):232–4.
30. Righini M, Van Es J, Den Exter PL, et al. Age-adjusted D-dimer cutoff levels to rule out pulmonary embolism: the ADJUST-PE study. JAMA 2014;311(11):1117–24.
31. Kline JA, Williams GW, Hernandez-Nino J. D-dimer concentrations in normal pregnancy: new diagnostic thresholds are needed. Clin Chem 2005;51(5):825–9.
32. Kovac M, Mikovic Z, Rakicevic L, et al. The use of D-dimer with new cutoff can be useful in diagnosis of venous thromboembolism in pregnancy. Eur J Obstet Gynecol Reprod Biol 2010;148(1):27–30.
33. Johnson SA, Stevens SM, Woller SC, et al. Risk of deep vein thrombosis following a single negative whole-leg compression ultrasound: a systematic review and meta-analysis. JAMA 2010;303(5):438–45.

34. Adhikari S, Zeger W, Thom C, et al. Isolated deep venous thrombosis: implications for 2-point compression ultrasonography of the lower extremity. Ann Emerg Med 2015;66(3):262–6.
35. Guideline developed in collaboration with the American College of Radiology, Society of Pediatric Radiology, Society of Radiologists in Ultrasound. AIUM practice guideline for the performance of peripheral venous ultrasound examinations. J Ultrasound Med 2015;34(8):1–9.
36. Pomero F, Dentali F, Borretta V, et al. Accuracy of emergency physician-performed ultrasonography in the diagnosis of deep-vein thrombosis: a systematic review and meta-analysis. Thromb Haemost 2013;109(1):137–45.
37. Hunter F, Thomson K. Towards evidence based emergency medicine: best BETs from the Manchester Royal Infirmary. BET 1: Emergency physician performed 2-point bedside compression ultrasound for deep venous thrombosis. Emerg Med J 2014;31(11):944–6.
38. Kearon C, Akl EA, Comerota AJ, et al. Antithrombotic therapy for VTE disease: antithrombotic therapy and prevention of thrombosis, 9th ed: American College of Chest Physicians evidence-based clinical practice guidelines. Chest 2012; 141(2 Suppl):e419S–494.
39. Kearon C, Akl EA, Ornelas J, et al. Antithrombotic therapy for VTE disease: CHEST guideline and expert panel report. Chest 2016;149(2):315–52.
40. Prins MH, Hutten BA, Koopman MM, et al. Long-term treatment of venous thromboembolic disease. Thromb Haemost 1999;82(2):892–8.
41. Decousus H, Leizorovicz A, Parent F, et al. A clinical trial of vena caval filters in the prevention of pulmonary embolism in patients with proximal deep-vein thrombosis. Prévention du Risque d'Embolie Pulmonaire par Interruption Cave Study Group. N Engl J Med 1998;338(7):409–15.
42. Brighton TA, Eikelboom JW, Mann K, et al. Low-dose aspirin for preventing recurrent venous thromboembolism. N Engl J Med 2012;367(21):1979–87.
43. Becattini C, Agnelli G, Schenone A, et al. Aspirin for preventing the recurrence of venous thromboembolism. N Engl J Med 2012;366(21):1959–67.
44. Becattini C, Agnelli G. Aspirin for prevention and treatment of venous thromboembolism. Blood Rev 2014;28(3):103–8.
45. Antithrombotic Trialists' Collaboration. Collaborative meta-analysis of randomised trials of antiplatelet therapy for prevention of death, myocardial infarction, and stroke in high risk patients. BMJ 2002;324(7329):71–86.
46. Collaborative overview of randomised trials of antiplatelet therapy–III: reduction in venous thrombosis and pulmonary embolism by antiplatelet prophylaxis among surgical and medical patients. Antiplatelet Trialists' Collaboration. BMJ 1994; 308(6923):235–46.
47. Tsai AW, Cushman M, Rosamond WD, et al. Cardiovascular risk factors and venous thromboembolism incidence: the longitudinal investigation of thromboembolism etiology. Arch Intern Med 2002;162(10):1182–9.
48. Sørensen HT, Horvath-Puho E, Søgaard KK, et al. Arterial cardiovascular events, statins, low-dose aspirin and subsequent risk of venous thromboembolism: a population-based case-control study. J Thromb Haemost 2009;7(4):521–8.
49. Becattini C, Agnelli G. Treatment of venous thromboembolism with new anticoagulant agents. J Am Coll Cardiol 2016;67(16):1941–55.
50. Prevention of pulmonary embolism and deep vein thrombosis with low dose aspirin: Pulmonary Embolism Prevention (PEP) trial. Lancet 2000;355(9212): 1295–302.

51. Anderson DR, Dunbar MJ, Bohm ER, et al. Aspirin versus low-molecular-weight heparin for extended venous thromboembolism prophylaxis after total hip arthroplasty: a randomized trial. Ann Intern Med 2013;158(11):800–6.
52. Barritt DW, Jordan SC. Anticoagulant drugs in the treatment of pulmonary embolism. A controlled trial. Lancet 1960;1(7138):1309–12.
53. Boey JP, Gallus A. Drug treatment of venous thromboembolism in the elderly. Drugs Aging 2016;33(7):475–90.
54. Hirsh J, Warkentin TE, Shaughnessy SG, et al. Heparin and low-molecular-weight heparin: mechanisms of action, pharmacokinetics, dosing, monitoring, efficacy, and safety. Chest 2001;119(1 Suppl):64S–94S.
55. Warkentin TE, Levine MN, Hirsh J, et al. Heparin-induced thrombocytopenia in patients treated with low-molecular-weight heparin or unfractionated heparin. N Engl J Med 1995;332(20):1330–5.
56. Gould MK, Dembitzer AD, Doyle RL, et al. Low-molecular-weight heparins compared with unfractionated heparin for treatment of acute deep venous thrombosis. A meta-analysis of randomized, controlled trials. Ann Intern Med 1999; 130(10):800–9.
57. Erkens PM, Prins MH. Fixed dose subcutaneous low molecular weight heparins versus adjusted dose unfractionated heparin for venous thromboembolism. Cochrane Database Syst Rev 2010;(9):CD001100.
58. Pettilä V, Leinonen P, Markkola A, et al. Postpartum bone mineral density in women treated for thromboprophylaxis with unfractionated heparin or LMW heparin. Thromb Haemost 2002;87(2):182–6.
59. Finazzi G, Marchioli R, Brancaccio V, et al. A randomized clinical trial of high-intensity warfarin vs. conventional antithrombotic therapy for the prevention of recurrent thrombosis in patients with the antiphospholipid syndrome (WAPS). J Thromb Haemost 2005;3(5):848–53.
60. Crowther MA, Ginsberg JS, Julian J, et al. A comparison of two intensities of warfarin for the prevention of recurrent thrombosis in patients with the antiphospholipid antibody syndrome. N Engl J Med 2003;349(12):1133–8.
61. Hyers TM, Agnelli G, Hull RD, et al. Antithrombotic therapy for venous thromboembolic disease. Chest 2001;119(1 Suppl):176S–93S.
62. Nieto JA, Solano R, Ruiz-Ribó MD, et al. Fatal bleeding in patients receiving anticoagulant therapy for venous thromboembolism: findings from the RIETE registry. J Thromb Haemost 2010;8(6):1216–22.
63. Middeldorp S, Hutten BA. Long-term vs short-term therapy with vitamin K antagonists for symptomatic venous thromboembolism. JAMA 2015;314(1):72–3.
64. Chan NC, Eikelboom JW, Weitz JI. Evolving treatments for arterial and venous thrombosis: role of the direct oral anticoagulants. Circ Res 2016;118(9):1409–24.
65. Yeh CH, Gross PL, Weitz JI. Evolving use of new oral anticoagulants for treatment of venous thromboembolism. Blood 2014;124(7):1020–8.
66. Gómez-Outes A, Lecumberri R, Suárez-Gea ML, et al. Case fatality rates of recurrent thromboembolism and bleeding in patients receiving direct oral anticoagulants for the initial and extended treatment of venous thromboembolism: a systematic review. J Cardiovasc Pharmacol Ther 2015;20(5):490–500.
67. Kakkos SK, Kirkilesis GI, Tsolakis IA. Editor's choice - efficacy and safety of the new oral anticoagulants dabigatran, rivaroxaban, apixaban, and edoxaban in the treatment and secondary prevention of venous thromboembolism: a systematic review and meta-analysis of phase III trials. Eur J Vasc Endovasc Surg 2014; 48(5):565–75.

68. Schulman S, Kakkar AK, Goldhaber SZ, et al. Treatment of acute venous thromboembolism with dabigatran or warfarin and pooled analysis. Circulation 2014; 129(7):764–72.
69. Schulman S, Kearon C, Kakkar AK, et al. Dabigatran versus warfarin in the treatment of acute venous thromboembolism. N Engl J Med 2009;361(24):2342–52.
70. Desai J, Kolb JM, Weitz JI, et al. Gastrointestinal bleeding with the new oral anticoagulants–defining the issues and the management strategies. Thromb Haemost 2013;110(2):205–12.
71. Ray B, Keyrouz SG. Management of anticoagulant-related intracranial hemorrhage: an evidence-based review. Crit Care 2014;18(3):223.
72. EINSTEIN Investigators, Bauersachs R, Berkowitz SD, Brenner B, et al. Oral rivaroxaban for symptomatic venous thromboembolism. N Engl J Med 2010;363(26): 2499–510.
73. EINSTEIN–PE Investigators, Büller HR, Prins MH, Lensin AW, et al. Oral rivaroxaban for the treatment of symptomatic pulmonary embolism. N Engl J Med 2012; 366(14):1287–97.
74. Agnelli G, Buller HR, Cohen A, et al. Apixaban for extended treatment of venous thromboembolism. N Engl J Med 2013;368(8):699–708.
75. Hokusai-VTE Investigators, Büller HR, Décousus H, Grosso MA, et al. Edoxaban versus warfarin for the treatment of symptomatic venous thromboembolism. N Engl J Med 2013;369(15):1406–15.
76. Giugliano RP, Ruff CT, Braunwald E, et al. Edoxaban versus warfarin in patients with atrial fibrillation. N Engl J Med 2013;369(22):2093–104.
77. Watson L, Broderick C, Armon MP. Thrombolysis for acute deep vein thrombosis. Cochrane Database Syst Rev 2014;(1):CD002783.
78. Bashir R, Zack CJ, Zhao H, et al. Comparative outcomes of catheter-directed thrombolysis plus anticoagulation vs anticoagulation alone to treat lower-extremity proximal deep vein thrombosis. JAMA Intern Med 2014;174(9): 1494–501.
79. Galanaud J-P, Monreal M, Kahn SR. Predictors of the post-thrombotic syndrome and their effect on the therapeutic management of deep vein thrombosis. J Vasc Surg Venous Lymphat Disord 2016;4(4):531–4.
80. Onuoha CU. Phlegmasia cerulea dolens: A rare clinical presentation. Am J Med 2015;128(9):e27–8.
81. Tung CS, Soliman PT, Wallace MJ, et al. Successful catheter-directed venous thrombolysis in phlegmasia cerulea dolens. Gynecol Oncol 2007;107(1):140–2.
82. Oguzkurt L, Ozkan U, Demirturk OS, et al. Endovascular treatment of phlegmasia cerulea dolens with impending venous gangrene: manual aspiration thrombectomy as the first-line thrombus removal method. Cardiovasc Intervent Radiol 2011;34(6):1214–21.
83. Heit JA, Silverstein MD, Mohr DN, et al. Predictors of survival after deep vein thrombosis and pulmonary embolism: a population-based, cohort study. Arch Intern Med 1999;159(5):445–53.
84. Iorio A, Kearon C, Filippucci E, et al. Risk of recurrence after a first episode of symptomatic venous thromboembolism provoked by a transient risk factor: a systematic review. Arch Intern Med 2010;170(19):1710–6.
85. Baglin T, Luddington R, Brown K, et al. Incidence of recurrent venous thromboembolism in relation to clinical and thrombophilic risk factors: prospective cohort study. Lancet 2003;362(9383):523–6.
86. Prandoni P, Lensing AW, Cogo A, et al. The long-term clinical course of acute deep venous thrombosis. Ann Intern Med 1996;125(1):1–7.

87. Agnelli G, Prandoni P, Santamaria MG, et al. Three months versus one year of oral anticoagulant therapy for idiopathic deep venous thrombosis. Warfarin Optimal Duration Italian Trial Investigators. N Engl J Med 2001;345(3):165–9.
88. Lip GYH, Frison L, Halperin JL, et al. Comparative validation of a novel risk score for predicting bleeding risk in anticoagulated patients with atrial fibrillation: the HAS-BLED (Hypertension, Abnormal Renal/Liver Function, Stroke, Bleeding History or Predisposition, Labile INR, Elderly, Drugs/Alcohol Concomitantly) score. J Am Coll Cardiol 2011;57(2):173–80.
89. Wells PS, Forgie MA, Simms M, et al. The outpatient bleeding risk index: validation of a tool for predicting bleeding rates in patients treated for deep venous thrombosis and pulmonary embolism. Arch Intern Med 2003;163(8):917–20.
90. Lee AYY, Levine MN, Baker RI, et al. Low-molecular-weight heparin versus a coumarin for the prevention of recurrent venous thromboembolism in patients with cancer. N Engl J Med 2003;349(2):146–53.
91. Lassen MR, Raskob GE, Gallus A, et al. Apixaban versus enoxaparin for thromboprophylaxis after knee replacement (ADVANCE-2): a randomised double-blind trial. Lancet 2010;375(9717):807–15.
92. Edoxaban (Savaysa)–The fourth new oral anticoagulant. JAMA 2015;314(1):76–7.
93. Eikelboom JW, Wallentin L, Connolly SJ, et al. Risk of bleeding with 2 doses of dabigatran compared with warfarin in older and younger patients with atrial fibrillation: an analysis of the randomized evaluation of long-term anticoagulant therapy (RE-LY) trial. Circulation 2011;123(21):2363–72.
94. Chai-Adisaksopha C, Crowther M, Isayama T, et al. The impact of bleeding complications in patients receiving target-specific oral anticoagulants: a systematic review and meta-analysis. Blood 2014;124(15):2450–8.
95. Hu TY, Vaidya VR, Asirvatham SJ. Reversing anticoagulant effects of novel oral anticoagulants: role of ciraparantag, andexanet alfa, and idarucizumab. Vasc Health Risk Manag 2016;12:35–44.
96. Rivosecchi RM, Durkin J, Okonkwo DO, et al. Safety and efficacy of warfarin reversal with four-factor prothrombin complex concentrate for subtherapeutic INR in intracerebral hemorrhage. Neurocrit Care 2016;25(3):359–64.
97. Sarode R, Milling TJ, Refaai MA, et al. Efficacy and safety of a 4-factor prothrombin complex concentrate in patients on vitamin K antagonists presenting with major bleeding: a randomized, plasma-controlled, phase IIIb study. Circulation 2013;128(11):1234–43.

Vascular Access Complications

An Emergency Medicine Approach

Erica Marie Simon, DO, MHA*, Shane Matthew Summers, MD

KEYWORDS

- Central venous catheterization • Arterial catheterization • Vascular hemorrhage
- Central line infection • Dialysis access complications
- Central catheterization and anticoagulation

KEY POINTS

- Central venous catheterizations and arterial catheterizations are frequently used in the emergency setting to establish invasive hemodynamic monitoring, perform acute resuscitation, and facilitate the initiation of specialty-directed therapies (hemodialysis and extracorporeal membranous oxygenation).
- Morbidity and mortality associated with vascular access attempts occur secondary to infection, thrombosis, embolism, and iatrogenic injury.
- As the prevalence of chronic kidney disease continues to increase, emergency physicians must be aware of complications associated with hemodialysis vascular access.
- When obtaining central venous access or arterial access in an anticoagulated patient, experts recommend catheterization of a directly compressible vessel.
- Vascular access complications may be limited by the employment of aseptic technique, choice of appropriate cannulation site, operator training, and the utilization of ultrasound.

INTRODUCTION

Approximately 8% of individuals presenting to United States emergency departments (EDs) require invasive vascular access procedures during their initial evaluation or subsequent hospitalization.[1] Today central venous cannulation and arterial catheterization are commonly used in the emergency setting to allow for resuscitation, administration of noxious medications, cardiac pacing, extracorporeal therapies, hemodialysis (HD), and hemodynamic monitoring. Because infectious and noninfectious

The authors have nothing to disclose.
Emergency Department, San Antonio Uniformed Services Health Education Consortium, San Antonio Military Medical Center, SAMMC, MCHE-EMR, 3551 Roger Brooke Drive, JBSA Fort Sam Houston, TX 78234-6200, USA
* Corresponding author.
E-mail address: emsimon85@gmail.com

Emerg Med Clin N Am 35 (2017) 771–788
http://dx.doi.org/10.1016/j.emc.2017.06.004
0733-8627/17/Published by Elsevier Inc.

complications related to vascular access are associated with increased patient morbidity and mortality, their prevention and early identification are vital to limiting personal and organizational costs, reducing inpatient hospital days, and improving quality of care.

CENTRAL VENOUS ACCESS

In the United States, physicians insert approximately 5 million central venous catheters (CVCs) annually.[2,3] Although CVCs are highly useful for hemodynamic monitoring, the administration of sclerosing medications, the performance of emergent dialysis, and so forth, the placement of these devices is associated with infectious, thrombotic, and mechanical complications.[2–4]

Infectious Complications

Central line–associated bloodstream infections (CLABSIs), or catheter-related bloodstream infections (CRBSIs), occur in 0.5% to 1.2% of patients having CVC, a number drastically reduced after the widespread use of sterile precautions.[5] Although the incidence of CLABSIs is variable across health care facilities, current ICU and ED studies report an average 30,000 catheter-related infections per year, with an associated 30-day hospital readmission rate of 37.1%.[2,4] Treatment costs associated with CVC infection range from $3700 to $36,000 per episode, representing $670 million to $2.68 billion in health care spending annually.[6]

Risk factors

Risk factors for CLABSIs are patient related, catheter related, and operator related. Patient risk factors include immunosuppression, medical comorbidities (peripheral atherosclerosis, diabetes, and recent surgery), increasing severity of illness, and concomitant bacteremia.[7,8] Catheter-associated risk factors center on the type of catheter used and the site chosen for cannulation.[2,9,10] In randomized trials, antiseptic impregnated CVCs (chlorhexidine and silver sulfadiazine or minocycline and rifampin) consistently demonstrate lower rates of CLABSIs compared with their nonimpregnated counterparts.[2,9,10] As an example, a study of 453 CVCs, performed by Maki and colleagues,[10] identified a 5-fold reduction in catheter-associated blood stream infections (1.6 compared with 7.6 infections per 1000 catheter days; relative risk 0.21 [CI, 0.03–0.95]; $P = .03$) with the utilization of antiseptic catheters. In terms of cannulation site, research has demonstrated subclavian venous catheterization (infection rate of 0.5%) as associated with fewer infectious complications compared with jugular venous and femoral venous access (infection rates of 1.4% and 1.2%, respectively).[5] Risk of infection greatly increases if sterile precautions are not used. Current evidence also suggests that subclavian venous cannulation is less likely to result in an infectious complication compared with catheterization of the internal jugular vein; however, randomized, controlled trials are needed.[2,9] As with any medical procedure, complication rates are intimately associated with operator experience.[2] Practitioner implementation of sterile barrier precautions, including mask, cap, sterile gown, and sterile gloves and the employment of cutaneous antiseptics have been shown to save approximately $167 per CVC inserted (estimated funds allocated to CLABSI treatment measures in the setting of poor sterile precautions).[2,11]

Identification and treatment of a central line–associated bloodstream infections

In an effort to improve heath surveillance efforts, the Centers for Disease Control and Prevention (CDC) has formally defined a CLABSI/CRBSI as a laboratory-confirmed bloodstream infection occurring in the presence of a CVC or within 48 hours of the

CVC removal.[4,12] CLABSIs/CRBSIs are associated with significant attributable mortality (5%–25%[4]) and substantial economic burden (increasing average length of stay by 14 days; associated with an additional cost of $2002 per patient).[13]

A CLABSI or CRBSI should be suspected in patients with CVCs presenting with signs and symptoms of a systemic inflammatory response (ie, temperature less than 36°C or greater than 38°C, heart rate greater than 90 beats per minute, respiratory rate greater than 20 breaths per minute, or white blood cell count less than 4000/μL or greater than 12,000/μL). All sites of central venous cannulation should be inspected for erythema, induration, fluctuance, skin maceration, and purulent drainage. Assessment for a CLABSI or CRBSI should include the removal of the CVC, culture of the catheter tip, 2 peripheral blood cultures, and initiation of antimicrobial therapy.[7,8] Common pathogens causing CLABSIs/CRBSIs include *Staphylococcus aureus*, *Pseudomonas aeruginosa*, coagulase-negative staphylococci, and gram-negative bacilli.[7,8] The initiation of antibiotics targeting these organisms is advised.[7,8] Antifungals targeting *Candida* spp should be administered for all patients receiving total parenteral nutrition, because this glucose-rich medium predisposes to CLABSI and systemic fungemia.[14]

Initiatives to reduce the incidence of central line–associated bloodstream infections/catheter-related bloodstream infections

Several agencies have released evidence-based guidelines for the reduction of CLABSIs/CRBSIs. The most recent, a publication by the CDC Healthcare Infection Control Practices Advisory Committee, offers a systematic review of 12 years of CVC research data, identifying best practices proven to reduce CLABSIs/CRBSIs.[15]

Recommendations contained within the CDC's Making Healthcare Safer (supported by metrics regarding declines in infections rates with the use of hand washing prior to CVC placement, the use of sterile barrier precautions, chlorhexidine for skin antisepsis, and so forth), when used in conjunction with the CDC National Healthcare Safety Network CLABSI/CRBSI surveillance program, have allowed thousands of medical facilities across the nation to improve CVC insertion and reduce the morbidity and mortality associated with infectious complications (50% decrease in CLABSIs between 2008 and 2014; 3655 acute care facilities across the United States reporting).[4]

Thrombotic Complications

Although reports vary widely according to study design, duration of follow-up, and screening modality, catheter-related thrombosis (CRT) is estimated to occur in 0.5% to 1.4% of patients after central venous cannulation.[5] Insertion of a CVC results in local vascular injury and the mechanical obstruction of blood flow.[16] In this setting, fibrin deposition occurs within hours of catheter placement and may result in the formation of a pericatheter sheath (fibrin sleeve), catheter lumen thrombus, or deep vein thrombosis.[16,17] Although a majority of thrombi associated with CVCs are asymptomatic, the presence of CRT predisposes to bacterial colonization and catheter-related sepsis as well as thromboembolic events.[18,19]

Risk factors

CRT risk factors are related to patient and catheter characteristics.[16,20] Individuals with a history of inherited thrombophilia or malignancy, acquired hypercoagulability (heparin-induced thrombocytopenia), those undergoing chemotherapy or receiving treatment with erythropoiesis-stimulating agents, or those with a history of CRT or CLABSI are at an increased risk for developing CRT.[16] Features of CVCs associated with increased risk of CRT include larger catheter size[21] and site used for placement.[16] In randomized trials, routine studies to assess for venous thrombosis after catheter placement have identified increased risk of CRT associated with femoral and internal jugular venous cannulation compared with subclavian cathterization.[2,3,16,22]

Identification and treatment of thrombosis

Because examination is not sensitive or specific for CRT, patients presenting with ipsilateral extremity edema, or those with localized tenderness, edema, or erythema at the CVC site should undergo formal evaluation with Doppler ultrasonography (US).[16,23] US evaluation is also indicated in the event that samples cannot be withdrawn, or infusions delivered, through the CVC.[16] The use of contrasted CT and MRI should be considered for patients suspected of having an intrathoracic CRT with normal or nondiagnostic US.[16]

The management of CRT centers on reducing symptoms, limiting extension of thrombosis, and preventing chronic venous occlusion. To date, however, no randomized controlled trials of acute or long-term therapies for CRT have been undertaken.[16,24–26] Because current evidence has failed to demonstrate improvement in patient outcomes after CVC removal in the setting of CRT, experts recommend that the catheter remain in place unless it is nonfunctional, infected, or no longer needed.[16,24,25] If a catheter-related thrombus is identified, the American College of Chest Physicians recommends therapeutic anticoagulation during CVC and for a duration of 3 months after CVC removal.[16,26] Because studies regarding the safety and efficacy of various anticoagulant therapies (vitamin K antagonists, direct thrombin inhibitors, and factor Xa inhibitors) in the treatment of CRT are ongoing, current recommendations regarding therapy are lacking.[16] Today case studies report the comparative safety of catheter-directed thrombolysis in addressing upper extremity CRT; therefore, consultation should be considered in this setting.[16,25–27]

A thrombus isolated to a catheter lumen may be managed with removal and replacement of the CVC versus instillation of a thrombolytic.[28] Both alteplase and tenecteplase have been shown to relieve 80% to 90% of catheter occlusions within 1 hour to 2 hours of instillation.[18,28,29]

Prevention of thrombotic complications

Strategies previously proposed to limit the incidence of thrombotic complications after CVC include cannulation of the subclavian vein, proper placement of subclavian and internal jugular CVCs, the employment of catheter flushes, and thromboprophylaxis.[16] Regarding appropriate placement, a 2011 meta-analysis of 5 randomized controlled trials and 7 prospective studies (n = 5636 subjects) revealed an increased risk of CRT for catheter tips placed outside of the junction of the superior vena cava and right atrium (odds ratio [OR] 1.92; CI, 1.22–3.01).[30] Thus, emergency physicians should examine postprocedure radiographs to localize the catheter tip. With regard to the other proposed strategies, routine heparin and saline flushes have failed to demonstrate a reduction in the incidence of CRTs.[16,31] Because numerous meta-analyses have failed to demonstrate a benefit of thromboprophylaxis in the prevention of CRTs, clinical practice guidelines currently recommend against the routine use of prophylactic anticoagulation in patients with a CVC.[16,25,32–35]

Mechanical Complications

Mechanical complications associated with CVC occur in 0.7% to 2.1%[5] of catheterization attempts and include arterial injury, pneumothorax, hemothorax, air embolism, and cardiac dysrhythmia.[2,5,36,37] Arterial puncture is a well-documented complication of central venous cannulation. Arterial cannulation (occurring during 4.2% to 9.3% of all line placements[38]) is encountered most often during femoral catheterization attempts.[2] Inadvertent arterial puncture can lead to uncontrolled hemorrhage, hematoma formation, pseudoaneurym, arteriovenous (AV) fistula, and embolic phenomenon.[37]

Pneumothorax complicates approximately 1% of CVC placements and is most often related to subclavian cannulation.[2,39,40] Hemothorax is associated with 0.4% to 0.6% of subclavian catheterization attempts.[2] Air emboli are rare, but depending on the volume of air instilled, may result in complete cardiovascular collapse due to limitations in left ventricular diastolic filling and decreased coronary perfusion.[41] Cerebral air emboli, occurring in patients with a patent foramen ovale, have a mortality rate of 23%.[42,43] Cardiac dysrhythmias may occur during CVC from guide wire contact with the right atrium, most frequently manifesting as premature atrial and ventricular contractions.[37,39,44] Prolonged guide wire stimulation of the atrioventricular node may result in supraventricular tachycardias predisposing to fatal dysrhythmias.[37,39,44]

Risk factors

Mechanical complications have been shown to increase with repeated cannulation attempts.[2,3,45] Similar to infectious complications of CVC placement, the risks of arterial injury, hemothorax, and pneumothorax vary according to the site chosen for cannulation.[2] Placement of a subclavian central line is more likely to be complicated by pneumothorax and hemothorax compared with internal jugular catheterization, and, as discussed previously, placement of a femoral central line is more commonly associated with arterial injury.[2] Patients with bleeding diathesis or those taking anticoagulants experience increasing morbidity and mortality secondary to vascular injury.[38]

Air emboli may occur with inappropriate patient positioning, failure of hub occlusion during line placement, or the delivery of air with line flushing.[37,39] Individuals with atrial or ventricular septal defects may transmit air emboli into systemic circulation leading to hemodynamic compromise.[38] As discussed previously, patients with a patent foramen ovale may suffer from cerebral air emboli.[37,42,43]

Identification and treatment of mechanical complications

Arterial puncture, often identified by pulsatile blood flow from the catheterization site, may be difficult to identify in a critically ill, septic, or hypoxemic patient.[38,40] If questions regarding arterial cannulation exist, experts recommend blood gas analysis or the placement of single-lumen catheter over guide wire followed by connection to a transducing system to identify arterial waveforms.[2,37,38] Although catheter removal and the application of direct pressure are appropriate interventions the setting of femoral arterial puncture, current studies indicate increased risk of expanding hematoma causing airway obstruction, stroke, and pseudoaneursym when this method is applied to cervicothoracic arterial injury.[37,46] In this scenario, consultation for endovascular repair is indicated.[37,46] If concern for arterial puncture with resultant hematoma formation in a noncompressible anatomic location (ie, intrathoracic or retroperitoneal) exists, advanced imaging should be considered, and consultation with a cardiothoracic, vascular, or interventional radiologist performed as appropriate.[4]

Large pnemothoraces occurring as a result of CVC placement may rapidly be identified due to patient hemodynamic instability and hypoxia, thereby necessitating emergent tube thoracostomy. Postprocedural chest radiographs (CXRs) demonstrate poor sensitivity (31%) in the detection of pneumothoraces.[47] CT remains the gold standard for diagnosis of a pneumothorax. Compared with a CXR, US demonstrates increased sensitivity (88.1%–95.3%[47,48]) and may be used as an expedient method of evaluation. Supplemental oxygen therapy and hemodynamic monitoring is indicated for pneumothoraces involving less than 15% of the involved lung volume; all others require tube thoracostomy.[37]

Studies identify CXR and US as demonstrating comparable sensitivity in the detection of hemothoraces (92%–96.2% and 81%–97.5%, respectively[49–52]). Similar to pneumothoraces, CT is the definitive diagnostic modality. All hemothoraces require treatment with tube thoracostomy to prevent the later complications of empyema and fibrothorax. In cases of massive hemothorax, urgent surgical consultation and transfusion of blood products may be required.[53]

Telemetry monitoring during the placement of subclavian and internal jugular CVCs is useful because it allows for the prompt identification of dysrhythmias caused by atrioventricular nodal irritation. Catheter repositioning on identification of premature contractions is recommended.[39] Although a majority of air emboli are subclinical,[41,42] patients receiving a large volume of air delivered to the vasculature may present with dyspnea, tachypnea, hypoxia (pulmonary air emboli), cardiovascular compromise (untreated atrial septal defect or ventricular septal defect), or neurologic sequelae (patent foramen ovale).[37,42] The diagnosis of air embolism is clinical as advanced imaging (CT pulmonary angiography/echocardiography) is commonly without diagnostic finding. If suspected, treatment with high-flow oxygen should be initiated immediately.[37] In extreme cases, depending on the duration and severity of symptoms, hyperbaric oxygen therapy may be required.[37]

Prevention of mechanical complications

Meta-analyses demonstrate significant risk reduction of arterial puncture, hematoma, pneumothorax, and hemothorax with the use of US-guided CVC compared with landmark methods (reducing complications rates previously as high as 11.8% to 4%–7%).[3,4,36,39,45,54,55]

Operator experience is paramount in CVC placement, because the number of unsuccessful cannulation attempts is the greatest predictor of mechanical complications.[44] The complication of cardiac dysrhythmias may be reduced with anticipation and knowledge of guide wire depth.[37]

ARTERIAL ACCESS

Approximately 8 million peripherally inserted arterial catheters are placed in the United States annually, partly due to their utility in hemodynamic monitoring.[56,57] The majority of arterial access is obtained through the radial artery, owing to ease and speed of placement and high success rate of cannulation; however, percutaneous arterial access may also be achieved through cannulation of the brachial, axillary, or femoral arteries.[56,57] Although it is a procedure often performed in the emergency setting, data regarding arterial catheterization are described primarily in cardiology and anesthesiology literature.[57] These sources detail the well-known complications of arterial cannulation: transient vascular occlusion, hematoma, hemorrhage, infection, pseudoaneurysm, air embolism, and neurologic injury.[58]

Complications of Arterial Access

Frequently associated with radial artery cannulation (mean incidence 19.7% of all radial attempts[59–61]), transient vascular occlusion may result from mechanical obstruction and subsequent thrombosis.[56] In contrast, axillary and femoral artery cannulation are much less likely to result in vascular occlusion (0.20% and 1.45%, respectively[56]), likely secondary to increased vessel diameter.[56,59,60] Hematoma formation occurs in approximately 6% of all femoral access attempts.[59] The most feared complication of femoral arterial access, retroperitonal hemorrhage, occurs in 0.15%[62] of all femorally placed CVCs. Retroperitoneal hematoma and hemorrhage are associated with significant morbidity and mortality.[62,63] In patients undergoing cardiac catheterization, retroperitoneal hematoma has been associated with increased risk of infection/sepsis (17.43% vs 3.00%, *P*<.0001) and increased in-hospital mortality (6.64% vs 1.07%, *P*<.0001).[64] Retroperitoneal hemorrhage in this population carries an attributable mortality of 4% to 12%.[63]

Rates of local and systemic infections associated with arterial catheter placement have been estimated as 10% to 20% and 0.4% to 5%, respectively.[57] Arterial line blood stream infections are associated with pseudoaneurysm, thromboarteritis, and arterial rupture.[64] As discussed previously, CRBSI/CLABSI definitions also apply to infections related to arterial access.[7] Similar to central venous CRBSI/CLABSI, data regarding the incidence of this complication is reported to the CDC NHSN.[7] Although femoral access has historically been implicated as the arterial access site associated with a majority of arterial-catheter related bloodstream infections, a recent analysis of more than 4932 ICU patients demonstrated similar infection rates with catheterization of radial and femoral sites.[59,65,66]

Iatrogenic pseudoaneurysms predominately occur after cannulation of the radial artery (incidence of 0.09%[59]) and femoral artery (incidence 0.1%–0.2%[67]). Although rare, pseudoaneurysm rupture, distal embolization, and compression neuropathy may result in significant morbidity.[68]

Air embolism is an infrequently reported complication of radial and axillary artery cannulation but may inadvertently occur with flushing of the line.[59] Because axillary artery catheterization is also associated hematoma formation and subsequent brachial plexopathy, cannulation is not recommended in an ED.[58,66,68]

Risk Factors

Numerous risk factors have been identified for arterial vascular occlusion: increased catheter size compared with vessel diameter, number of access attempts, duration of cannulation, and patient hemodynamic status (hypotension or the requirement for inotropes or vasopressors).[56,63,65] Risk of retroperitoneal hematoma and hemorrhage increases when cannulation is attempted at an anatomic location superior to the inguinal ligament.[62] Access attempts at this location increase the risk of uncontrolled bleeding, given the inability to achieve hemostasis through direct compression.[62] Women are predisposed to retroperitoneal hematoma and hemorrhage with femoral access attempts. Experts attribute this fact to the smaller diameter and shorter length of femoral arteries in women compared with their male counterparts, making femoral access increasingly challenging and contributing to the need for multiple attempts.[63,69,70] Smaller body surface area (associated with a smaller diameter femoral artery) is also a risk factor for retroperitoneal hemorrhage and hematoma.[63]

Poor aseptic technique during placement and prolonged duration of cannulation (>96 hours) increase the rates of systemic and local infection occurring as a result of arterial access.[14,59,60] Risk factors for pseudoaneurysm formation include number of access attempts and coagulopathy.[71] Risk factors for air embolism are similar to those seen with CVC: failure of catheter hub occlusion and the inadvertent delivery of air with flushing.[53] Direct nerve injury has been reported with improper needle placement, and hematoma formation has been associated with multiple cannulation attempts.[68]

Identification and Treatment of Complications

A majority of identified cases of radial artery vascular occlusion remain asymptomatic secondary to collateral circulation.[72–74] Rare complications, including distal limb ischemia and clot embolization, occur in less than 0.01% of all documented cannulation attempts.[56,59] Patients experiencing extremity pain, paresthesias, or pulse deficit (a late finding) should undergo evaluation by Doppler US. In the setting of concern for distal limb ischemia, angiography should be considered as appropriate. In severe cases, expert consultation may be required for the performance of thrombectomy.[56] All patients with identified arterial thrombosis should undergo arterial line removal.[31] Although recannulation of an occluded artery occurs spontaneously, this may take up to 75 days; therefore, systemic anticoagulation is indicated.[31,59,72,73]

Hemorrhage is a feared complication of femoral artery cannulation.[67] Common complaints associated with retroperitoneal hematoma and hemorrhage include lower abdominal, back, or flank pain and abdominal fullness.[62] Hypotension and bradycardia may be late findings.[62] In the setting of retroperitoneal hemorrhage, emergency physicians should consider urgent consultation with vascular surgery or interventional radiology, because operative intervention or embolization may be required. In the setting of hemodynamic instability, resuscitation with the transfusion of blood products may be necessary as a temporizing measure.[62]

Similar to patients with CVCs, CRBSI/CLABSI should be suspected in patients with arterial catheters presenting with systemic inflammatory response syndrome criteria/sepsis or those with erythema, induration, fluctuance, or purulent drainage from access sites.[7,8,14] After blood cultures and line removal, antibiotic/antifungal (if total parenteral nutricion) therapy is advised.[9,10,14]

Hematoma and pseudoaneurysm formation secondary to vascular access both commonly present with localized pain. Pseudoaneurysm may be detected with the new onset of a thrill or bruit.[67] If a patient is reports pain in a nerve root distribution or if a neurologic deficit is elicited on examination, Doppler US should be performed to rule out hematoma or pseudoaneursym.[59,67]

Depending on the volume and speed of air delivered, patients with air emboli often detail the sudden onset of chest pain, palpitations, shortness of breath, or new neurologic symptoms.[59,75] Electrocardiogram may demonstrate tachycardia, acute ST segment changes, or evidence of right heart strain.[41] All patients with suspected arterial air emboli should receive supplemental oxygen therapy via a nonrebreather mask to maximize end-organ oxygenation. CT angiography may be used to assess emboli burden; however, as discussed previously, this study may be nondiagnostic.[76] In the setting of hemodynamic instability or significant neurovascular symptoms, hyperbaric oxygen therapy should be considered within 6 hours of insult (studies demonstrating improved neurologic outcomes when initiated within this time frame).[41,76]

Prevention of Arterial Access Complications

As discussed previously, thrombus formation and subsequent arterial occlusion result from direct tissue injury and the mechanical obstruction of blood flow.[15,16,59] Although clinically significant thrombi localized to the brachial, axillary, and femoral arteries are rare, those localized to the radial artery more commonly result in the sequelae detailed previously.[57] To minimize the risk for clinically significant radial arterial thrombi, a 20-gauge catheter should be used during cannulation (the incidence of radial obstruction increases as the catheter lumen diameter more closely approximates the vessel lumen diameter).[74] Limiting the duration of radial catheterization has also been demonstrated to decrease the occurrence of arterial thrombi.[59,74]

Similar to CVC, the use of sterile technique, preparation, and occlusion of the catheter hub during placement and a working knowledge of anatomy significantly reduce the risk of hemorrhage, infection, and air emboli.[14,59,60,71]

Finally, several studies have identified the benefits of US-guided arterial access. These include increased accuracy of vessel cannulation, reduced number of attempts, increased patient comfort, and reduced risk of complications, such as hemorrhage, hematoma formation, pseudoaneurysm, and neurologic injury.[77,78]

SPECIAL POPULATIONS

Because 300,000 to 400,000 chronic kidney disease patients residing in the United States are maintained on HD, and greater than 2.6 million Americans use anticoagulation therapy for the acute and long-term prevention and management of thromboembolic disorders, a discussion of these patient populations is warranted.[79–83]

Complications of Vascular Access in the Hemodialysis Patient

Approximately 16% to 25% of HD patients are hospitalized annually secondary to complications associated with vascular access.[84–86] The process of HD requires CVC or the surgical placement of an AV graft or fistula. Because complications of CVC have been previously addressed, this section focuses on complications arising from the repetitive cannulation of graft and fistula sites. These complications include infection, stenosis, thrombosis, aneurysm or pseudoaneurysm formation, and hemorrhage. Given their significant morbidity and mortality (average 5-year survival rate for an HD patient: 25%–27%[81]), recognition and treatment of these conditions are paramount.

Infection represents the cause of death in 9% to 36% of HD patients.[81] A study of more than 5000 patients demonstrated mortality secondary to infection as occurring most commonly in patients receiving HD through CVCs and least frequently in those undergoing HD through AV fistula access (relative risk CVC 1.54, $P<.002$; relative risk AV graft 1.41, $P<.003$ compared with AV fistula).[82] In addition, infection is the most common cause of AV graft loss in HD patients (representing 35% of grafts lost).[87–89] Stenosis and thrombosis are the most common complications of AV fistulas and are even more common in AV grafts. A study performed by the Dialysis Access Consortium identified 77% of patients with newly placed AV grafts as developing stenosis or thrombosis within a year after placement.[89,90] AV graft and AV fistula aneurysms and pseudoaneurysms form secondary to repetitive cannulation. The incidence of these conditions (occurring in 5%–60% of patients with AV grafts or fistulas[91]) is highly variable, owing to the lack of a standardized classification system.[92] According to CDC data, from 2000 to 2006, 1654 HD patients died secondary to vascular access hemorrhage (known as fatal vascular access hemorrhage), representing 0.4% of HD patient deaths during that time frame.[86]

Risk Factors

Risk factors for infection are similar to those encountered in patients undergoing central venous and arterial access and include poor antiseptic technique during access attempts and repetitive cannulation.[82,86,93,94] Patients undergoing dialysis are also predisposed to infection given altered humoral and cell-mediated immunity occurring in the setting of chronic uremia.[87] Patients with stenotic lesions may experience an increased incidence in aneurysm formation due to abnormal hemodynamics (arterial or venous hypertension).[94,95] Cannulation in the presence of local site infection also predisposes to pseudoaneurym formation.[92] Risk factors associated with hemorrhage include the presence of an AV graft, local site infection, and stenosis resulting in arterial or venous hypertension.[86]

Identification and Treatment of Complications

AV fistula or graft infection may be difficult to identify on examination. Patients often lack localized erythema, induration, and warmth at the site and present reporting only fever or myalgias.[88] Laboratory studies are often significant for leukocytosis, although this may not be present.[88] Suspected access site infection should be managed aggressively with blood cultures and parenteral antibiotic therapy. Because a majority of graft and fistula infections occur secondary to *Staphylococcus aureus*, *Staphylococcus epidermidis,* and gram-negative bacteria, vancomycin and gentamycin are recommended.[82,88] HD patients with presumed vascular access site infection should be hospitalized until blood cultures are resulted.[88] Doppler US is indicated in hemodynamically stable patients to assess for the presence of a thrombus or localized abscess.[96]

Patients experiencing graft or fistula stenosis often present with distress secondary to extremity pain.[82] Graft or fistula stenosis should be suspected in HD patients in which the physical examination is notable for extremity edema, presence of collateral veins, or alteration in the bruit or thrill.[94] If localized to the upper extremity, failure of the graft or fistula site to collapse on arm elevation is indicative of venous outflow stenosis.[94,97] Doppler US may be used for the evaluation of stenosis. If a stenotic lesion is identified, vascular surgery consultation is appropriate because percutaneous transluminal angioplasty is the treatment of choice.[89] Thrombosis should be suspected in patients presenting with limb pain in the hours after HD.[98] Physical examination of a patient with AV fistula or graft thrombosis is notable for the absence of a bruit or thrill.[85,99] In the case of thrombosis, vascular surgery should be consulted immediately, because management options include surgical thrombectomy versus thrombolysis with or without angioplasty.[85] Doppler US may confirm the diagnosis but should not delay consultation.[84]

Patients experiencing aneurysms secondary to repetitive cannulation may present to an ED reporting extremity pain, motor or sensory dysfunction secondary to aneurysmal impingement of surrounding nerves, superficial skin erosion, or hemorrhage due to skin erosion.[82,99] Patients suffering from pseudoaneurysms are more likely to present with bleeding secondary to skin ulceration or signs and symptoms of infection.[84] Both aneurysms and pseudoaneurysms are detectable through the use of Doppler US.[82] Vascular surgery should be consulted, because operative repair is frequently required.[82,86,99]

Individuals presenting with hemorrhage should be instructed on the application of direct pressure to the access site for 5 minutes to 10 minutes.[82,86] Topical hemostatic agents, including gel foam, chitosan, and recombinant human thrombin, may be considered.[82,87] Persistent oozing or bleeding in the hours after HD should prompt consideration of supratherapeutic anticoagulation and the administration of protamine sulfate. Experts recommend a dose of 1 mg for every 100 mg heparin given during dialysis, or if the amount of heparin administered is unknown, 10 mg to 20 mg total (estimated sufficient to reverse an average dose of 1000–2000 units of heparin).[82] Parenteral desmopressin has been demonstrated to decrease the activated partial thromboplastin and bleeding times in uremic patients and is a treatment option that may be used.[100,101] Given its diuretic effect, however, this therapy should be avoided in patients with hyponatremia and unstable angina and used with caution in patients previously diagnosed with congestive heart failure (when presenting with signs of symptoms of intravascular volume depletion).[82,100] If bleeding is refractory to the aforementioned therapies and seems life-threatening, vascular surgery should be consulted for immediate intervention and a tourniquet applied. It is recommended that in patients in whom hemostasis is achieved, monitoring in the ED should be continued for a minimum of 2 hours to evaluate for rebleed.[82]

Prevention of Vascular Access Complications in Hemodialysis Patients

In 2001, the National Kidney Foundation launched a "Fistula First Breakthrough Initiative" with the goal of reducing the morbidity and mortality associated with HD-related infections by increasing the rates of fistula placement for all prevalent and incident cases of HD dependent ESRD.[85] Data collection to assess the efficacy of this program is currently under way. In addition, the Foundation advocates the use of aseptic technique for all CVC, AV graft, and AV fistula access attempts to limit infectious complications.[85]

Because a majority of patients with AV grafts and fistulas experience stenosis and thrombosis throughout their HD treatment course, National Kidney Foundation guidelines dictate a protocol for flow assessment, which includes monthly physical evaluation of the access site by a trained practitioner, monthly surveillance using diagnostic imaging (Doppler US, magnetic resonance angiography, fistulagram, and so forth), and an assessment of flow during HD sessions (low-flow state predisposing to thrombosis).[85] These techniques are also useful in identifying venous and arterial hypertension (risk factors for aneurysm and pseudoaneurysm formation) and for identifying the presence of vessel irregularities.[85] Patient education and compliance is, therefore, key to limiting sequelae associated with stenosis, thrombosis, aneurysms, and pseudoaneurysms.

Patients with chronic kidney disease commonly experience platelet dysfunction (secondary to uremia) and transient thrombocytopenia (the pathophysiology of which remains controversial).[102–104] To date, there are no published, prospective, randomized trials to support or negate the theory that platelet level should be greater than 50×10^9/L at the time of central venous or arterial catheterization.[102,103] A prospective study assessing the outcome CVC in 105 patients with variable platelet counts less than 50×10^9/L, ranging from 50×10^9/L to 100×10^9/L, and greater than 100×10^9/L, revealed no bleeding complications secondary to catheterization requiring intervention; however, patients with a platelet count of less than 50×10^9/L received platelet transfusions during cannulation.[104]

If a patient is thrombocytopenic and requires arterial or venous access, a directly compressible cannulation site should be used and US employed. If there is evidence of prolonged bleeding from the cannulation site, it is recommended that direct pressure be applied for approximately 15 minutes and that consideration be made (in consultation with a nephrologist of vascular surgeon) for a platelet transfusion to attain a platelet count greater than 50×10^9/L.[104]

Complications of Vascular Access in the Anticoagulated Patient

Anticoagulants are commonly prescribed to address conditions, including chronic atrial fibrillation, venous thromboembolism, and pulmonary embolism. In the United States, more than 30 million prescriptions for warfarin are written annually.[84] Prescriptions for novel oral anticoagulants (NOACs) are also on the rise: from 2012 to 2013, 62% of patients with a new diagnosis of atrial fibrillation were given a NOAC as initial therapy.[105]

Risk Factors

Anticoagulated patients are at significant risk of increased morbidity and mortality secondary to the complications of hematoma and hemorrhage during attempts at venous and arterial cannulation. As discussed previously, risk factors for these complications include operator inexperience (arterial injury during CVC placement, venous puncture and subsequent hematoma formation secondary to inaccurate anatomic location, and retroperitoneal hematoma formation secondary to cannulation attempts above the inguinal ligament) and number of cannulation attempts.[44,58,62,63]

Identification and Treatment of Complications

Patient presentation may range from extremity pain secondary to hematoma formation and compression of surrounding neurovascular structures, to chest pain, dyspnea, or hypoxia (hemothorax) or refractory hypotension (retroperitoneal hematoma secondary to vascular injury).[53,59,60,67] If concern for vascular injury with resultant hemorrhage or hematoma formation in a noncompressible anatomic location (ie, intrathoracic or retroperitoneal) exists, advanced imaging should be considered and consultation with a cardiothoracic, vascular, or interventional radiologist performed as appropriate.[4]

Preventions of Vascular Access Complications in Anticoagulated Patients

Although anticoagulation is not a contraindication to attaining arterial or venous access, in patients taking NOACs or vitamin K antagonists, the risk and benefits associated with cannulation should be weighed carefully and discussed with both patients and applicable consultants. In emergent situations, the femoral vein or internal jugular vein is recommended for venous access. Subclavian venous cannulation should be avoided in patients taking anticoagulants, because the site is difficult to compress, and iatrogenic arterial puncture may be missed secondary to bleeding into the pleural cavity.[105,106] Femoral venous catheterization should be performed below the level of the inguinal ligament to avoid retroperitoneal hemorrhage secondary to external iliac artery puncture.[107]

Again, as discussed previously, the use of US guidance has been demonstrated to reduce the total number of cannulation attempts during arterial and venous catheterization and to reduce the complications of hemorrhage and hematoma formation.[3,4,36,39,45,54,55]

SUMMARY

CVCs and arterial catheterizations are frequently performed to aid in resuscitation and establish advanced hemodynamic monitoring. An understanding of the complications associated with these procedures is vital for emergency physicians, because subsequent evaluation and treatment contribute to prolonged hospital stays and increased costs of care. HD patients warrant special attention, because complications associated with vascular access represent 16% to 25% of annual hospital admissions among this population.[82] As the prevalence of anticoagulant therapy in the United States is increasing,[84] physicians must weigh individuals risks and benefits of vascular access attempts. Emergency physicians can mitigate complications associated with vascular access through the use of sterile technique, antimicrobial impregnated catheters, and cuffs; employment of US guidance during cannulation; and occlusion of catheter hubs during central line placement.

REFERENCES

1. Ruesch S, Walder B, Tramer M. Complications of central venous catheters: internal jugular versus subclavian access – a systematic review. Crit Care Med 2002; 30(2):454.
2. McGee D, Gould M. Preventing complications of central venous catheterization. N Engl J Med 2003;348:1123–33.

3. Merrer J, De Jonghe B, Golliot F, et al. Complications of femoral and subclavian venous catheterization in critically ill patients: a randomized controlled trial. JAMA 2001;286(6):700–7.
4. CDC National and State Healthcare-Associated Infections Progress Report. 2014. Available at: www.cdc.gove/HAI/pdfs/progress-report/hai-progress-report.pdf. Accessed November 28, 2016.
5. Parienti J, Mongardon N, Megarbane B, et al. Intravascular complications of central venous catheterization by insertion site. N Engl J Med 2015;373(13):1220–9.
6. Scott R. The Direct Medical Costs of Healthcare-Associated Infections in U.S. Hospitals and the Benefits of Prevention. 2009. Available at: http://www.cdc.gov/hai/pdfs/hai/scott_costpaper.pdf. Accessed November 28, 2016.
7. Shah H, Bosch W, Thompson K, et al. Intravascular catheter-related bloodstream infection. Neurohospitalist 2013;3(3):144–51.
8. Fletcher S. Catheter-related bloodstream infection. Cont Educ Anaesth Crit Care Pain 2005;5(2):49–51.
9. Mckinley S, Mackenzie A, Finfer S, et al. Incidence and predictors of central venous catheter related infection in intensive care patients. Anaesh Intensive Care 1999;27:164–9.
10. Maki D, Stolz S, Wheeler S, et al. Prevention of central venous catheter-related bloodstream infection by use of an antiseptic-imp regnated catheter: a randomized, controlled trial. Ann Intern Med 1997;127:257–66.
11. Raad I, Hohn D, Gilbreath B, et al. Prevention of central venous catheter-related infections by using maximal sterile barrier precautions during insertion. Infect Control Hosp Epidemiol 1994;15:231–8.
12. CDC Bloodstream Infection Event (Central Line-Associated Bloodstream Infection and non-central line-associated Bloodstream Infection). 2014. Available at: https://www.cdc.gov/nhsn/pdfs/pscmanual/4psc_clabscurrent.pdf. Accessed December 13, 2016.
13. Stone P, Braccia D, Larson E. Systematic review of economic analysis of health care-associated infections. Am J Infect Control 2005;33(9):501–9.
14. O'Grady N, Alexander M, Burns L, et al. Guidelines for the Prevention of Intravascular Catheter-Related Infections, 2011. Centers for Disease Control and Prevention. Available at: https://www.cdc.gov/hicpac/pdf/guidelines/bsi-guidelines-2011.pdf. Accessed December 15, 2016.
15. Chopra V, Krein S, Olmstead R, et al. Making healthcare safer ii: an updated critical analysis of the evidence of patient safety practices. Washington, DC: Agency for Healthcare Research and Quality; 2013. Available at: https://www.ncbi.nlm.nih.gov/books/NBK133364.
16. Geerts W. Central venous catheter-related thrombosis. ASH Education Book 2014;1:306–11.
17. Forauer A, Throharis C, Dasika N. Jugular vein catheter placement: histologic features and development of catheter-related (fibrin) sheaths in a swine model. Radiology 2006;240(2):427–34.
18. Itkin M, Mondshin J, Stavropoulous S, et al. Peripherally inserted central catheter thrombosis—reverse tapered versus nontapered catheters: a randomized controlled study. J Vasc Interv Radiol 2014;25(1):85–91.e1.
19. Raad I, Luna M, Khalil S, et al. The relationship between the thrombotic and infectious complications of central venous catheters. JAMA 1994;271(13):1014–6.
20. Crawford J, Liem T, Moneta G. Management of catheter-associated upper extremity deep venous thrombosis. J Vasc Surg Venous Lymphat Disord 2016; 4(3):375–9.

21. Nifong T, McDevitt T. The effect of catheter to vein ratio on blood flow rates in a simulated model of peripherally inserted central venous catheters. Chest 2011; 140(1):48–53.
22. Timsit J, Farkas J, Boyer J, et al. Central vein catheter-related thrombosis in intensive care patients: incidence, risk factors, and relationship with catheter-related sepsis. Chest 1998;114(1):207–13.
23. Grant J, Stevens S, Woller S, et al. Diagnosis and management of upper extremity deep-vein thrombosis in adults. Thromb Haemost 2012;108(6):1097–108.
24. Hirsch D, Ingenito E, Goldhaber S. Prevalence of deep venous thrombosis among patients in medical intensive care. JAMA 1995;274:335–7.
25. Debourdeau P, Farge D, Beckers M, et al. International clinical practice guidelines for the treatment and prophylaxis of thrombosis associated with central venous catheters in patients with cancer. J Thromb Haemost 2013;11(1):71–80.
26. Kearon C, Akl E, Comerota A, et al. Antithrombotic therapy for VTE disease: Antithrombotic therapy and prevention of thrombosis, 9th ed: American college of chest physicians evidence-based clinical practice guidelines. Chest 2012;141(2 Suppl):e419S–494.
27. Baskin J, Reiss U, Wilimas J, et al. Thrombolytic therapy for central venous catheter occlusion. Haematologica 2012;97(5):641–50.
28. Baskin J, Pui C, Reiss U, et al. Management of occlusion and thrombosis associated with long-term indwelling central venous catheters. Lancet 2009; 374(9684):159–69.
29. Tebbi C, Costanzi J, Shulman R, et al. A phase III, open-label, single-arm study of tenecteplase for restoration of function in dysfunctional central venous catheters. J Vasc Interv Radiol 2011;22(8):1117–23.
30. Saber W, Moua T, Williams E, et al. Risk factors of catheter-related thrombosis (CRT) in cancer patients: a patient-level data (IPD) meta-analysis of clinical trials and prospective studies. J Thromb Haemost 2011;9(2):312–9.
31. Mitchell M, Anderson B, Williams K, et al. Heparin flushing and other interventions to maintain patency of central venous catheters: a systematic review. J Adv Nurs 2009;65(10):2007–21.
32. Akl E, Vasireddi S, Gunukula S, et al. Anticoagulation for patients with cancer and central venous catheters. Cochrane Database Syst Rev 2011;(4):CD006468.
33. Young A, Billingham L, Begum G, et al. Warfarin thromboprophylaxis in cancer patients with central venous catheters (WARP): an open-label randomized trial. Lancet 2009;373(9663):567–74.
34. Schiffer C, Manqu P, Wade J, et al. Central venous catheter care for the patient with cancer: American Society of Clinical Oncology clinical practice guideline. J Clin Oncol 2013;31(10):1357–70.
35. Kahn S, Lim W, Dunn A, et al. Prevention of VTE in nonsurgical patients: Antithrombotic Therapy and Prevention of Thrombosis, 9th ed: American College of Chest Physicians Evidence-Based Clinical Practice Guidelines. Chest 2012; 141(2 Suppl):e195S–226.
36. Mansfield P, Hohn D, Fornage B, et al. Complications and failures of subclavian-vein catheterization. N Engl J Med 1994;331:1735–8.
37. Kornbau C, Lee K, Hughes G, et al. Central line compilcations. Int J Crit Illn Inj Sci 2015;5(3):170–8.
38. Bowdle A. Vascular complications of central venous catheter placement: evidence-based methods for prevention and treatment. J Cardiothorac Vasc Anesth 2014;28(2):358–68.

39. Bhutta S, Culp W. Evaluation and management of central venous access complications. Tech Vasc Interv Radiol 2011;14(4):217–24.
40. Vats H. Complications of catheters: tunneled and nontuneled. Adv Chronic Kidney Dis 2012;19(3):188–94.
41. Gordy S, Rowell S. Vascular air embolism. Int J Crit Illn Inj Sci 2013;3(1):73–6.
42. Brockmeyer J, Johnson E. Cerebral air embolism following removal of central venous catheter. Mil Med 2011;176(2):i.
43. Brockmeyer J, Simon T, Seery J, et al. Mil Med 2009;174(8):878–81.
44. Kusminsky RE. Complications of central venous catheterization. J Am Coll Surg 2007;204:681–96.
45. Randolph AG, Cook DJ, Gonzales CA, et al. Ultrasound guidance for placement of central venous catheters: a meta-analysis of the literature. Crit Care Med 1996;24:2053–8.
46. Guilbert M, Elkouri S, Bracco D, et al. Arterial trauma during central venous catheter insertion: Case series, review and proposed algorithm. J Vasc Surg 2008;48(4):918–25.
47. Nagarsheth K, Kurek S. Ultrasound detection of pneumothorax compared with chest X-ray and computed tomography scan. Am Surg 2011;77(4):480–4.
48. Lichtenstein D, Meziere G, Biderman P, et al. The 'comet-tail artifact': An ultrasound sign ruling out pneumothorax. Intensive Care Med 1999;25:383–8.
49. Ma O, Mateer J. Trauma ultrasound examination versus chest radiography in the detection of hemothorax. Ann Emerg Med 1997;29(3):312–5.
50. Sisley A, Rozycki G, Ballard R, et al. Rapid detection of traumatic effusion using surgeon-performed ultrasonography. J Trauma 1998;44(2):291–7.
51. Noble V, Nelson P. Manual of emergency and critical care ultrasound. New York: Cambridge University Press; 2011.
52. Abboud P, Kendall J. Emergency department ultrasound for hemothorax after blunt traumatic injury. J Emerg Med 2003;25(3):181–4.
53. Bernardin B, Troquet J. Initial management and resuscitation of severe chest trauma. Emerg Med Clin North Am 2012;30:377–400.
54. Koh D, Gowardman J, Rickard C, et al. Prospective study of peripheral arterial catheter infection and comparison with concurrently sited central venous catheters. Crit Care Med 2008;36(2):397–402.
55. Wu S, Ling Q, Cao L, et al. Real-time two-dimensional ultrasound guidance for central venous cannulation: a meta-analysis. Anesthesiology 2013;118(2):361–75.
56. Cousins T, O'Donnell J. Arterial cannulation: a critical review. AANA J 2004;72(4):267–71.
57. LeMaster C, Agrawal A, Hou P, et al. Systematic review of emergency department central venous and arterial catheter infection. Int J Emerg Med 2010;3(4):409–23.
58. Gardner R. Direct arterial pressure monitoring. Curr Anaesh Crit Care 1990;1:239–46.
59. Scheer B, Perel A, Pfeiffer U. Clinical review: Complications and risk factors of peripheral arterial catheters used for haemodynamic monitoring in anaesthesia and intensive care medicine. Crit Care 2002;6(3):199–204.
60. Soderstrom C, Wasserman D, Dunham C, et al. Superiority of the femoral artery of monitoring. A prospective study. Am J Surg 1982;144(3):309–12.
61. Bedford R. Wrist circumference predicts the risk of radial-arterial occlusion after cannulation. Anesthesiology 1978;48(5):377–8.

62. Sajnani N, Bogart D. Retroperitoneal hemorrhage as a complication of percutaneous intervention: report of 2 cases and review of the literature. Open Cardiovasc Med J 2013;7:16–22.
63. Trimarchi S, Smith D, Share D, et al. Retroperitoneal hematoma after percutaneous coronary intervention: prevalence, risk factors, management, outcomes, and predictors of mortality: a report from the BMC2 (Blue Cross Blue Shield of Michigan Cardiovascular Consortium) registry. J Am Coll Cardiol 2010;3(8): 845–50.
64. Safdar N, O'Horo J, Maki D. Arterial catheter-related bloodstream infection: incidence, pathogenesis, risk factors and prevention. J Hosp Infect 2013;85(3): 189–95.
65. Frezza E, Mezghebe H. Indications and complications of arterial catheter use in surgical or medical intensive care units: analysis of 4932 patients. Am Surg 1998;64(2):127–31.
66. Ranganath A, Hanumanthaiah D. Radial artery pseudo aneurysm after percutaneous cannulation using Seldinger technique. Indian J Anaesh 2011;55(3): 274–6.
67. Lenartova M, Tak T. Iatrogenic pseudoaneurysm of femoral artery: case report and literature review. Clin Med Res 2003;1(3):243–7.
68. Bryan-Brown C, Kwun K, Lumb P, et al. The axillary artery catheter. Heart Lung 1983;12:492–7.
69. Kennedy A, Grocott M, Schwartz M, et al. Medial nerve injury: an underrecognised complication of brachial artery cathterisation? J Neurol Neurosurg Psychiatry 1997;63:542–6.
70. Schnyder G, Sawhney N, Whisenant B, et al. Common femoral artery anatomy is influenced by demographics and comorbidity: implications for cardiac and peripheral invasive studies. Catheter Cardiovasc Interv 2001;53(3):289–95.
71. Band J, Maki D. Infections caused by arterial catheters used for hemodynamic monitoring. Am J Med 1979;67(5):735–41.
72. Ganchi P, Wilhelmi B, Fujita K, et al. Ruptured pseucoaneurysm complicating an infected radial artery catheter: case report and review of the literature. Ann Plast Surg 2001;46(6):647–50.
73. Abadir A, Ung K. Complications of radial artery cannulation. Anesthesiol Rev 1980;7:11–6.
74. Bedford R. Radial arterial function following percutaneous cannulation with 18- and 20-gauge catheters. Anesthesiology 1977;47(1):37–9.
75. Bedford R. Long-term radial artery cannulation: effects on subsequent vessel formation. Crit Care Med 1978;6:64–7.
76. McCarthy C, Behravesh S, Naidu S, et al. Air embolism: practical tips for prevention and treatment. J Clin Med 2016;5(11):93.
77. Blanc P, Boussuges A, Henriette K, et al. Iatrogenic cerebral air embolism: importance of an early hyperbaric oxygenation. Intensive Care Med 2002; 28(5):559–63.
78. Seto A, Abu-Fadel M, Sparling J, et al. Real-time ultrasound guidance facilitates femoral arterial access and reduces vascular complications: FAUST (femoral arterial access with ultrasound trial. J Am Coll Cardiol 2010;3(7):751–8.
79. Zochlos V, Wilkinson J, Dasgupta K. The role of ultrasound as an adjunct to arterial catheterization in critically ill surgical and intensive care unit patients. J Vasc Access 2014;15(1):1–4.

80. Soi V, Moore C, Kumar L, et al. Prevention of catheter-related bloodstream infections in patients on hemodialysis: challenges and management strategies. Int J Nephrol Renovasc Dis 2016;9:95–103.
81. Leake A, Winger D, Leers S, et al. Management and outcomes of dialysis access-associated steal syndrome. J Vasc Surg 2015;61(3):754–60.
82. Dhingra R, Young E, Hulbert-Shearon T, et al. Type of vascular access and mortality in US hemodialysis patients. Kidney Int 2001;60(4):1443–51.
83. Hodde L, Sandroni S. Emergency department evaluation and management of dialysis patient complications. J Emerg Med 1992;10:317–34.
84. NA. National action plan for adverse drug event prevention: Section 5 Anticoagulants. 2015. Available at: https://health.gov/hcq/pdfs/ADE-Action-Plan-Anticoagulants.pdf. Accessed December 27, 2016.
85. KDOQI clinical practice guidelines and clinical practice recommendations for 2006 updates: hemodialysis adequacy, peritoneal dialysis adequacy and vascular access. Am J Kidney Dis 2004;48:S1–322.
86. United States Renal Data System (USRDS) Annual Data Report. Epidemiology of kidney disease in the United States. 2015. Available at: https://www.usrds.org/adr.aspx. Accessed December 28, 2016.
87. Ball L. Fatal vascular access hemorrhage: reducing the odds. Nephrol Nurs J 2013;40(4):297–303.
88. Tintinalli J. Tintinalli's emergency medicine: a comprehensive study guide. New York: McGraw-Hill; 2011.
89. Schutte W, Helmer S, Salazar L, et al. Surgical treatment of infected prosthetic dialysis arteriovenous grafts: total versus partial graft excision. Am J Surg 2007;193:385–8.
90. Dixon B, Beck G, Vazquez M, et al. Effect of dipyridamole plus aspirin on hemodialysis graft patency. N Engl J Med 2009;360(21):2191.
91. Pirozzi N, Garcia-Medina J, Hanoy M. Stenosis complicating vascular access for hemodialysis: indications for treatment. J Vasc Access 2014;15(2):76–82.
92. Pasklinsky G, Meisner R, Labropoulos N, et al. Management of true aneurysms of hemodialysis access fistulas. J Vasc Surg 2011;53(5):1291–7.
93. Mudoni A, Cornacchiari M, Gallieni M, et al. Aneurysms and pseudoaneurysms in dialysis access. Clin Kidney J 2015;8(4):363–7.
94. Padberg F, Calligaro K, Sidawy A. Complications of arteriovenous hemodialysis access: recognition and management. J Vasc Surg 2008;48(5 Suppl):55S–80S.
95. A clinical update on the management of infected arteriovenous graft access (AVG) for the hemodialysis patient. National Kidney Foundation; 2014. Available at: https://www.kidney.org/sites/default/files/02-10-6071_GBD_Infected_AVG-Cryolife.pdf. Accessed December 15, 2016.
96. Mickley V. Stenosis and thrombosis in haemodialysis fistulae and grafts: the surgeon's point of view. Nephrol Dial Transplant 2004;19(2):309–11.
97. Hammes M. Medical complications in hemodialysis patients requiring vascular access radiology procedures. Semin Intervent Radiol 2004;21(2):105–10.
98. Vachharajani T. Diagnosis of arteriovenous fistula dysfunction. Semin Dial 2012;25(4):445–50.
99. Wolfson A, Singer I. Hemodialysis-related emergencies-part I. J Emerg Med 1987;5(6):533–43.
100. Siedlecki A, Barker J, Allon M. Aneurysm formation in arteriovenous grafts: associations and clinical significance. Semin Dial 2007;20(1):73–7.
101. Mannucci P, Remuzzi G, Pusineri F, et al. Deamino-8-D-arginine vasopressin shortens the bleeding time in uremia. N Engl J Med 1983;308:8–12.

102. Dorgalaleh A, Mahmudi M, Taibibian S, et al. Anemia and thrombocytopenia in acute and chronic renal failure. Int J Hematol Oncol Stem Cell Res 2013;7(4):34–9.
103. Bishop L, Dougherty L, Bodenham A, et al. Guidelines on the insertion and management of central venous access devices in adults. Int J Lab Hematol 2007;29:261–78.
104. Ray C, Shenoy S. Patients with thrombocytopenia: outcome of radiological placement of central venous access devices. Radiology 1997;204:97–9.
105. Alpert J. The NOACs (novel oral anticoagulants) have landed! Am J Med 2014;127(11):1027–8.
106. Evans S. Surgical pitfalls: prevention and management. Section 8. Philadelphia: Saunders Elsevier; 2009. p. 113.
107. Timsit J. What is the best site for central venous catheter insertion in critically ill patients? Crit Care 2003;7(6):397–9.

Penetrating Vascular Injury

Diagnosis and Management Updates

Richard Slama, MD, LT*, Frank Villaume, MD, LCDR

KEYWORDS

- Vascular injury • Hemorrhage control • Damage control resuscitation
- Extremity hemorrhage • Junctional hemorrhage • Noncompressible hemorrhage
- Hemostatic dressing • Junctional tourniquet

KEY POINTS

- Penetrating vascular injury is increasing and becoming more important in emergency medicine (EM). The extent of a projectile injury depends on mass, velocity, and characteristics.
- Hard signs are usually treated operatively. Soft signs or asymptomatic patients warrant further workup. There are numerous diagnostic modalities; computed tomography angiography is the gold standard.
- Direct pressure is the most important hemorrhage control but others are reviewed.
- Resuscitation of these patients should focus on balance component therapy, prevention of coagulopathy, and permissive hypotension when allowable.
- There are numerous complications other than the vascular injury alone and EM physicians must be cognizant of these. Always thoroughly document a neurovascular examination.

INTRODUCTION

Penetrating vascular injury has become a topic of increased interest in the United States with the recent rise in gun violence. Much of the treatment has been derived from trauma research during wartime. Although the Joint Trauma System (JTS) Clinical Practice Guidelines are widely adopted in the military, the translation into the civilian

---

Disclosure Statement: Both authors have no financial or commercial conflicts of interest to disclose. The views expressed in this article are those of the authors and do not necessarily reflect the official policy or position of the Department of the Navy, Department of Defense, or the United States Government.

620 John Paul Jones Circle, Portsmouth, VA 23708, USA
* Corresponding author.
E-mail address: Rslama1@gmail.com

Emerg Med Clin N Am 35 (2017) 789–801
http://dx.doi.org/10.1016/j.emc.2017.06.005
0733-8627/17/Published by Elsevier Inc.

sector has been limited. This article outlines these guidelines and the latest research in the United States to help emergency medicine physicians best manage penetrating vascular trauma.

EPIDEMIOLOGY

Approximately 300 people per day sustain gunshot wounds from all causes combined in the United States. Of these, 90 will die because of the inflicted wounds. There were approximately 125,000 assaults with knives and 140,000 cases of assaults with firearms in 2014 according to the Federal Bureau of Investigation.[1] This does not include other mass casualty events, including the Boston Marathon bombings, the Fort Hood Texas shootings, the Charleston Emanuel African Methodist Episcopal Church shootings, and numerous others. However, firearms are not the only causes for vascular injury. Other modalities include crush injuries, animal bites, and other traumatic forces that can either completely or partially obstruct vascular structures.[2]

PATHOPHYSIOLOGY

When addressing penetrating vascular trauma it is important to talk about the physics involved.[3]

$$KE = \frac{1}{2}mv^2$$

The kinetic energy (KE) is directly proportional to the mass (m) of the object and exponentially proportional to the velocity (v) of the object. Weapons can be divided into low, medium, and high energy (**Table 1**). As the velocity of the weapon increases, the size of the temporary cavitation on entry increases to almost 25 times the diameter of the missile. This is in part why high velocity weapons are so much more dangerous than medium or low energy. All 3 types create damage in the path of their trajectory; however, the indirect damage from cavitation is significantly larger in the high-energy weapons. There are some other factors that can make particular weapons more dangerous than others.

The profile of an object also affects its transfer of energy. Therefore, an object that has a greater surface area has the ability to transfer more energy to the object it is striking (a good example of this is a hollow point bullet vs a regular bullet). The characteristics of the missile equally affect how much damage is given. Tumble describes the changing of an angle of a missiles angle when it enters the body (bullets with offset centers of mass tend to tumble through the object they strike, causing greater damage). Fragmentation is simply when an object breaks into many others to increase the surface area and the damage dealt. The most important point to take away is that neither the velocity or missile characteristics can independently predict the amount of damage caused; it is more often a combination of both.[4]

Table 1
Weapon classification

Weapon Type	Feet per second	Examples
Low-energy	Not applicable	Knives, daggers, ice picks
Medium-energy	~1000 ft/s	Common handguns
High-energy	>2000 ft/s	AK47, M16

FEATURES AND PRESENTATION

Most vascular injuries are obvious on presentation; however, some are subtle and attention to detail is required.[5] When classifying vascular injury, it is helpful to look for both hard and soft signs of injury. This allows the clinician to determine the next best step in managing the patient. In general, patients with hard signs of vascular injury will need immediate intervention, whereas those with soft signs should receive diagnostic testing to better illicit the type of injury (**Table 2**).

Although these signs are helpful, their absence does not exclude a serious vascular injury. Ten percent of injuries will manifest with hard signs, but many will have only soft signs, delayed presentation, or be completely asymptomatic.[6,7] Therefore, the emergency department (ED) physician must maintain a high index of suspicion when caring for any patient with increased likelihood of these injuries.

Classification of injuries is also important, especially when considering treatment modalities. For the purpose of this discussion, vascular injuries are divided into peripheral or extremity, junctional, and noncompressible truncal or torso hemorrhage (NCTH).

Extremity hemorrhage, as its name suggests, is any injury to the vasculature of the extremities resulting in hemorrhage. Although these injuries are generally smaller vasculature and are more likely to have a better outcome than junctional or NCTH, they can still result in morbidity and mortality if not addressed early. These injuries are amendable to tourniquets and usually respond well to direct compression (see later discussion).

A junctional hemorrhage is defined as a hemorrhage in which an extremity meets the torso, which precludes the effective use of a tourniquet to control bleeding.[8] Examples of junction hemorrhage include the groin proximal to the inguinal ligament, the buttocks, the gluteal and pelvic areas, the perineum, the axilla and shoulder girdle, and the base of the neck. By definition, junctional trauma is compressible and, therefore, technically able to be controlled if personnel are trained appropriately.

NCTH is the leading cause of death in battle field and is defined as trauma to torso vessels, pulmonary parenchyma, solid abdominal organs, and disruption of the bony pelvis.[9] As the name implies, these are injuries that are not amenable to tourniquets, not amendable to compression, and overall have a very high mortality rate due to the rate of bleeding. These are by far among most complex types of injuries and much of trauma research is now dedicated to them.

DIFFERENTIAL DIAGNOSIS

Differential diagnosis includes arterial injury, venous injury, nerve injury, fracture, dislocation, compartment syndrome, thrombosis, and dissection.

Table 2
Hard versus soft signs of vascular injury

Hard Signs	Soft Signs
Absent distal pulse	Subjective reduction in pulse
Expanding or pulsatile hematoma	Large nonpulsatile hematoma
Bruit or thrill	Neural injury
Active hemorrhage	Large hemorrhage on scene
	High-risk orthopedic injuries

Diagnosis

1. Usually, visual inspection may be enough to diagnose vascular injury; however, there are some useful tools aside from visual inspection. Many of these presentations can appear subtly or as normal and so caution must be taken not to anchor on a patient's initial presentation.
2. Injured extremity index (IEI) is a test that is almost identical to performing an ankle brachial index with the exception that this is used to compare opposite extremities as opposed to upper and lower. The first step is to determine the pressure at which the arterial Doppler signal returns in the injured extremity as the cuff is deflated, which is the numerator in the equation. Next the cuff and Doppler are moved to the uninjured extremity, ideally an uninjured upper extremity, and again the pressure at which the arterial Doppler signal returns as the cuff is deflated is recorded as the denominator in the ratio. An injured extremity index greater than 0.90 is normal and has a high sensitivity for excluding major extremity vascular injury.[10] The negative predictive value of an IEI greater than 0.90 can be as high as 96%.[11] Due to IEI's ease of use, rapidity, and noninvasiveness, it is an ideal test that emergency medicine physicians should use in the care of patients with suspected vascular injury.
   a. Case example: A 24-year-old man is shot in the right medial aspect of the forearm. The blood pressure cuff is applied to the injured arm and inflated until the Doppler signal is no longer audible and then deflated until there is a return of arterial waveform; the pressure is 90. This is repeated in the uninjured arm and found to be 150. For this particular patient, the IEI would be 90/150 = 0.6; this is concerning for a peripheral vascular injury.
3. Computed tomography angiography remains the gold standard for the diagnosis of vascular injuries because of its accuracy, cost, and rapidity.[12,13] Examples of penetrating vascular injuries are seen in **Fig. 1**.[14]
4. Duplex ultrasound has been evaluated in the diagnosis of this condition, but it does not have high enough sensitivity to exclude these injuries.[15,16] To the authors' knowledge there have been no randomized studies on the use of point-of-care ultrasound (POCUS) for the evaluation of penetrating vascular injuries. Therefore, POCUS can only be recommended as an adjunct in the evaluation of these patients.

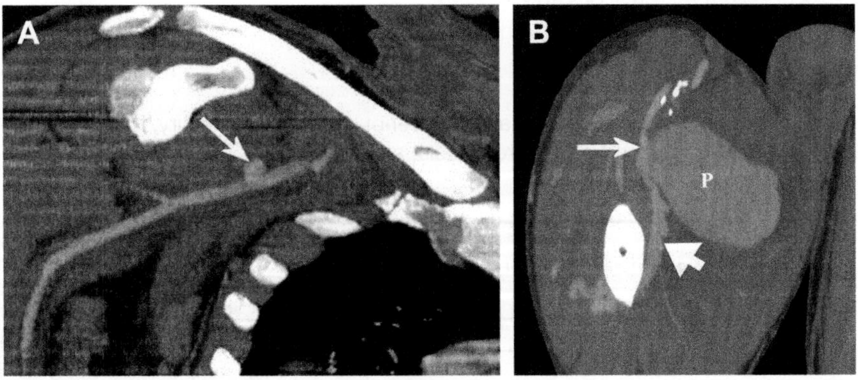

Fig. 1. (*A*) Contrast extravasation (*arrow*) after arterial injury. (*B*) Arteriovenous fistula formation (*arrow*) after gunshot wound (*arrowhead*) to the thigh. (*From* Miller-Thomas MM, West OC, Cohen AM. Diagnosing traumatic arterial injury in the extremities with CT angiography: pearls and pitfalls. RadioGraphics 2005;25:S133-42.)

MANAGEMENT

Most of the management of these conditions has been derived from the JTS guidelines. ED management includes

- Hemorrhage control (direct pressure, tourniquet, or topical hemostatic agent) should be first-line therapy and, if there are hard signs of vascular injury with shock, the patient should be taken immediately to the operating room for further exploration.[5] The emphasis should be on direct pressure as the first and most important step in hemorrhage control. Avoidance of ligation should be avoided by emergency physicians. A summary of the proposed management of penetrating vascular injuries is outlined in **Fig. 2**.
- Damage control resuscitation (DCR; see later discussion).

Review of Modalities for Extremity Hemorrhage Control

Although surgery is the definitive answer for most severe penetrating vascular injury, the first principle in the initial management should be hemorrhage control. Direct pressure over the area of bleeding is the first and most important step. After this, there are numerous other modalities available for control of bleeding.

When deciding how to control hemorrhage, one must first recognize the type of injury. For most extremity injuries with active hemorrhage, tourniquets are a cheap, readily available, and efficacious method to control bleeding. Tourniquets, for the most part, had fallen out of favor until their reemergence in Operation Iraqi Freedom. There have been multiple studies to date showing favorable outcomes when tourniquets have been applied in the battlefield setting.[17–19] Because of favorable survivability data, tourniquets have become an integral part of the Trauma Combat Casualty Care (TCCC) course taught to almost all military medics, corpsmen, physicians, nurses, and even dentists. Although there are multiple facets to the TCCC guidelines, the basic premise for use is early application of a tourniquet to a bleeding extremity as high and tight as possible until hemorrhage control is obtained.[20]

Initially tourniquet use in the civilian setting was relatively limited, but in recent years they have become more popular equipment for most prehospital personnel. In addition, there are now numerous centers in the United States that are beginning to study the prehospital use of tourniquets.[21] The longstanding debate and controversy is whether these devices cause more harm than good.[22] Although the injuries incurred during wartime are different than those in the civilian setting, the same principles can still be applied so long as appropriate use is followed (**Box 1**). There are complications that can occur from tourniquets, including compartment syndrome, neuropraxia, nerve paralysis, and limb ischemia.[23] Although most of these complications have been noted at greater than 2 hours, a tourniquet should not be removed if hemorrhage cannot be controlled by other means. In the civilian setting, prolonged tourniquet use should not be as much of an issue as on the battlefield where definitive care is not always immediately available.

In injuries not amendable to tourniquet placement or when tourniquets are not available, direct pressure over the wound should be the next viable option.[10] Clamping and ligation may be performed by a surgeon when indicated, but the initial recommendation for ED management is to avoid these maneuvers when at all possible because this may hinder future vessel repair.

There are numerous hemostatic agents and dressings on the market that are used to crosslink red blood cells or activate the clotting cascade. Some of the most commonly available agents are listed in **Table 3**, although this list is continually

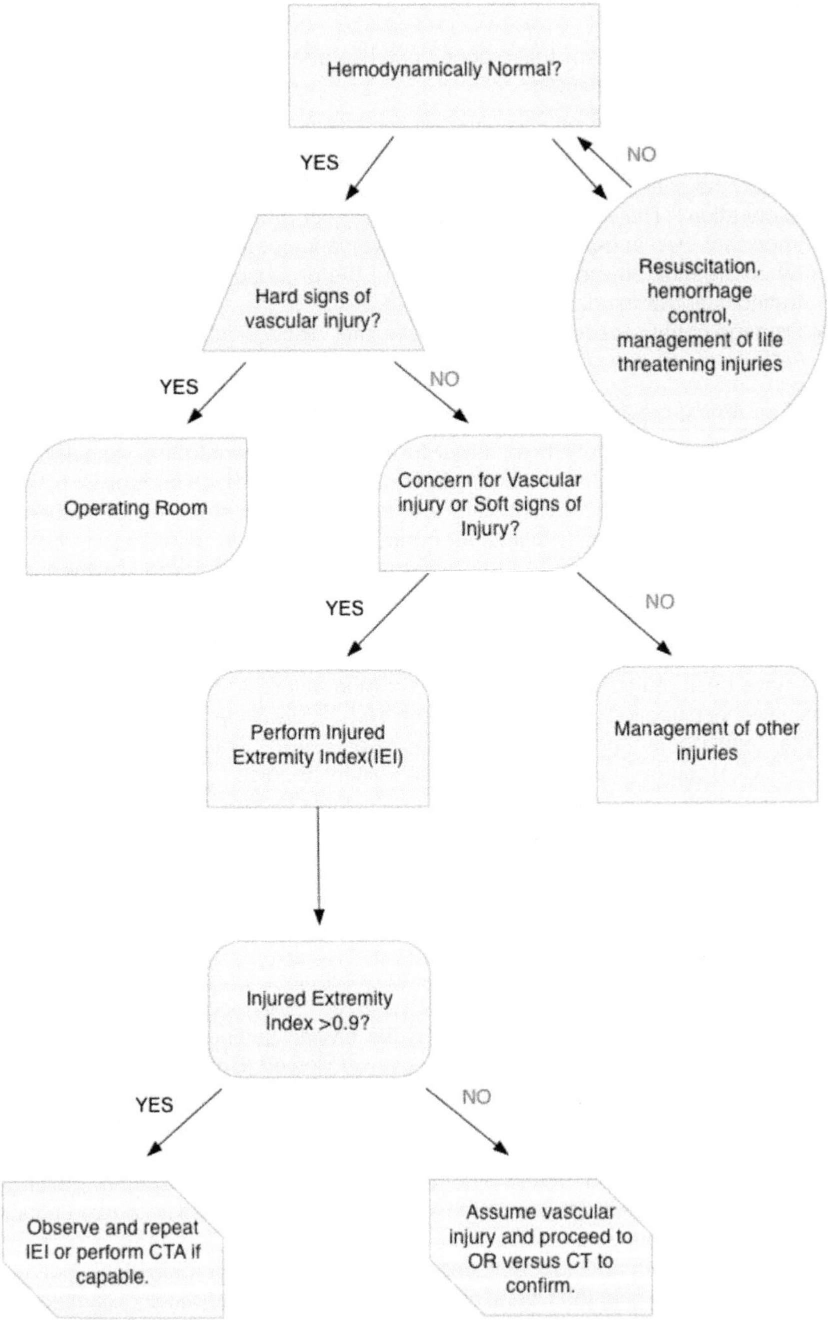

Fig. 2. Management of penetrating vascular injury. CT, computed tomography, CTA, computed tomography angiography; OR, operating room. (*Adapted from* the Joint Trauma System clinical practice guideline. Available at: http://www.usaisr.amedd.army.mil/cpgs/Vascular_Injury_12_Aug_2016.pdf.)

Box 1
Guidelines for appropriate tourniquet use based on Trauma Combat Casualty Care guidelines

- Identify that patient has sustained a vascular injury.
- If on an extremity, it is likely amendable to tourniquet use.
- Apply the tourniquet over the patients' uniform or clothing initially and if bleeding is not identified, place the tourniquet as high and tight as possible.
- If the first tourniquet does not work, apply a second tourniquet side by side with the first.
- Tourniquet should be converted to a compression dressing as soon as possible if the following criteria are met:
  - No evidence of shock
  - The wound can be monitored for bleeding
  - The tourniquet is not being used to control bleeding from an amputated extremity.
- When possible, tourniquets should be converted to compression dressings within 2 hours.
- Tourniquets in place for greater than 6 hours should only be removed if there is adequate monitoring of the patients vitals, bleeding, and laboratory tests.

Adapted from TCCC-MP guidelines and curriculum. Available at: http://www.naemt.org/education/TCCC/guidelines_curriculum.

growing.[24] These agents have been shown to be superior to standard nonhemostatic dressings in numerous studies.[25] However, a recent study that emulated severe penetrating vascular injury in areas not amendable to tourniquet placement showed that standard gauze without hemostatic agent compared equally well to hemostatic agents in the swine model.[26] Therefore, hemostatic agents may confer benefit to some specific types of wounds. The most important aspect of hemorrhage control is direct pressure over the area of vascular injury, regardless of dressing type.

Review of Modalities to Control Junctional and Truncal Hemorrhage

Any vascular injury can be life-threatening, but junctional and truncal hemorrhage can be exceedingly difficult to control, even for the most experienced clinician. There are no randomized controlled trials that give an algorithmic approach to controlling these types of hemorrhage. Therefore, many of the methods presented here are controversial or upcoming, and should only be used if approved by one's institution.

After the TCCC guidelines began to recommend tourniquets as a first-line treatment for extremity trauma, deaths from peripheral vascular injuries dropped and those from junctional injuries became the leading cause of mortality. To date, there is no definitive

Table 3
Commercially available hemostatic dressings

Agent	Mechanism	Form	Cost in United States $
Combat gauze	Activates intrinsic pathway	Gauze	55
Celox gauze	Crosslinks red blood cells	Gauze	41
ChitoGauze	Crosslinks red blood cells	Gauze	50
Modified rapid deployable hemostat	Vasoconstriction, red blood cell agglutination, platelet activation	4 × 4 inch dressing	500+

approach to controlling junctional hemorrhage; therefore, most of the recommendations presented are either from case reports, cadaveric studies, or animal models. As previously outlined, a junctional injury is compressible by definition. Therefore, when treating a patient with this type of injury, the most important aspect of care is direct compression with either mechanical force or a junctional tourniquet device.[8] Junctional tourniquets are prevalent in the military; however, they are much less prevalent in prehospital, or even hospital, settings in the United States. There are multiple different devices that are currently approved by the US Food and Drug Administration, none of which has been proven to be superior or undergone a randomized prospective study (**Table 4**).

NCTH is a unique entity that still poses a challenge in terms of management. It is defined as hemorrhage arising from trauma to the torso vessels, pulmonary parenchyma, solid abdominal organs, and disruption of the bony pelvis.[9] Some examples include portal vein injury, inferior vena cava injury, and aortic injury. Aside from exploratory laparotomy with proximal and distal control, there are few if any treatments that have any true benefit for these patients. The main issue is that when these injuries occur and hemorrhage control does not occur expeditiously, the patients expire quickly from exsanguination. This has, in particular, become a problem for the battlefield where definitive care is rarely available on the scene. One popular modality for control of hemorrhage that is up and coming is resuscitative endovascular balloon occlusion of the aorta (REBOA). REBOA is not a new concept and has been around since the 1950s.[9] The basic idea behind this procedure is to use a percutaneously introduced endovascular balloon to occlude different areas of the aorta based on the desired effect. The benefit to performing this procedure is cessation of bleeding and subsequent increased cardiac and cerebral perfusion.[27]

The classic approach to control of NCTH usually involves an emergent thoracotomy followed by crossclamping of the thoracic aorta. Although there are current

Table 4
Commercially available junctional tourniquets

Name	Mechanism	Indication	Cost in United States $
Abdominal aortic tourniquet	Compresses the abdominal aorta	Inguinal or lower extremity bleeds not amenable to tourniquets	572
Combat-ready clamp	Directly compresses over junctional injury	Inguinal, axilla, and proximal extremity bleeds not amendable to tourniquets	512
Junctional emergency treatment tool	Directly compresses over junctional injury	Inguinal or lower extremity bleeds not amenable to tourniquets	225
SAM junctional tourniquet	Directly compresses over junctional injury	Inguinal, axilla bleeds, pelvic fracture and extremity wounds in which tourniquet not effective	279

guidelines for the use of resuscitative thoracotomy, the use of this modality in conjunction with aortic crossclamping is not as well-defined.[28] This is obviously a very invasive procedure that can be fraught with numerous complications.[29] This is, in part, why REBOA has been suggested as an alternate modality to aortic crossclamping, although it also has numerous complications of its own. These include but are not limited to accessing the wrong vascular tree, misplacement of the wire or balloon within the arterial system, aortic dissection, arterial injury, retroperitoneal hemorrhage, lactic acidosis, organ dysfunction, clotting, or limb ischemia.[30] Although these are serious complications, overall REBOA is less invasive than thoracic aortic crossclamping and theoretically has less complications. REBOA is undoubtedly gaining more popularity, and there are starting to be more randomized trials evaluating its efficacy. In a recent prospective study performed in the United States, when compared with aortic crossclamping, REBOA was found to be comparable in terms of morbidity and mortality.[27] Further research is undoubtedly needed on this particular topic, but it does provide a unique and less invasive technique for an injury that was once unsurvivable.

DAMAGE CONTROL RESUSCITATION

In an ideal situation, unstable patients with penetrating vascular trauma would be transported immediately to the operating room. This is not always the case when caring for trauma patients because there are many factors than can delay operative intervention (eg, surgical consultant not in house, multiple casualties necessitating triage). Because of these factors, it is imperative for the emergency physician to be knowledgeable on how to appropriately resuscitate a patient with active hemorrhage. Although Advanced Trauma Life Support (ATLS) provides an excellent basis and systematic approach to trauma patients, there are some aspects of these algorithms that are falling out of favor and less applicable to patients with massive hemorrhage. For example, previous versions of ATLS recommended initial crystalloid resuscitation, which in both military and civilian settings has been associated with poor outcomes including multiorgan failure, death, and abdominal compartment syndrome.[31]

DCR is very broadly defined as a resuscitative strategy in which hemorrhage is controlled while preventing coagulopathy through dilution of clotting factors.[32] The basic underlying principles of DCR are as follows:

- Permissive hypotension: In patients without central nervous system injury, it is reasonable to allow a lower blood pressure before surgical intervention. This target, in general, should be around a blood pressure of 90 systolic with the use of minimal, if any, crystalloid and resuscitation with blood products.[33]
- Balanced component therapy: Most severe traumas will receive massive transfusion protocol, defined as greater than or equal to 10 units of blood in 24 hours. The principle of balanced component therapy is the use of blood, fresh frozen plasma, and platelets in a 1:1:1 ratio. The ratio has been shown beneficial in terms of outcomes in multiple trials but probably most notably in the The Pragmatic, Randomized Optimal Platelet and Plasma Ratios (PROPPR) and PRospective, Observational, Multicenter, Major Trauma Transfusion (PROMMTT) studies.[34–36]
- Prevention of coagulopathy: This is very often multifactorial and can, in part, be prevented by balanced component therapy. The classic teaching of preventing the vicious cycle of coagulopathy aims at prevention of the lethal triad of trauma. This triad consists of hypothermia, acidosis, and coagulopathy. All of these processes attenuate each other, leading to worsening outcomes.[37] Simple

measures, such as rewarming, prevention of tissue hypoperfusion, and hemorrhage control, can go a long way in reducing development of the lethal triad.

Tranexamic acid (TXA) is an agent that prevents the degradation of the fibrin mesh network by binding to plasmin. The Clinical Randomisation of an Antifibrinolytic in Significant Head-2 trial showed a decreased in mortality in trauma patients who received this drug within 3 hours of major trauma.[38] This should be strongly considered for trauma patients likely to receive massive transfusions. The caveat to TXA is that administration past 3 hours from the initial injury may actually increase mortality, so caution must be taken.

COMPLICATIONS

Although there are numerous complications from penetrating vascular injury, most of these are delayed and occur after initial evaluation and repair. Although these are more applicable to the inpatient team, they include limb ischemia, wound infection, and vascular graft or repair thrombosis. There are some complications that the emergency medicine provider should be aware of. Most severe penetrating vascular trauma will involve large vessels and, by the principles of anatomy, these vessels most usually run in neurovascular bundles. Therefore, it is exceedingly important to at least consider concomitant vein and nerve injury when evaluating arterial injury. Although the immediate management may not differ, the importance of performing and documenting a thorough neurovascular examination cannot be emphasized enough.

The documentation and monitoring of the neurovascular examination also becomes important when monitoring for compartment syndrome. Briefly, compartment syndrome is a mismatch between the volume and contents of a muscular compartment, leading to tissue hypoxia and ischemia.[39] This can be from many different causes, but the basic concepts are increased contents, decreased volume, or external compression. This pressure overcomes the venous and eventually arterial blood supply, leading to pulselessness, paresthesias, pallor, pain, and eventually tissue death. Although management of this condition is ultimately surgical, expeditious diagnosis and treatment is paramount to preventing complications such as contractures.

DISPOSITION

Patients with major vascular injury will usually require admission and repair by a vascular surgeon. The difficulty comes in the patients with penetrating trauma to areas not always in need of vascular repair. Forearm injuries with either radial or ulnar artery injury do not need to be repaired unless there are hard signs of vascular injury or if both arteries are disrupted. In the lower leg, arterial injuries below the trifurcation of the popliteal artery do not need to be repaired unless there are hard signs of vascular injury or 2 out of 3 arteries are occluded on computed tomography angiography.[2] Nonetheless, both the lower leg and the forearm must be monitored closely for development of compartment syndrome.

SUMMARY

Penetrating vascular injuries are serious and common presenting complaints in the ED. They are associated with significant morbidity and mortality if not addressed early and cared for in the appropriate manner. The management of these patients has improved dramatically thanks to research and clinical practice guidelines implemented during wars, most recently in Iraq and Afghanistan. The TCCC and JTS clinical practice guidelines are evidence-based and have proven effective in decreasing mortality from injuries sustained in wartime. As gun violence increases and these concepts translate into the prehospital and hospital settings in the United States, emergency physicians will be an integral part of the care of patients with penetrating vascular trauma.

REFERENCES

1. FBI UCR. 2014. Available at: https://ucr.fbi.gov/crime-in-the-u.s/2014/crime-in-the-u.s.-2014/tables/table-15. Accessed December 15, 2016.
2. Newton EJ, Arora S. Peripheral Vascular Injury. Rosen's Emerg Med - Concepts Clin Pract 2-Volume Set. 2014:500–510.e3.
3. McSwain N, et al. The kinematics of trauma, . Prehospital trauma life support (PHTLS). 8th edition. Burlington (NJ): Jones & Barlett; 2016. p. 70–113.
4. Fackler ML. Civilian gunshot wounds and ballistics: dispelling the myths. Emerg Med Clin North Am 1998;16(1):17–28.
5. Van Waes OJ. Treatment of penetrating trauma of the extremities: ten years' experience at a Dutch level 1 trauma center. Scand J Trauma Resusc Emerg Med 2013;21(2):1–6.
6. Frykberg ER, Dennis JW, Bishop K, et al. The reliability of physical examination in the evaluation of penetrating extremity trauma for vascular injury: results at one year. J Trauma 1991;31(4):502–11.
7. Sekharan J, Dennis JW, Veldenz HC, et al. Continued experience with physical examination alone for evaluation and management of penetrating zone 2 neck injuries: results of 145 cases. J Vasc Surg 2000;32(3):483–9.
8. Kotwal RS, Butler FK, Gross KR, et al. Management of Junctional Hemorrhage in Tactical Combat Casualty Care: TCCC Guidelines? Proposed Change 13-03. J Spec Oper Med 2013;13(4):85–93. Available at: http://www.ncbi.nlm.nih.gov/pubmed/24227566.
9. Resuscitative Endovascular Balloon Occlusion of the Aorta (REBOA) for Hemorrhagic Shock. Jt Theater Trauma Syst Clin Pract Guidel 2012;1–18. Available at: http://www.usaisr.amedd.army.mil/cpgs/Vascular_Injury_12_Aug_2016.pdf. Accessed July 31, 2017.
10. Stockinger CZ, Antevil CDRJ, White LTCC, et al. Joint Trauma System Clinical Practice Guideline- Vascular Injury. 2016.
11. Lynch K, Johansen K. Can Doppler pressure measurement replace "exclusion" arteriography in the diagnosis of occult extremity arterial trauma? Ann Surg 1991;214(6):737–41. Available at: http://www.ncbi.nlm.nih.gov/pmc/articles/PMC1358501/.
12. Ivatury RR, Anand R, Ordonez C. Penetrating extremity trauma. World J Surg 2015;39(6):1389–96.
13. Wallin D, Yaghoubian A, Rosing D, et al. Computed tomographic angiography as the primary diagnostic modality in penetrating lower extremity vascular injuries: a level I trauma experience. Ann Vasc Surg 2011;25(5):620–3.
14. Miller-Thomas MM, West OC, Alan M. Diagnosing Traumatic Arterial Injury in the Extremities with CT Angiography: Pearls and pitfalls. Radiographics 2005;25:133–43.
15. Patterson BO, Holt PJ, Cleanthis M, et al. Imaging vascular trauma. Br J Surg 2012;99(4):494–505.
16. Mollberg NM, Wise SR, Banipal S, et al. Color-flow duplex screening for upper extremity proximity injuries: a low-yield strategy for therapeutic intervention. Ann Vasc Surg 2013;27(5):594–8.

17. Kragh JF, Littrel ML, Jones JA, et al. Battle casualty survival with emergency tourniquet use to stop limb bleeding. J Emerg Med 2011;41(6):590–7.
18. Kragh JFJ, Dubick MA, Aden JK, et al. U.S. Military use of tourniquets from 2001 to 2010. Prehosp Emerg Care Off J Natl Assoc EMS Physicians Natl Assoc State EMS Dir 2015;19(2):184–90.
19. Beekley AC, Sebesta JA, Blackbourne LH, et al. Prehospital tourniquet use in Operation Iraqi Freedom: effect on hemorrhage control and outcomes. J Trauma 2008;64(2 Suppl):S28–37 [discussion: S37].
20. NAEMT. Tactical Combat Casualty Care Guidelines for Medical Personnel. 2015; (June). Available at: https://www.naemt.org/education/TCCC/tccc-ac. Accessed December 15, 2016.
21. Passos E, Dingley B, Smith A, et al. Tourniquet use for peripheral vascular injuries in the civilian setting. Injury 2014;45(3):573–7.
22. Mayo Clinic. The return of tourniquets - For Medical Professionals - Mayo Clinic. Available at: http://www.mayoclinic.org/medical-professionals/clinical-updates/trauma/combat-tested-tourniquets-save-lives-limbs. Accessed December 15, 2016.
23. Dayan L, Zinmann C, Stahl S, et al. Complications associated with prolonged tourniquet application on the battlefield. Mil Med 2008;173(1):63–6.
24. Bennett BL, Littlejohn L. Review of new topical hemostatic dressings for combat casualty care. Mil Med 2014;179(5):497–514.
25. Clay JG, Grayson JK, Zierold D. Comparative testing of new hemostatic agents in a swine model of extremity arterial and venous hemorrhage. Mil Med 2010; 175(4):280–4.
26. Littlejohn LF, Devlin JJ, Kircher SS, et al. Comparison of Celox-A, Chitoflex, WoundStat, and combat gauze hemostatic agents versus standard gauze dressing in control of hemorrhage in a swine model of penetrating trauma. Acad Emerg Med 2011;18(4):340–50.
27. DuBose JJ, Scalea TM, Brenner M, et al. The AAST prospective Aortic Occlusion for Resuscitation in Trauma and Acute Care Surgery (AORTA) registry. J Trauma Acute Care Surg 2016;81(3):409–19.
28. Rhee PM, Acosta J, Bridgeman A, et al. Survival after emergency department thoracotomy: review of published data from the past 25 years. J Am Coll Surg 2000;190(3):288–98.
29. Mollberg NM, Wise SR. Appropriate use of emergency department thoracotomy. J Am Coll Surg 2012;214(5):870–1.
30. Qasim Z, Brenner M, Menaker J, et al. Resuscitative endovascular balloon occlusion of the aorta. Resuscitation 2015;96(2015):275–9.
31. Balogh Z, McKinley BA, Cocanour CS, et al. Supranormal trauma resuscitation causes more cases of abdominal compartment syndrome. Arch Surg 2003; 138(6):633–7.
32. Joint Theater Trauma System Clinical Practice Guideline. Damage Control Resuscitation CPG. 2012. p. 1–34.
33. Duke MD, Guidry C, Guice J, et al. Restrictive fluid resuscitation in combination with damage control resuscitation: time for adaptation. J Trauma Acute Care Surg 2012;73(3):674–8.
34. Duchesne JC, Barbeau JM, Islam TM, et al. Damage control resuscitation: from emergency department to the operating room. Am Surg 2011;77(2):201–6.
35. Holcomb JB, Tilley BC, Baraniuk S, et al. Transfusion of plasma, platelets, and red blood cells in a 1:1:1 vs a 1:1:2 ratio and mortality in patients with severe trauma: the PROPPR randomized clinical trial. JAMA 2015;313(5):471–82.

36. Holcomb JB, del Junco DJ, Fox EE, et al. The PRospective, Observational, Multi-center, Major Trauma Transfusion (PROMMTT) study: comparative effectiveness of a time-varying treatment with competing risks. JAMA Surg 2013;148(2): 127–36.
37. Jansen JO, Thomas R, Loudon MA, et al. Damage control resuscitation for patients with major trauma. BMJ 2009;338:b1778.
38. Williams-Johnson JA, McDonald AH, Strachan GG, et al. Effects of tranexamic acid on death, vascular occlusive events, and blood transfusion in trauma patients with significant haemorrhage (CRASH-2) a randomised, placebo-controlled trial. Lancet 2010;376(6):23–32.
39. Geiderman JM, Katz D. General Principles of Orthopedic Injuries. Rosen's Emerg Med - Concepts Clin Pract 2-Volume Set. 2014. p. 511–533.e2.

Subarachnoid Hemorrhage

Updates in Diagnosis and Management

Brit Long, MD[a,*], Alex Koyfman, MD[b], Michael S. Runyon, MD, MPH[c]

KEYWORDS

- Subarachnoid hemorrhage • Computed tomography • Lumbar puncture
- Angiography • Cerebral aneurysm • Xanthochromia • Vasospasm • Rebleed

KEY POINTS

- Subarachnoid hemorrhage (SAH) is deadly, with 25% dying within 24 hours and an overall mortality rate of 50%.
- Outside of trauma, SAH most commonly arises from aneurysmal rupture (80%) but may be due to peri-mesencephalic bleed or other less common causes.
- Most patients will present with sudden, maximal headache, associated with nausea/vomiting, neck pain, and exertion. The headache is usually different than patients' baseline headaches.
- Diagnosis centers on head noncontrast computed tomography (CT). If conducted within 6 hours of headache onset, this test is reliable. If it is negative but patients present after 6 hours, lumbar puncture and/or CT angiography should be used.
- Management requires rapid neurologic assessment, monitoring for intracranial pressure elevation, nimodipine, blood pressure management, analgesia, seizure treatment, and coagulopathy correction.

INTRODUCTION

Subarachnoid hemorrhage (SAH) is a neurologic emergency and is defined by bleeding in the subarachnoid space, which lies between the arachnoid and pia mater. This area is normally filled with cerebrospinal fluid (CSF). Trauma is the most common cause of SAH.[1–3] Most nontraumatic SAH, approximately 80%, is due to ruptured aneurysm.[1–3] The causes of nonaneurysmal SAH are diverse, and the mechanism may not be identified.[4,5]

Disclosure statement: This review does not reflect the views or opinions of the US government, Department of Defense, SAUSHEC EM Program, or US Air Force.

[a] Department of Emergency Medicine, San Antonio Military Medical Center, 3841 Roger Brooke Drive, Fort Sam Houston, TX 78234, USA; [b] Department of Emergency Medicine, The University of Texas Southwestern Medical Center, 5323 Harry Hines Boulevard, Dallas, TX 75390, USA; [c] Department of Emergency Medicine, Carolinas HealthCare System, Medical Education Building, Third floor, 1000 Blythe Boulevard, Charlotte, NC 28203, USA
* Corresponding author.
E-mail address: Brit.long@yahoo.com

Emerg Med Clin N Am 35 (2017) 803–824
http://dx.doi.org/10.1016/j.emc.2017.07.001
0733-8627/17/Published by Elsevier Inc.

EPIDEMIOLOGY

Headache accounts for approximately 2% of emergency department (ED) visits, with SAH occurring in 1% to 3% of these patients.[1,6–8] The incidence is approximately 7 to 10 per 100,000, with mortality approaching 50%.[6–8] SAH is the most common form of intracranial hemorrhage in trauma.[1–5] Close to 15% of patients will die before they reach the hospital, with 25% dying within 24 hours and 45% of patients dying within 30 days.[9–12] Morbidity is also severe, with only one-third of patients demonstrating full recovery after treatment.[9]

Prognosis is predicted by level of consciousness and neurologic examination on initial evaluation, patient age (younger patients experience better outcome), and amount of hemorrhage on initial imaging (increased hemorrhage associated with worse outcome).[13–15] For patients who reach the hospital, early complications of SAH account for most mortality, including rebleeding, vasospasm, seizures, increased intracranial pressure (ICP), and cardiac complications.

PATHOPHYSIOLOGY

Aneurysmal

Most nontraumatic SAHs are due to aneurysmal rupture, and these aneurysms are usually not congenital. Most never rupture and arise at sites of arterial branching, specifically the circle of Willis in the anterior circulation.[1–6] Saccular aneurysms account for 90%, and the overall prevalence of cerebral aneurysm ranges from 0.5% to 6.0% depending on the population.[4,5,16–19] A systematic review including more than 56,000 patients from 23 studies found an incidence of 2.3%.[18] Risk factors include a family history of SAH or aneurysm, smoking, hypertension, and heavy alcohol use.[1–3]

Nonaneurysmal

Peri-mesencephalic SAH is characterized by localized blood on computed tomography (CT) without aneurysm.[4,5,20] These bleeds are defined by hemorrhage restricted to the cisterns around the brainstem with absence of aneurysm on vascular imaging, such as CT angiography (CTA) and magnetic resonance angiography (MRA).[4,5,20] This type has a much better prognosis than aneurysmal SAH. Other causes include vascular malformation, intracranial dissection, sickle cell disease with intracerebral hemorrhage, pituitary apoplexy, cerebral amyloid angiopathy, central nervous system tumor, cocaine use, and cerebral venous thrombosis.[20–28]

Traumatic

SAH is a common form of intracranial bleeding in trauma. It results from disruption of the parenchyma and subarachnoid vasculature and often presents with headache, meningeal signs, and photophobia.[1–4,29] This finding is one of the most common CT findings in patients with moderate to severe traumatic brain injury, and traumatic SAH is associated with a 3-fold increase in mortality.[1–4,29]

FEATURES AND PRESENTATION

Most patients with SAH experience abrupt headache, often thunderclap in nature, defined by a headache that reaches maximal intensity within 1 minute.[30] However, 10% to 25% of patients with thunderclap headache have SAH.[31–34] Most of these headaches are atypical in nature and different from patients' prior headaches. The headache may begin or worsen with exertion, and it may lateralize to the side of the bleed in 30% of patients.[31,34] Key historical features are shown in **Table 1**.

Table 1
Key historical features of subarachnoid hemorrhage

Feature	Question
Onset	Did the headache reach maximal intensity suddenly rather than gradually (over 1 h or more)? • Sudden onset is suggestive.
Severity/ quality	Have you had headaches before? How does this compare? • Different or new headache is concerning.
Other symptoms	Are there other symptoms, including seizure, syncope, neck stiffness, focal neurologic deficit, vomiting, or change in vision? • New or different symptoms are concerning.

Sentinel bleeding may occur weeks before the maximal bleeding. Approximately 30% to 50% of patients experience this sentinel headache, which most commonly precedes a major bleed by 1 to 3 weeks.[31,34] Close to 70% of patients present with headache and no neurologic deficit. Nausea and vomiting may occur in 77% of patients, though vomiting is not predictive.[35,36] Carpenter and colleagues[37] conducted a recent meta-analysis evaluating the diagnostic accuracy of history, physical examination, imaging, and lumbar puncture (LP). The key findings of this study are demonstrated in **Table 2**. Of note, the absence of the *worst headache of life* and onset of headache that is more than 1 hour possess likelihood ratios (LRs) that are less than 1, though confidence intervals (CIs) cross 1.[37] Other findings, such as family history of cerebral aneurysm, lethargy, history of headache, scotomata, and diplopia, demonstrate LRs with CIs crossing 1.[37]

Seizure at the time of onset is predictive of bleeding. Seizures occur in less than 20% of patients during or shortly after SAH.[5,38,39] Loss of consciousness affects approximately 25% to 53% of patients; neck stiffness, or meningismus, may occur

Table 2
Key findings of Carpenter study on subarachnoid hemorrhage

Evaluated Characteristic	Likelihood Ratio (95% CI)
Neck pain history	4.12 (2.24–7.59)
Neck stiffness on examination	6.59 (3.95–11.00)
Absence of worst headache of life	0.36 (0.01–14.22)
Onset of headache more than 1 h	0.06 (0–0.95)
Noncontrast head CT within 6 h positive for SAH	230 (6–8700)
Noncontrast head CT within 6 h negative for SAH	0.01 (0–0.04)
Noncontrast head CT beyond 6 h negative for SAH	0.07 (0.01–0.61)
CSF analysis: RBC count $\geq$1000 $\times$ 10^6/L	5.7 (1.4–23.0)
CSF analysis: RBC count <1000 $\times$ 10^6/L	0.21 (0.03–1.7)
Visible xanthochromia	Present: 24.67 (12.13–50.14) Absent: 0.22 (0.09–0.54)

Abbreviations: CI, confidence interval; RBC, red blood cell.

Data from Carpenter CR, Hussain AM, Ward MJ, et al. Spontaneous subarachnoid hemorrhage: a systematic review and meta-analysis describing the diagnostic accuracy of history, physical examination, imaging, and lumbar puncture with an exploration of test thresholds. Acad Emerg Med 2016;23(9):963–1003.

in 35% of patients after several hours as a reaction to blood in the subarachnoid space.[3,5,32,36] Cranial nerve III palsy is due to direct local pressure from an aneurysm arising from the posterior communicating artery. Up to 50% of patients will have neurologic abnormalities on examination, ranging from mental status change to focal deficit.[3,5,32–39]

Patients may present with a combination of symptoms that suggest another diagnosis. Isolated neck pain, fever, headache, nausea and vomiting, elevated blood pressure, or electrocardiogram (ECG) changes (deep T-wave inversions or ST changes) may occur.[40] ECG changes may be due to catecholamine surge or autonomic vascular tone increase.[40] Some patients may experience cardiac arrest. All of these make the diagnosis more difficult, especially in comatose patients.

DIFFERENTIAL DIAGNOSIS

Although the classic presentation of SAH is sudden severe headache, SAH may present with vague headache and normal neurologic status. However, many other conditions may present with headache, including some with significant morbidity and mortality. This differential is demonstrated in **Table 3**.

DIAGNOSIS

Diagnosis centers on several investigations including imaging and laboratory analysis such as CSF. Misdiagnosis most commonly arises from 3 errors: failure to appreciate the full clinical spectrum of SAH, failure to obtain initial cerebral imaging, and failure to perform LP in the correct settings.[41,42] Particularly in alert, neurologically normal patients, this diagnosis can be difficult, with up to 53% of patients with SAH missed on initial presentation.[1,41,42] Missed diagnosis can result in mortality that approaches 50%, increasing to 70% in patients with rebleed.[43–45]

The American College of Emergency Physicians' (ACEP) clinical policy on the evaluation and management of adult patients with headache provides a level B recommendation for lumbar puncture (LP) in patients who present with sudden-onset, severe headache and negative noncontrast head CT.[46] Likewise, the American Heart Association (AHA) gives a level B recommendation for LP following negative head CT noncontrast.[47] The AHA guidelines also give a level C recommendation for CTA as a follow-up test when a noncontrast head CT is nondiagnostic in patients with suspected SAH.[47]

NONCONTRAST HEAD COMPUTED TOMOGRAPHY

Noncontrast head CT is the primary means of diagnosis; however, early generation scanners had the potential to miss 5% of cases.[48–50] Thus, LP has traditionally been advocated for those patients with suspected SAH and a negative noncontrast CT. CT technology is rapidly improving. First-generation scanners demonstrated sensitivity of 92% within 24 hours of headache onset, but more advanced-generation scanners approach a sensitivity of 100% if completed within 6 hours of symptom onset.[37,42,48–50] **Fig. 1** displays SAH on CT.

A study of nearly 3000 patients by Perry and colleagues[42] found a sensitivity of 100% for noncontrast head CT performed within 6 hours in patients with the worst ever headache, when the CT was performed on a third-generation, or newer, scanner and interpreted by a neuroradiologist. A subsequent study of 137 patients in 2012 found a sensitivity of 98.5% for noncontrast head CT performed within 6 hours, though the one miss was due to a bleeding cervical arteriovenous malformation that presented without headache.[50] With exclusion of this patient, sensitivity for SAH was

Table 3
Differential of sudden-onset, severe headache

	History and Physical Examination Findings
Deadly Causes	
Hypertensive encephalopathy	Severe hypertension with altered consciousness
Cervical or cranial artery dissection	Neck and/or face pain, usually abrupt onset, several variations of neurologic deficit
Cerebral venous and dural sinus thrombosis	Headache with focal deficit or seizure with risk factors, including hypercoagulable state, pregnancy, tobacco use
Carbon monoxide poisoning	Headache, nausea, and vomiting; often with multiple patients affected with similar symptoms
Idiopathic intracranial hypertension	Obese females with papilledema, may have cranial nerve VI deficit
Meningitis or encephalitis	Fever, headache, stiff neck in meningitis; encephalitis may present with focal deficits or seizure
Giant cell arteritis	Commonly in patients aged >50 y, decreased pulse in temporal artery, temporal artery tenderness, ESR elevation, may have vision loss
Acute angle closure glaucoma	Painful eye with decreased vision, corneal edema, pupil midposition
Spontaneous intracranial hypotension	Headache worse when upright and improves when supine
Mass lesion (tumor, abscess, cyst)	Neurologic deficit common, commonly focal; may have altered mental status
Pituitary apoplexy	Headache with visual deficit, sudden onset; patient commonly with pituitary tumor
Posterior reversible encephalopathy syndrome	Recurrent sudden-onset headache with nausea, vomiting, altered mental status, visual field changes; may have seizure; patients often with history of hypertension and renal disease
Stroke: hemorrhagic	Sudden-onset headache with neurologic deficit, altered mental status; patients often hypertensive
Benign Causes	
Migraine, tension, cluster, exertional, cough, viral sinusitis	

Abbreviation: ESR, erythrocyte sedimentation rate.

100%. Therefore, it is reasonable to assume that CT sensitivity approaches 100% with at least third-generation scanners when an experienced radiologist interprets a scan obtained within 6 hours of headache onset. A negative head CT noncontrast within 6 hours of onset possesses a negative LR of 0.01.[37] Beyond 6 hours the sensitivity is approximately 95%, which decreases with time to less than 90% as the time from headache onset approaches 24 hours.[48–50] One important aspect is the CT should be interpreted by an experienced radiologist.[51] With experienced radiologist interpretation, a systematic review and meta-analysis finds overall sensitivity more than 99.0%, with specificity of 99.9%, for CT obtained within 6 hours of headache onset.[52] The pooled LR of SAH with negative CT within 6 hours is 0.010.[37,52] If the scanner is an older generation and an experienced radiologist is not available, further evaluation may be considered.

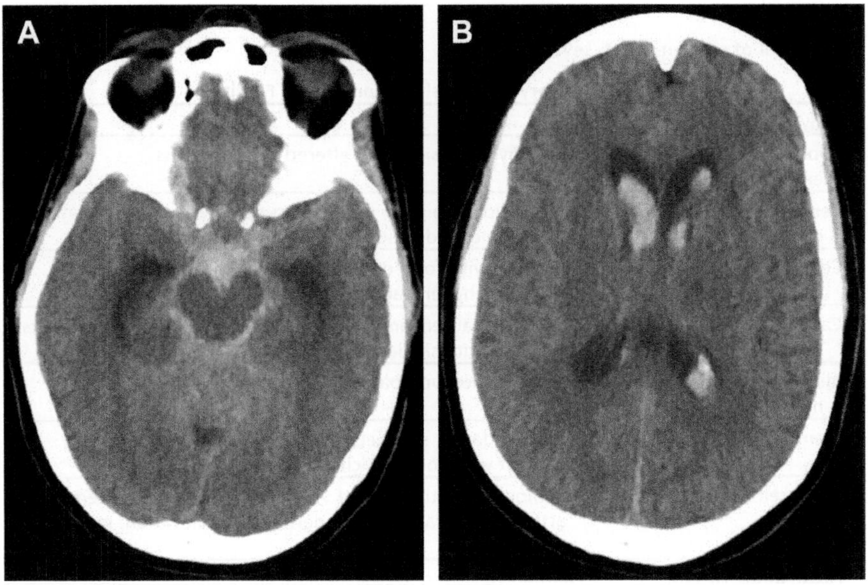

Fig. 1. (*A, B*) Noncontrast-enhanced CT of the head; a classic example of SAH with intraventricular extension. Note the starfish appearance of the hyperdensity caused by the blood in the subarachnoid space. (*Courtesy of* Michael Abraham, MD, MS, Baltimore, MD.)

Limitations of CT include anemia (sensitivity decreases when the hematocrit is <30%), smaller hemorrhage volume, CT quality, radiologist experience, and image artifacts.[43,51–54] High-quality CT within 6 hours of headache onset interpreted by an experienced radiologist provides a risk of missing SAH with negative CT of less than 1.0% and a negative LR of 0.01.[37,51]

COMPUTED TOMOGRAPHY ANGIOGRAPHY

The AHA's guidelines give a level C recommendation for CTA to follow nondiagnostic noncontrast head CT.[47] CTA can rapidly identify an aneurysm, classically with a sensitivity of 77% to 100% and specificity of 87% to 100%.[55–61] A recent meta-analysis of CTA found a pooled sensitivity of 98% (95% CI: 97%–99%) and pooled specificity of 100% (95% CI: 97%–100%) for the detection of aneurysm.[59] However, sensitivity is significantly lower for aneurysms less than 3 to 4 mm, though most aneurysms that rupture are more than 5 mm.[57,62] Notably, approximately 0.6% to 5.0% of the general population will have an aneurysm on CTA, with most being asymptomatic.[18]

Potential advantages of CTA over noncontrast head CT followed by LP include patient comfort and improved diagnostic ability to detect aneurysm. A negative noncontrast head CT and negative CTA indicate a relatively benign clinical course.[37,51,55–59] Patients with negative noncontrast head CT and negative CTA have a post-test probability for aneurysmal SAH of less than 0.3%, and this combination of tests has a negative predictive value more than 99%.[60] The potential problem with the CT/CTA approach without LP is that visualizing an aneurysm on CTA does not confirm the diagnosis of aneurysmal SAH. There is a possibility that the aneurysm is an incidental finding that will prompt unnecessary intervention, placing patients at increased risk of complications.[37,60,61] However, patients with aneurysm and headache may be at an 8-fold higher rate of aneurysm rupture when compared with asymptomatic patients with an aneurysm.[18] Complication rates of CTA range from 0.25% to 1.8% and include nephrotoxicity, increased radiation exposure, and allergic reaction.[31,37,63]

CTA can provide a benefit in patients whereby LP would be difficult or not feasible (obesity, inability to cooperate, decline LP). The test will consistently show aneurysms greater than 3 to 4 mm in size, if present.

MRI/MAGNETIC RESONANCE ANGIOGRAPHY

A recent meta-analysis of MRI with MRA demonstrated a pooled sensitivity of 95% (95% CI: 89%–98%) and pooled specificity of 89% (95% CI: 80%–95%) for identification of cerebral aneurysms.[64] This modality is also effective in subacute (3 days after headache onset) or chronic SAH.[37,64,65] MRA in conjunction with MRI can diagnose aneurysms greater than 3 mm in size with more than 95% sensitivity. MRI may diagnose other conditions, such as neoplasm, multiple sclerosis, posterior reversible encephalopathy syndrome, and encephalitis.[64–66] This modality does not require radiation, though several limitations exist, including limited availability in the ED, the time required for scanning, the potential for inducing claustrophobia, and the need for specialist interpretation. False-negative and false-positive aneurysms detected on MRA are often located at the skull base or the middle cerebral artery.[37,64–66] MRI/MRA is optimal for patients who present in a subacute or chronic timeframe.

LUMBAR PUNCTURE

Traditionally, LP followed nondiagnostic head CT in cases of suspected SAH. LP after negative CT is a level B recommendation by the ACEP.[46] Of note, the ACEP's guidelines predate the work of Perry and colleagues[42] on the sensitivity of CT obtained within 6 hours of headache onset. However, many patients fear LP because of its painful and invasive nature as well as the risk of post-LP headache, which approaches 30%.[67] Other issues include the time and potential difficulty of performing the test as well as the yield, which may be complicated by a traumatic tap.[67–72] Contraindications include bleeding disorder or coagulopathy and increased ICP.[73] Interestingly, less than half of patients with negative CT and acute headache undergo LP; in these studies, less than 1% of LPs are true positive when a third-generation scanner is used.[68–70]

LP can add important clinical information for other diagnoses, including meningitis, spontaneous intracranial hypotension, and idiopathic intracranial hypertension. Unfortunately, LP cannot diagnose pituitary apoplexy, cerebral venous sinus thrombosis, arterial dissection, or unruptured aneurysm.[70,73] Brunell and colleagues[72] found that LP provides an alternative diagnosis in 3% of cases, though findings altered management in less than 0.5%. More than 250 LPs are required to diagnose one additional SAH missed by CT per Carpenter and colleagues'[37] meta-analysis.

There are several controversies in the interpretation of CSF results.[37,70] Traumatic LP may occur in 15% of cases.[37,70] Classically in traumatic LP, red blood cell (RBC) clearing is seen when tubes 1 and 4 are compared, with no RBCs in tube 4.[70,71,74] However, the complete absence of RBCs in tube 4 is rare, resulting in difficulty with interpretation. Using the CSF RBC count to distinguish SAH and traumatic LP can be complex. Perry and colleagues[75] used a threshold of 2000×10^6/L in the final tube and found a sensitivity of 93% (95% CI: 66%–98%) and specificity of 93% (95% CI: 91%–95%) for aneurysmal SAH. Czuczman and colleagues[71] found an LR for the diagnosis of SAH of 0 (95% CI: 0–0.3) with an RBC count less than 100 in the final tube and 1.6 (95% CI: 1.1–2.3) with an RBC count less than

$10{,}000 \times 10^6$/L. Combining data from these studies and a threshold of 1000×10^6/L demonstrates a pooled sensitivity of 76% and specificity of 88%.[37,70,71]

XANTHOCHROMIA

Xanthochromia is due to the in vivo breakdown of hemoglobin by normal enzymatic action, creating a yellow color in CSF. Appearance of xanthochromia takes several hours after bleeding begins (20% of patients at 6 hours) and lasts for up to 2 weeks.[36,69,70,75–77] The sensitivity for the diagnosis of SAH approaches 90% at 12 hours after symptom onset, though classically it was thought to be 100%.[75–77]

Two methods of assessment are available. The first is visual inspection, whereby the CSF is compared with water against a white background. Visible inspection possesses a pooled sensitivity of 85%, with specificity 97% based on meta-analysis.[37] Multiwavelength spectrophotometry has poor specificity (29%–75%) but sensitivity approximately more than 95%; however, it is available in approximately 1% of US EDs.[77–80] Xanthochromia in the setting of SAH greatly reduces the likelihood of traumatic LP, with a negative LR of 0.22.[37] Physicians should consider that only 20% of those receiving an LP within 6 hours of headache onset will have positive xanthochromia.[77–79,81]

COMBINATION OF CEREBROSPINAL FLUID, RED BLOOD CELL, AND XANTHOCHROMIA

The use of CSF RBC count and xanthochromia together has been advocated. One prospective cohort demonstrated that the combination of absence of visual xanthochromia with less than 2000 RBCs may rule out SAH.[75] A cutoff of 2000 RBCs has a sensitivity of 93% alone. When xanthochromia is added to this, the sensitivity was 100% (95% CI: 75%–100%), though this finding requires further validation in other populations.[75]

OPENING PRESSURE

CSF pressure can provide valuable information in the setting of suspected SAH. Pressures greater than 20 cm H_2O are defined as elevated, which can be found in approximately 60% of patients with SAH. Elevated pressures may also be found in cerebral venous thrombosis, idiopathic intracranial hypertension, and meningitis.[37,70,82,83] Low pressure may be seen with spontaneous intracranial hypotension. Of note, pressure measurements must be taken with patients in the lateral recumbent position.[70]

TEST THRESHOLD

The test threshold is the pretest probability of disease that balances the risks of missing a diagnosis with the harms imposed by (1) the diagnostic strategy itself and (2) the treatment of those with a false-positive diagnosis.[37,70] In the setting of SAH, potential evaluation and treatment entail angiography, CT, LP, and neurosurgical intervention. A meta-analysis by Carpenter and colleagues[37] used pooled estimates of diagnostic accuracy, risks, and benefits to estimate the test threshold for the performance of LP after a negative head CT. Investigators suggest LP benefits patients with negative CT if the pre-LP probability of SAH is 5% or if the pre-CT probability of SAH is 20%.[37] Per this meta-analysis, a 1 in 10 pre-CT probability of SAH, while assuming CT sensitivity of 95%, results in a 1 in 180 chance of missing a ruptured aneurysm.[37]

MANAGEMENT

Management involves several key steps, shown later. Neurosurgical consultation is required to arrange for definitive therapy.[46,47,84–87] ED management must focus on management of the airway, hemodynamic monitoring, supportive care, and management and prevention of complications, demonstrated in **Box 1**. A multidisciplinary team specialized in the care of these patients can improve outcomes, and patients may benefit from transfer to a specialized center for further care.[46,47,84–87]

INITIAL RESUSCITATION

Patients with SAH, traumatic and nontraumatic, are at risk for severe complications resulting in hemodynamic compromise and neurologic decompensation.[47,84–94] Pulmonary edema and dysrhythmia may occur in 23% and 35% of SAH, respectively, within the first 24 hours of admission.[84–86,95] Neurologic decompensation occurs in up to 35% of patients within 24 hours.[84,85] Most interventions target initial stabilization and avoidance of these complications. Airway intervention may be needed for airway protection or anticipated clinical decompensation. Indications for intubation include Glasgow Coma Scale (GCS) less than 8, signs of elevated ICP (posturing), impaired oxygenation or ventilation, and need for sedation and paralysis.[47,86] The most important prognostic factors for SAH include level of consciousness at the time of hospital admission, age, and amount of blood on initial head CT.[13–15,47,86] Several physiologic derangements that are common and may worsen brain injury and increase mortality include serum glucose greater than180 mg/dL, troponin elevation, fever (>100.4°F), acidosis with serum bicarbonate less than 20 mmol/L, hypoxemia with arterio-alveolar gradient greater than 125 mm Hg, blood pressure instability (mean arterial pressure [MAP] <70 or >130 mm Hg), and hypothalamic pituitary dysfunction.[47,85–94] There are several grading scales that assess the severity of SAH; as each score increases, mortality increases.[96–98] These scales are shown in **Box 2**.

Box 1
Subarachnoid hemorrhage management considerations

- Closely evaluate for need for airway protection/endotracheal intubation
- Monitor for signs of increased ICP: decline in neurologic status, posturing, altered mental status
- Treat pain and anxiety: short-acting IV analgesics, such as fentanyl
- Treat nausea/vomiting
- Evaluate and monitor closely for complications, including decline in mental status, herniation, seizure, ECG changes, pulmonary edema
- BP management should target SBP less than 160 mm Hg or MAP less than 110 mm Hg
- Maintain normothermia; avoid fever
- Correct any coagulopathy
- Treat any seizure
- Provide nimodipine to decrease vasospasm risk

Abbreviations: BP, blood pressure; IV, intravenous; MAP, mean arterial pressure; systolic blood pressure.

Box 2
Subarachnoid hemorrhage grading/severity scales

Hunt and Hess Severity Scale

- Grade 1: Asymptomatic, mild headache
- Grade 2: Moderate to severe headache, nuchal rigidity, no focal deficit other than cranial nerve palsy
- Grade 3: Mild mental status change, mild focal neurologic deficit
- Grade 4: Stupor or moderate to severe hemiparesis
- Grade 5: Comatose or decerebrate rigidity

World Federation of Neurologic Surgeons

- Grade 1: GCS 15, no motor deficit
- Grade 2: GCS 13 to 14, no motor deficit
- Grade 3: GCS 13 to 14, motor deficit present
- Grade 4: GCS 7 to 12, motor deficit may be present or absent
- Grade 5: GCS 3 to 6, motor deficit may be present or absent

Fisher Scale (based on CT)

- Group 1: No blood
- Group 2: Diffuse deposits of SAH blood but no clots or layers of blood >1 mm
- Group 3: Local clots or vertical layers on blood >1 mm thickness
- Group 4: Diffuse or no SAH but intracerebral or intraventricular clot present

Data from Refs.[96–98]

GENERAL CARE

Patients must be provided adequate analgesia, antiemetics, and sedation, if needed. Weight-based fentanyl boluses (0.5–1.0 μg/kg intravenous [IV]) allow for rapid pain relief.[47,86] Nausea and vomiting are common in these patients; an antiemetic, such as ondansetron or metoclopramide, can be beneficial. Stool softeners should be provided to reduce risk of further straining and ICP increase.[4,86,92–94,99] Cardiac monitoring is vital to evaluate for dysrhythmia.[86–88] Head of bed elevation to 30° can facilitate venous drainage and decrease elevated ICP. Reevaluation of mental status, pupillary size and reactivity, and motor function is warranted, at minimum every hour. Critically ill patients may require more frequent reassessment. Patients should be given nothing by mouth until the treatment plan is determined.[47,86]

IV fluid administration should target euvolemia and normal electrolytes.[47,86,93,94] Normal saline is recommended over hypo-osmotic fluids, such as 5% dextrose in water or albumin. Hypovolemia and hypervolemia can worsen outcomes.[93,94]

Blood pressure control may be required, though the optimal target is not clear.[47,86,93,99–101] A definitive target has been the subject of several studies, many with conflicting results. One study of 134 patients found an 18% decrease in the rebleed rate when systolic blood pressure (SBP) was reduced to 100 mm Hg, though the cerebral infarction rate doubled (40% from 22%) in the treatment group.[99] The American Stroke Association's 2012 guidelines recommend maintaining the SBP at less than 160 mm Hg.[47] However, recent studies have not demonstrated a change in outcome with specific blood pressure targets in intracerebral hemorrhage.[102–104] Although reducing blood pressure can decrease the risk of rebleed, it can also worsen infarction. Cerebral perfusion pressure (CPP) is equal to MAP minus ICP. The CPP should be maintained at greater than 70 mm Hg.[5,47,86,103,104] Blood pressure management should be discussed with the neurosurgery and neurocritical care teams. An SBP of 160 mm Hg is likely safe in patients with hypertension.[47,86,101–105] Antihypertensive agents include labetalol, nicardipine, clevidipine, nitroprusside, and nitroglycerin.[47,86,106–109] Both nitroprusside and nitroglycerin should be avoided because of the increase in ICP and long-term decrease in cerebral perfusion. Nicardipine and clevidipine are calcium channel blocking agents with rapid time of onset and short half-life, allowing for easy titration to avoid hypotension.[107–109] Nicardipine can be started as an infusion of 5 mg/h IV, with titration by 2.5 mg/h every 5 minutes to a maximum of 15 mg/h. Once "the SBP target is reached", the infusion is decreased to 3 mg/h. Labetalol has greater heart rate control when compared with vasodilation effects (1:7 alpha to beta activity), with initial dosing of 10 to 20 mg IV.[47,86,106,107] This dose can be doubled every 10 minutes to a maximum 300 mg IV. Arterial catheter placement may be required for continuous blood pressure monitoring during administration of vasoactive medications.[5,47,86]

If patients are anticoagulated, rapid reversal should be completed. Four factor prothrombin complex concentrates (PCCs) and IV vitamin K are recommended for reversal of vitamin K antagonists, such as coumadin.[47,86,106,110] Heparin may be reversed with protamine. IV idarucizumab may reverse the anticoagulant effects of dabigatran.[111] The other target-specific oral anticoagulants, including apixaban, edoxaban, and rivaroxaban, can be difficult to reverse; 4-factor PCC administration may be beneficial.[111] Previously, patients taking antiplatelet medications with hemorrhage, including SAH, received platelet transfusion and/or desmopressin. However, the recent PATCH Platelet transfusion versus standard care after acute stroke due to spontaneous cerebral haemorrhage associated with antiplatelet therapy (PATCH) trial suggests platelet transfusion in these patients may be harmful; at this time, platelets cannot be recommended in these patients.[47,106,110,112]

Antifibrinolytic agents, such as tranexamic acid and aminocaproic acid, may have potential in treatment.[47,106,110,113] The American Stroke Association recommends use of these agents for less than 72 hours if definitive treatment is delayed and there are no contraindications.[47] These agents may reduce rebleeding, though no benefit in mortality or neurologic outcome has been demonstrated.[113–115]

DEFINITIVE MANAGEMENT

Two primary approaches exist for aneurysm repair, which include microvascular neurosurgical clipping or endovascular coiling. Many surgeons seek to repair abnormalities within 72 hours of the event.[47,86] Endovascular coiling has demonstrated better outcomes when compared with clipping, though not all patients are suitable for coiling.[5,47,116,117] The approach is determined by the aneurysm anatomy, clinician experience, and comorbidities.

COMPLICATIONS

Rebleeding

Rebleeding is a devastating consequence of SAH, accounting for significant morbidity and mortality that occurs in 8% to 23% of patients.[47,86,118,119] Up to 90% of rebleeding occurs within the first 6 hours after initial hemorrhage.[118,119] Patients with severe SAH, large aneurysm, sentinel bleed, longer time to surgery, and those undergoing catheter angiography have a higher risk of rebleeding.[47,86,118,119] Rebleeding may manifest as a worsening or acute headache, change in mental status, posturing, seizure, or cardiac arrest. Early repair is the only therapy currently associated with prevention of rebleeding.[47,86] Blood pressure management and antifibrinolytic therapy with aminocaproic acid or tranexamic acid may be beneficial. These therapies may reduce bleeding without causing secondary ischemia.[5,47,113] However, they are not associated with improving neurologic outcome or reducing the risk of death.

Vasospasm

Cerebral vessel vasospasm is a delayed complication that occurs within the first 2 weeks, most commonly 3 to 10 days after the initial bleed.[2,47,84–86,120,121] The incidence is related to the amount of blood present in the CSF. The pathogenesis is not well understood, but it is thought to occur because of spasmogenic substances released during RBC lysis.[120,121] The presentation varies from no symptoms to hemiplegia or reduced level of consciousness. From 30% to 70% of patients will not experience symptoms, whereas 30% can experience significant neurologic decompensation.[2,47,86,120] However, when vasospasm does occur with symptoms, it is associated with significant morbidity.

Nimodipine is an oral calcium channel blocker that reduces vasospasm and the risk of secondary ischemia.[2,47,86,120,121] Multiple studies support its use; a Cochrane review demonstrated a risk ratio of 0.67 (95% CI 0.55–0.81) for reducing secondary ischemia, with trends toward reducing mortality, as have other studies.[122–124] Other calcium channel blockers have not displayed this ability to improve outcomes. Dosing includes 60 mg orally every 4 hours. Patients unable to take medications by mouth can be given nimodipine through a nasogastric tube.[47,86,118] Nicardipine has also been associated with decreased vasospasm, though with no improvement in neurologic outcome.[123,125] Magnesium sulfate IV has been used, though it has not demonstrated efficacy in preventing vasospasm.[126] Statins have shown promise, but they do not affect neurologic outcome or mortality. The American Stroke Society states statin therapy is reasonable to prevent vasospasm.[47,86] Statins may affect cerebral vascular stability through several different mechanisms, but meta-analyses have not demonstrated improved clinical outcomes.[47,118] Pravastatin 40 mg orally or simvastatin 80 mg orally can be provided within 48 hours of hemorrhage; however, this can be completed in the intensive care unit and not the ED.[47,118,127,128]

If symptoms of vasospasm occur, often with focal deficit or change in mental status 3 to 10 days after the initial hemorrhage, aggressive therapy is warranted.[5,46,47,84–86,118] CTA is needed for definitive diagnosis and differentiation from rebleeding or hydrocephalus.[5,47,118] Previously hemodynamic augmentation, or triple-H therapy, consisting of hemodilution, induced hypertension, and hypervolemia, was recommended, with goals to increase MAP and cerebral perfusion.[47,86,129,130] Perfusion is often achieved with crystalloid fluids and vasopressor agents, though the data on the efficacy of this approach are mixed; outcomes may be worse with hemodynamic augmentation through these means.[5,47,129,130] Balloon angioplasty is often the mainstay of treatment, though intra-arterial vasodilator therapy can be used for diffuse vasospasm.[130,131]

Hydrocephalus

Hydrocephalus may occur in up to 30% of patients within the first 3 days, most commonly in those with severe bleeds, and may be asymptomatic.[132,133] Physicians should consider this complication in patients with sudden neurologic decline, motor posturing, or change in mental status.[47,132,133] Management includes placement of an external ventricular drain, which allows for CSF drainage and precise monitoring of ICP.[47]

Increased Intracranial Pressure

SAH can commonly lead to increased ICP due to hydrocephalus and hyperemia after hemorrhage.[134–136] Head of bed elevation, followed by hypertonic saline (3.0% 150–250 mL, or 23.4% 30 mL) or 20% mannitol (1 g/kg IV) is warranted to decrease ICP. Both can also improve cerebral perfusion pressure. If hypotensive, hypertonic saline is more beneficial.[5,47,134–136]

For intubated patients with concern of elevated ICP, analgesia (such as fentanyl) followed by sedation with propofol can reduce ICP.[5,47,118] Hyperventilation should be used with caution, as utilization of this measure for extended periods will reduce cerebral perfusion.[5,47,118] In patients with hydrocephalus and elevated ICP, ventriculostomy allows drainage of CSF and measurement of ICP. Decompressive craniectomy may be needed for ICP control with cerebral edema if other measures are not effective.[118,137,138]

Hyponatremia

Hyponatremia is a common occurrence due to inappropriate secretion of antidiuretic hormone (SIADH) or, more rarely, cerebral salt-wasting.[81,118,139] Patients with SIADH are euvolemic; though classic therapy for SIADH focuses on water restriction, this can cause vasospasm in SAH. Thus, isotonic saline or hypertonic saline is used in patients with SIADH. Cerebral salt-wasting is less common and is diagnosed in the setting of volume depletion. Isotonic saline infusions are needed, with the goal of euvolemia.[47,118,139]

Seizure

Seizures affect less than 20% of patients with SAH.[38,47,84–88] However, any seizure that occurs is associated with worse outcomes through the risk of further aneurysm damage and increased ICP.[38,47,87] Therefore, seizures must be diagnosed and managed rapidly with benzodiazepines followed by an anticonvulsant medication, such as levetiracetam. The AHA and the Neurocritical Care Society suggest anticonvulsant consideration in the immediate postbleed period for seizure prophylaxis, especially in patients with poor neurologic status and unsecured aneurysm.[47,106,118] However, this is controversial, as a Cochrane review states there is a lack of evidence that supports or refutes the use of prophylactic anticonvulsants.[140,141] Many neurosurgeons argue to treat seizures and withhold prophylaxis. If prophylactic anticonvulsants are given, levetiracetam or valproate may be used.[5,47,105,118] Once the aneurysm is secured, prophylactic antiepileptics may be stopped.[5,47,86,106,118]

NEW DIRECTIONS

Treatments currently being studied include corticosteroids for vasospasm.[142] Other investigational therapies for vasospasm prevention include intrathecal thrombolysis, lumbar drain placement, phosphodiesterase inhibitors, angioplasty, and endothelin receptor antagonists.[143–148] These measures target prevention of cerebral ischemia. Several studies have found cilostazol, eicosapentaenoic acid, heparin, steroids, and erythropoietin to show promise in smaller, nonrandomized studies.[149]

DISPOSITION

All patients with diagnosed SAH warrant admission.[5,47,118] Those with high-quality negative noncontrast head CT within 6 hours may be discharged home with pain control and referred for follow-up care. If studies are negative but the pain is refractory to

ED management, patients may require admission for pain control and further evaluation of other serious causes of their headache. If the physician has high suspicion for SAH after a negative noncontrast CT, further evaluation, such as LP or CTA, is indicated.

SUMMARY

SAH is a neurologic emergency, with mortality of 50%. It is due to bleeding into the subarachnoid space, which often presents in the form of headache, classically defined as maximal at onset and worst of life. Patients may demonstrate neck stiffness, nausea/vomiting, and altered mental status. Approximately 80% of nontraumatic SAH are due to aneurysmal rupture, with the remainder due to peri-mesencephalic bleed or other causes. Noncontrast head CT performed within 6 hours is reliable for diagnosis, though after 6 hours LP or CTA may be needed. Management of SAH includes initial resuscitation with intubation if needed, ongoing monitoring of neurologic status, analgesia, blood pressure management, coagulopathy correction, seizure treatment, and nimodipine to prevent vasospasm. Complications are common, including seizure, hydrocephalus, vasospasm, and rebleeding. Admission to a neurocritical care unit is recommended.

REFERENCES

1. Edlow JA, Malek AM, Ogilvy CS. Aneurysmal subarachnoid hemorrhage: update for emergency physicians. J Emerg Med 2008;34(3):237–51.
2. Fukuda T, Hasue M, Ito H. Does traumatic subarachnoid hemorrhage caused by diffuse brain injury cause delayed ischemic brain damage? Comparison with subarachnoid hemorrhage caused by ruptured intracranial aneurysms. Neurosurgery 1998;43(5):1040–9.
3. Suarez JI, Tarr RW, Selman WR. Aneurysmal subarachnoid hemorrhage. N Engl J Med 2006;354(4):387–96.
4. Watanabe A, Hirano K, Kamada M, et al. Perimesencephalic nonaneurysmal subarachnoid haemorrhage and variations in the veins. Neuroradiology 2002; 44(4):319–25.
5. van Gijn J, Kerr RS, Rinkel GJ. Subarachnoid haemorrhage. Lancet 2007; 369(9558):306–18.
6. Ingall T, Asplund K, Mahonen M, et al. A multinational comparison of subarachnoid hemorrhage epidemiology in the WHO MONICA stroke study. Stroke 2000; 31(5):1054–61.
7. Kozak N, Hayashi M. Trends in the incidence of subarachnoid hemorrhage in Akita prefecture, Japan. J Neurosurg 2007;106(2):234–8.
8. King JT Jr. Epidemiology of aneurysmal subarachnoid hemorrhage. Neuroimaging Clin N Am 1997;7(4):659–68.
9. Hop JW, Rinkel GJ, Algra A, et al. Case-fatality rates and functional outcome after subarachnoid hemorrhage: a systematic review. Stroke 1997;28(3):660–4.
10. Neil-Dwyer G, Lang D. 'Brain attack'–aneurysmal subarachnoid haemorrhage: death due to delayed diagnosis. J R Coll Physicians Lond 1997;31(1):49–52.
11. Broderick JP, Brott TG, Duldner JE, et al. Initial and recurrent bleeding are the major causes of death following subarachnoid hemorrhage. Stroke 1994; 25(7):1342–7.
12. Feigin VL, Lawes CM, Bennett DA, et al. Stroke epidemiology: a review of population-based studies of incidence, prevalence, and case-fatality in the late 20th century. Lancet Neurol 2003;2(1):43–53.

13. Hijdra A, van Gijn J, Nagelkerke NJ, et al. Prediction of delayed cerebral ischemia, rebleeding, and outcome after aneurysmal subarachnoid hemorrhage. Stroke 1988;19:1250.
14. Rosengart AJ, Schultheiss KE, Tolentino J, et al. Prognostic factors for outcome in patients with aneurysmal subarachnoid hemorrhage. Stroke 2007;38:2315.
15. Ko SB, Choi HA, Carpenter AM, et al. Quantitative analysis of hemorrhage volume for predicting delayed cerebral ischemia after subarachnoid hemorrhage. Stroke 2011;42:669.
16. Heiskanen O. Ruptured intracranial arterial aneurysms of children and adolescents. Surgical and total management results. Childs Nerv Syst 1989;5(2): 66–70.
17. Stehbens WE. Etiology of intracranial berry aneurysms. J Neurosurg 1989;70(6): 823–31.
18. Rinkel GJ, Djibuti M, Algra A, et al. Prevalence and risk of rupture of intracranial aneurysms: a systematic review. Stroke 1998;29(1):251–6.
19. Brown RD Jr, Broderick JP. Unruptured intracranial aneurysms: epidemiology, natural history, management options, and familial screening. Lancet Neurol 2014;13:393–404.
20. Schwartz TH, Solomon RA. Perimesencephalic nonaneurysmal subarachnoid hemorrhage: review of the literature. Neurosurgery 1996;39:433.
21. Jung JY, Kim YB, Lee JW, et al. Spontaneous subarachnoid haemorrhage with negative initial angiography: a review of 143 cases. J Clin Neurosci 2006;13: 1011.
22. Bikmaz K, Erdem E, Krisht A. Arteriovenous fistula originating from proximal part of the anterior cerebral artery. Clin Neurol Neurosurg 2007;109:589.
23. Suzuki S, Kayama T, Sakurai Y, et al. Subarachnoid hemorrhage of unknown cause. Neurosurgery 1987;21:310.
24. Oppenheim C, Domigo V, Gauvrit JY, et al. Subarachnoid hemorrhage as the initial presentation of dural sinus thrombosis. AJNR Am J Neuroradiol 2005; 26:614.
25. Karabatsou K, Lecky BR, Rainov NG, et al. Cerebral amyloid angiopathy with symptomatic or occult subarachnoid haemorrhage. Eur Neurol 2007;57:103.
26. Rogers LR. Cerebrovascular complications in cancer patients. Neurol Clin 2003; 21:167.
27. Sergides IG, Minhas PS, Anotun N, et al. Pituitary apoplexy can mimic subarachnoid haemorrhage clinically and radiologically. Emerg Med J 2007;24:308.
28. Quigley MR, Chew BG, Swartz CE, et al. The clinical significance of isolated traumatic subarachnoid hemorrhage. J Trauma Acute Care Surg 2013;74:581.
29. Rinkel GJ, van Gijn J, Wijdicks EF. Subarachnoid hemorrhage without detectable aneurysm. A review of the causes. Stroke 1993;24:1403.
30. Ducros A, Bousser MG. Thunderclap headache. BMJ 2013;346:e8557.
31. Linn FH, Wijdicks EF, van der Graaf Y, et al. Prospective study of sentinel headache in aneurysmal subarachnoid haemorrhage. Lancet 1994;344(8922):590–3.
32. Landtblom AM, Fridriksson S, Boivie J, et al. Sudden-onset headache: a prospective study of features, incidence and causes. Cephalalgia 2002;22(5): 354–60.
33. Morgenstern LB, Luna-Gonzales H, Huber JC Jr, et al. Worst headache and subarachnoid hemorrhage: prospective, modern computed tomography and spinal fluid analysis. Ann Emerg Med 1998;32(3 Pt 1):297–304.
34. Gorelick PB, Hier DB, Caplan LR, et al. Headache in acute cerebrovascular disease. Neurology 1986;36:1445.

35. Harling DW, Peatfield RC, Van Hille PT, et al. Thunderclap headache: is it migraine? Cephalalgia 1989;9(2):87–90.
36. Linn FH, Rinkel GJ, Algra A, et al. Headache characteristics in subarachnoid haemorrhage and benign thunderclap headache. J Neurol Neurosurg Psychiatry 1998;65(5):791–3.
37. Carpenter CR, Hussain AM, Ward MJ, et al. Spontaneous subarachnoid hemorrhage: a systematic review and meta-analysis describing the diagnostic accuracy of history, physical examination, imaging, and lumbar puncture with an exploration of test thresholds. Acad Emerg Med 2016;23(9):963–1003.
38. Schievink WI. Intracranial aneurysms. N Engl J Med 1997;336:28.
39. Butzkueven H, Evans AH, Pitman A, et al. Onset seizures independently predict poor outcome after subarachnoid hemorrhage. Neurology 2000;55:1315.
40. Chatterjee S. ECG changes in subarachnoid haemorrhage: a synopsis. Neth Heart J 2011;19(1):31–4.
41. Edlow JA, Caplan LR. Avoiding pitfalls in the diagnosis of subarachnoid hemorrhage. N Engl J Med 2000;342:29–36.
42. Perry JJ, Stiell IG, Sivilotti ML, et al. Sensitivity of computed tomography performed within six hours of onset of headache for diagnosis of subarachnoid haemorrhage: prospective cohort study. BMJ 2011;343:d4277.
43. Leblanc R. The minor leak preceding subarachnoid hemorrhage. J Neurosurg 1987;66:35–9.
44. Johansson A, Lagerstedt K, Asplund K. Mishaps in the management of stroke: a review of 214 com- plaints to a medical responsibility board. Cerebrovasc Dis 2004;18:16–21.
45. Duffy GP. The “warning leak” in spontaneous sub- arachnoid haemorrhage. Med J Aust 1983;1:514–6.
46. Edlow JA, Panagos PD, Godwin SA, et al. Clinical policy: critical issues in the evaluation and management of adult patients presenting to the emergency department with acute headache. Ann Emerg Med 2008;52(4):407–36.
47. Connolly ES, Rabinstein AA, Carhuapoma JR, et al. Guidelines for the management of aneurysmal subarachnoid hemorrhage: a statement for healthcare professionals from a special writing group of the Stroke Council, American Heart Association. Stroke 2012;43:1711–37.
48. Sames TA, Storrow AB, Finkelstein JA, et al. Sensitivity of new-generation computed tomography in subarachnoid hemorrhage. Acad Emerg Med 1996; 3(1):16–20.
49. Byyny RL, Mower WR, Shum N, et al. Sensitivity of non-contrast cranial computed tomography for the emergency department diagnosis of subarachnoid hemorrhage. Ann Emerg Med 2008;51(6):697–703.
50. Backes D, Rinkel GJ, Kemperman H, et al. Time-dependent test characteristics of head computed tomography in patients suspected of nontraumatic subarachnoid hemorrhage. Stroke 2012;43(8):2115–9.
51. Dubosh NM, Bellolio MF, Rabinstein AA, et al. Sensitivity of early brain computed tomography to exclude aneurysmal subarachnoid hemorrhage: a systematic review and meta-analysis. Stroke 2016 Mar;47(3):750–5.
52. Blok KM, Rinkel GJ, Majoie CB, et al. CT within 6 hours of headache onset to rule out subarachnoid hemorrhage in nonacademic hospitals. Neurology 2015;84: 1927–32.
53. van der Wee N, Rinkel GJ, Hasan D, et al. Detection of subarachnoid haemorrhage on early CT: is lumbar puncture still needed after a negative scan? J Neurol Neurosurg Psychiatry 1995;58(3):357–9.

54. Schriger DL, Kalafut M, Starkman S, et al. Cranial computed tomography interpretation in acute stroke: physician accuracy in determining eligibility for thrombolytic therapy. JAMA 1998;279(16):1293–7.
55. Agid R, Lee SK, Willinsky RA, et al. Acute subarachnoid hemorrhage: using 64-slice multidetector CT angiography to "triage" patients' treatment. Neuroradiology 2006;48(11):787–94.
56. Bederson JB, Awad IA, Wiebers DO, et al. Recommendations for the management of patients with unruptured intracranial aneurysms: a statement for healthcare professionals from the Stroke Council of the American Heart Association. Stroke 2000;31(11):2742–50.
57. Dammert S, Krings T, Moller-Hartmann W, et al. Detection of intracranial aneurysms with multislice CT: comparison with conventional angiography. Neuroradiology 2004;46(6):427–34.
58. Uysal E, Yanbuloglu B, Erturk M, et al. Spiral CT angiography in diagnosis of cerebral aneurysms of cases with acute subarachnoid hemorrhage. Diagn Interv Radiol 2005;11(2):77–82.
59. Westerlaan HE, van Dijk JM, Jansen-van der Weide MC, et al. Intracranial aneurysms in patients with subarachnoid hemorrhage: CT angiography as a primary examination tool for diagnosis–systematic review and meta-analysis. Radiology 2011;258:134–45.
60. McCormack RF, Hutson A. Can computed tomography angiography of the brain replace lumbar puncture in the evaluation of acute-onset headache after a negative noncontrast cranial computed tomography scan? Acad Emerg Med 2010;17(4):445–51.
61. Brennan JW, Schwartz ML. Unruptured intracranial aneurysms: appraisal of the literature and suggested recommendations for surgery, using evidence-based medicine criteria. Neurosurgery 2000;47:1359–71 [discussion: 1371–2].
62. Anderson GB, Findlay JM, Steinke DE, et al. Experience with computed tomographic angiography for the detection of intracranial aneurysms in the setting of acute subarachnoid hemorrhage. Neurosurgery 1997;41(3):522–7.
63. Cloft HJ, Joseph GJ, Dion JE. Risk of cerebral angiography in patients with subarachnoid hemorrhage, cerebral aneurysm, and arteriovenous mal- formation: a meta-analysis. Stroke 1999;30:317–20.
64. Sailer AM, Wagemans BA, Nelemans PJ, et al. Diagnosing intracranial aneurysms with MR angiography: systematic review and meta-analysis. Stroke 2014;45(1):119–26.
65. Wiesmann M, Mayer TE, Yousry I, et al. Detection of hyperacute subarachnoid hemorrhage of the brain by using magnetic resonance imaging. J Neurosurg 2002;96(4):684–9.
66. Pierot L, Portefaix C, Rodriguez-Regent C, et al. Role of MRA in the detection of intracranial aneurysm in the acute phase of subarachnoid hemorrhage. J Neuroradiol 2013;40(3):204–10.
67. Seupaul RA, Somerville GG, Viscusi C, et al. Prevalence of postdural puncture headache after ED performed lumbar puncture. Am J Emerg Med 2005;23: 913–5.
68. Perry JJ, Stiell IG, Sivilotti ML, et al. High risk clinical characteristics for subarachnoid haemorrhage in patients with acute headache: prospective cohort study. BMJ 2010;341:c5204.
69. Perry JJ, Stiell IG, Sivilotti ML, et al. Clinical decision rules to rule out subarachnoid hemorrhage for acute headache. JAMA 2013;310:1248–55.

70. Long B, Koyfman A. Controversies in the diagnosis of subarachnoid hemorrhage. J Emerg Med 2016;50(6):839047.
71. Czuczman AD, Thomas LE, Boulanger AB, et al. Interpreting red blood cells in lumbar puncture: distinguishing true subarachnoid hemorrhage from traumatic tap. Acad Emerg Med 2013;20:247–56.
72. Brunell A, Ridefelt P, Zelano J. Differential diagnostic yield of lumbar puncture in investigation of suspected subarachnoid haemorrhage: a retrospective study. J Neurol 2013;260:1631–6.
73. Eurle BD. Spinal puncture and cerebral spinal fluid examination. In: Roberts JR, Hedges JR, Custalow CB, et al, editors. Clinical procedures in emergency medicine. 5th edition. Philadelphia: Saunders-Else- vier; 2010. p. 1107–12.
74. Dupont SA, Wijdicks EF, Manno EM, et al. Thunderclap headache and normal computed tomographic results: value of cerebrospinal fluid analysis. Mayo Clin Proc 2008;83(12):1326–31.
75. Perry JJ, Alyahya B, Sivilotti ML, et al. Differentiation between traumatic tap and aneurysmal subarachnoid hemorrhage: prospective cohort study. BMJ 2015; 350:h568.
76. Barrows LJ, Hunter FT, Banker BQ. The nature and clinical significance of pigments in the cerebrospinal fluid. Brain 1955;78(1):59–80.
77. Edlow JA, Bruner KS, Horowitz GL. Xanthochromia. Arch Pathol Lab Med 2002; 126(4):413–5.
78. Arora S, Swadron SP, Dissanayake V. Evaluating the sensitivity of visual xanthochromia in patients with subarachnoid hemorrhage. J Emerg Med 2010;39: 13–6.
79. Petzold A, Keir G, Sharpe TL. Why human color vision cannot reliably detect cerebrospinal fluid xanthochromia. Stroke 2005;36(6):1295–7.
80. Perry JJ, Sivilotti ML, Stiell IG, et al. Should spectrophotometry be used to identify xanthochromia in the cerebrospinal fluid of alert patients suspected of having subarachnoid hemorrhage? Stroke 2006;37(10):2467–72.
81. Vermeulen M, Hasan D, Blijenberg BG, et al. Xanthochromia after subarachnoid haemorrhage needs no revisitation. J Neurol Neurosurg Psychiatry 1989;52: 826–8.
82. Schievink WI, Wijdicks EF, Meyer FB, et al. Spontaneous intracranial hypotension mimicking aneurysmal subarachnoid hemorrhage. Neurosurgery 2001; 48(3):513–6.
83. Perry JJ, Eagles D, Clement CM, et al. An international study of emergency physicians' practice for acute headache management and the need for a clinical decision rule. CJEM 2009;11(6):516–22.
84. Helbok R, Kurtz P, Vibbert M, et al. Early neurological deterioration after subarachnoid haemorrhage: risk factors and impact on outcome. J Neurol Neurosurg Psychiatry 2013;84:266.
85. Solenski NJ, Haley EC Jr, Kassell NF, et al. Medical complications of aneurysmal subarachnoid hemorrhage: a report of the multicenter, cooperative aneurysm study. Participants of the multicenter cooperative aneurysm study. Crit Care Med 1995;23:1007.
86. Findlay JM. Current management of aneurysmal subarachnoid hemorrhage guidelines from the Canadian Neurosurgical Society. Can J Neurol Sci 1997; 24(2):161–70.
87. Claassen J, Vu A, Kreiter KT, et al. Effect of acute physiologic derangements on outcome after subarachnoid hemorrhage. Crit Care Med 2004;32:832.

88. Zacharia BE, Ducruet AF, Hickman ZL, et al. Renal dysfunction as an independent predictor of outcome after aneurysmal subarachnoid hemorrhage: a single-center cohort study. Stroke 2009;40:2375.
89. Wartenberg KE, Mayer SA. Medical complications after subarachnoid hemorrhage. Neurosurg Clin N Am 2010;21:325.
90. Dorhout Mees SM, van Dijk GW, Algra A, et al. Glucose levels and outcome after subarachnoid hemorrhage. Neurology 2003;61:1132.
91. Fernandez A, Schmidt JM, Claassen J, et al. Fever after subarachnoid hemorrhage: risk factors and impact on outcome. Neurology 2007;68:1013.
92. Oddo M, Milby A, Chen I, et al. Hemoglobin concentration and cerebral metabolism in patients with aneurysmal subarachnoid hemorrhage. Stroke 2009; 40:1275.
93. Hoff R, Rinkel G, Verweij B, et al. Blood volume measurement to guide fluid therapy after aneurysmal subarachnoid hemorrhage: a prospective controlled study. Stroke 2009;40:2575.
94. Hasan D, Vermeulen M, Wijdicks EF, et al. Effect of fluid intake and antihypertensive treatment on cerebral ischemia after subarachnoid hemorrhage. Stroke 1989;20:1511.
95. Ciccone A, Celani MG, Chiaramonte R, et al. Continuous versus intermittent physiological monitoring for acute stroke. Cochrane Database Syst Rev 2013;(5):CD008444.
96. Hunt WE, Hess RM. Surgical risk as related to time of intervention in the repair of intracranial aneurysms. J Neurosurg 1968;28(1):14–20.
97. Teasdale GM, Drake CG, Hunt W, et al. A universal subarachnoid hemorrhage scale: report of a committee of the World Federation of Neurosurgical Societies. J Neurol Neurosurg Psychiatry 1988;51(11):1457.
98. Fisher CM, Kistler JP, Davis JM. Relation of cerebral vaso- spasm to subarachnoid hemorrhage visualized by computerized tomographic scanning. Neurosurgery 1980;6(1):1–9.
99. Wijdicks EF, Vermeulen M, Murray GD, et al. The effects of treating hypertension following aneurysmal subarachnoid hemorrhage. Clin Neurol Neurosurg 1990; 92:111.
100. Ohkuma H, Tsurutani H, Suzuki S. Incidence and significance of early aneurysmal rebleeding before neurosurgical or neurological management. Stroke 2001;32(5):1176–80.
101. Naidech AM, Janjua N, Kreiter KT, et al. Predictors and impact of aneurysm rebleeding after subarachnoid hemorrhage. Arch Neurol 2005;62(3):410–6.
102. Anderson CS, Heeley E, Huang Y, et al. Rapid blood-pressure lowering in patients with acute intracerebral hemorrhage. N Engl J Med 2013;368(25): 2355–65.
103. Qureshi AI, Palesch YY, Barsan WG, et al. Intensive blood-pressure lowering in patients with acute cerebral hemorrhage. N Engl J Med 2016;375:1033–43.
104. Naval NS, Stevens RD, Mirski MA, et al. Controversies in the management of aneurysmal subarachnoid hemorrhage. Crit Care Med 2006;34:511.
105. Schmidt JM, Ko SB, Helbok R, et al. Cerebral perfusion pressure thresholds for brain tissue hypoxia and metabolic crisis after poor-grade subarachnoid hemorrhage. Stroke 2011;42:1351.
106. Hemphill JC, Greenberg SM, Anderson CS, et al. Guidelines for the management of spontaneous intracerebral hemorrhage: a guideline for healthcare professionals from the American Heart Association/American Stroke Association. Stroke 2015;46(7):2032–60.

107. Liu-Deryke X, Janisse J, Coplin WM, et al. A comparison of nicardipine and labetalol for acute hypertension management following stroke. Neurocrit Care 2008;9:167–76.
108. Roitberg BZ, Hardman J, Urbaniak K, et al. Prospective randomized comparison of safety and efficacy of nicardipine and nitroprusside drip for control of hypertension in the neurosurgical intensive care unit. Neurosurgery 2008;63: 115–21.
109. Smith WB, Marbury TC, Komjathy SF, et al. Pharmacokinetics, pharmacodynamics, and safety of clevidipine after prolonged continuous infusion in subjects with mild to moderate essential hypertension. Eur J Clin Pharmacol 2012;68(10): 1385–94.
110. Christos S, Naples R. Anticoagulation reversal and treatment strategies in major bleeding: update 2016. West J Emerg Med 2016;17(3):264–70.
111. Pollack CV Jr, Reilly PA, Eikelboom J, et al. Idarucizumab for dabigatran reversal. N Engl J Med 2015;373:511–20.
112. Baharoglu M, Cordonnier C, Al-Shahi Salman R, et al. Platelet transfusion versus standard care after acute stroke due to spontaneous cerebral haemorrhage associated with antiplatelet therapy (PATCH): a randomised, open-label, phase 3 trial. Lancet 2016;387(10038):2605–13.
113. Roos YB, Rinkel GJ, Vermeulen M, et al. Antifibrinolytic therapy for aneurysmal subarachnoid haemorrhage. Cochrane Database Syst Rev 2003;(2):CD001245.
114. Roos Y. Antifibrinolytic treatment in subarachnoid hemorrhage: a randomized placebo-controlled trial. STAR Study Group. Neurology 2000;54:77.
115. Starke RM, Kim GH, Fernandez A, et al. Impact of a protocol for acute antifibrinolytic therapy on aneurysm rebleeding after subarachnoid hemorrhage. Stroke 2008;39:2617–21.
116. Brilstra EH, Algra A, Rinkel GJ, et al. Effectiveness of neurosurgical clip application in patients with aneurysmal subarachnoid hemorrhage. J Neurosurg 2002; 97:1036.
117. Pierot L, Wakhloo AK. Endovascular treatment of intracranial aneurysms: current status. Stroke 2013;44:2046–54.
118. Diringer MN, Bleck TP, Claude Hemphill J 3rd, et al. Critical care management of patients following aneurysmal subarachnoid hemorrhage: recommendations from the Neurocritical Care Society's Multidisciplinary Consensus Conference. Neurocrit Care 2011;15(2):211–40.
119. Larsen CC, Astrup J. Rebleeding after aneurysmal sub- arachnoid hemorrhage: a literature review. World Neurosurg 2013;79(2):307–12.
120. Kassell NF, Sasaki T, Colohan AR, et al. Cerebral vasospasm following aneurysmal subarachnoid hemorrhage. Stroke 1985;16:562.
121. Donahue RP, Abbott RD, Reed DM, et al. Alcohol and hemorrhagic stroke. The Honolulu heart program. JAMA 1986;255(17):2311–4.
122. Rabinstein AA, Friedman JA, Weigand SD, et al. Predictors of cerebral infarction in aneurysmal subarachnoid hemorrhage. Stroke 2004;35(8):1862–6.
123. Dorhout Mees SM, Rinkel GJ, Feigin VL, et al. Calcium antagonists for aneurysmal subarachnoid haemorrhage. Cochrane Database Syst Rev 2007;(3):CD000277.
124. Pickard JD, Murray GD, Illingworth R, et al. Effect of oral nimodipine on cerebral infarction and outcome after subarachnoid haemorrhage: British aneurysm nimodipine trial. BMJ 1989;298(6674):636–42.

125. Haley EC Jr, Kassell NF, Torner JC. A randomized controlled trial of high-dose intravenous nicardipine in aneurysmal subarachnoid hemorrhage. A report of the Cooperative Aneurysm Study. J Neurosurg 1993;78(4):537–47.
126. van den Bergh WM, Algra A, van Kooten F, et al. Magnesium sulfate in aneurysmal subarachnoid hemorrhage: a randomized controlled trial. Stroke 2005; 36(5):1011–5.
127. Liu Z, Liu L, Zhang Z, et al. Cholesterol-reducing agents for aneurysmal subarachnoid haemorrhage. Cochrane Database Syst Rev 2013;(4):CD008184.
128. Vergouwen MD, de Haan RJ, Vermeulen M, et al. Effect of statin treatment on vasospasm, delayed cerebral ischemia, and functional outcome in patients with aneurysmal subarachnoid hemorrhage: a systematic review and meta-analysis update. Stroke 2010;41:e47.
129. Frontera JA, Fernandez A, Schmidt JM, et al. Clinical response to hypertensive hypervolemic therapy and outcome after subarachnoid hemorrhage. Neurosurgery 2010;66:35.
130. Rabinstein AA, Wijdicks EF. Cerebral vasospasm in subarachnoid hemorrhage. Curr Treat Options Neurol 2005;7:99.
131. Polin RS, Coenen VA, Hansen CA, et al. Efficacy of transluminal angioplasty for the management of symptomatic cerebral vasospasm following aneurysmal subarachnoid hemorrhage. J Neurosurg 2000;92:284.
132. Graff-Radford NR, Torner J, Adams HP Jr, et al. Factors associated with hydrocephalus after subarachnoid hemorrhage. A report of the Cooperative Aneurysm Study. Arch Neurol 1989;46:744.
133. van Gijn J, Hijdra A, Wijdicks EF, et al. Acute hydrocephalus after aneurysmal subarachnoid hemorrhage. J Neurosurg 1985;63:355.
134. Nornes H, Magnaes B. Intracranial pressure in patients with ruptured saccular aneurysm. J Neurosurg 1972;36:537.
135. Heuer GG, Smith MJ, Elliott JP, et al. Relationship between intracranial pressure and other clinical variables in patients with aneurysmal subarachnoid hemorrhage. J Neurosurg 2004;101:408.
136. Heinsoo M, Eelmäe J, Kuklane M, et al. The possible role of CSF hydrodynamic parameters following in management of SAH patients. Acta Neurochir Suppl 1998;71:13.
137. Hellingman CA, van den Bergh WM, Beijer IS, et al. Risk of rebleeding after treatment of acute hydrocephalus in patients with aneurysmal subarachnoid hemorrhage. Stroke 2007;38:96.
138. Al-Rawi PG, Tseng MY, Richards HK, et al. Hypertonic saline in patients with poor-grade subarachnoid hemorrhage improves cerebral blood flow, brain tissue oxygen, and pH. Stroke 2010;41:122.
139. Woo CH, Rao VA, Sheridan W, et al. Performance characteristics of a sliding-scale hypertonic saline infusion protocol for the treatment of acute neurologic hyponatremia. Neurocrit Care 2009;11:228.
140. Marigold R, Günther A, Tiwari D, et al. Antiepileptic drugs for the primary and secondary prevention of seizures after subarachnoid haemorrhage. Cochrane Database Syst Rev 2013;(6):CD008710.
141. Naidech AM, Kreiter KT, Janjua N, et al. Phenytoin exposure is associated with functional and cognitive disability after subarachnoid hemorrhage. Stroke 2005; 36:583.
142. Mistry AM, Mistry EA, Ganesh Kumar N, et al. Corticosteroids in the management of hyponatremia, hypovolemia, and vasospasm in subarachnoid hemorrhage: a meta-analysis. Cerebrovasc Dis 2016;42:263–71.

143. Guo J, Shi Z, Yang K, et al. Endothelin receptor antagonists for subarachnoid hemorrhage. Cochrane Database Syst Rev 2012;(9):CD008354.
144. Senbokuya N, Kinouchi H, Kanemaru K, et al. Effects of cilostazol on cerebral vasospasm after aneurysmal subarachnoid hemorrhage: a multicenter prospective, randomized, open-label blinded end point trial. J Neurosurg 2013;118:121.
145. Zwienenberg-Lee M, Hartman J, Rudisill N, et al. Effect of prophylactic transluminal balloon angioplasty on cerebral vasospasm and outcome in patients with fisher grade III subarachnoid hemorrhage: results of a phase II multicenter, randomized, clinical trial. Stroke 2008;39:1759.
146. Kramer AH, Fletcher JJ. Locally-administered intrathecal thrombolytics following aneurysmal subarachnoid hemorrhage: a systematic review and meta-analysis. Neurocrit Care 2011;14:489.
147. Al-Tamimi YZ, Bhargava D, Feltbower RG, et al. Lumbar drainage of cerebrospinal fluid after aneurysmal subarachnoid hemorrhage: a prospective, randomized, controlled trial (LUMAS). Stroke 2012;43:677.
148. Macdonald RL, Higashida RT, Keller E, et al. Clazosentan, an endothelin receptor antagonist, in patients with aneurysmal subarachnoid haemorrhage undergoing surgical clipping: a randomised, double-blind, placebo-controlled phase 3 trial (CONSCIOUS-2). Lancet Neurol 2011;10:618.
149. Veldeman M, Hollig A, Stevanovic A, et al. Delayed cerebral ischaemia prevention and treatment after aneurysmal subarachnoid haemorrhage. Br J Anaesth 2016;117(1):17–40.

Spontaneous Intracerebral Hemorrhage

Stephen Alerhand, MD[a,*], Cappi Lay, MD[a,b]

KEYWORDS

- Intracerebral hemorrhage • Intracranial hemorrhage • Hemorrhagic stroke

KEY POINTS

- Poorly controlled hypertension is the most common risk factor for spontaneous intracerebral hemorrhage (ICH).
- Patients with spontaneous ICH may present with headache and vomiting, but are at risk for early deterioration including loss of consciousness, coma, and death.
- The location, appearance, and size of the hemorrhage on computed tomography scan, in conjunction with the clinical picture, can help point toward its etiology and prognosis.
- Once hemorrhage has occurred, management focuses on prevention of hematoma expansion, perihematoma edema, obstructive hydrocephalus, and brain herniation.
- Primary emergency management focuses on blood pressure and empiric intracranial pressure management, reversal of existing coagulopathies, and identification of indications for early neurosurgical intervention.

INTRODUCTION

Spontaneous intracerebral hemorrhage (ICH) is a medical emergency with potentially devastating morbidity and mortality. After ischemic stroke, ICH represents the second most common type of stroke (15%).[1] Bleeding within the brain can arise from multiple different etiologies (**Box 1**), each of which can be considered its own separate disease.

RISK FACTORS AND PATHOPHYSIOLOGY

Although several other risk factors exist, by far the greatest risk factor for spontaneous ICH is hypertension (**Box 2**).[2–7] Over the course of time, chronic stress on the vascular walls leads to the fragmentation, degeneration, and eventual rupture of small penetrating vessels within the brain parenchyma. Hypertensive hemorrhages tend to occur

[a] Department of Emergency Medicine, Icahn School of Medicine at Mount Sinai, 1 Gustave L. Levy Place, New York, NY 10029, USA; [b] Department of Neurocritical Care, Icahn School of Medicine at Mount Sinai, 1 Gustave L. Levy Place, New York, NY 10029, USA
* Corresponding author.
E-mail address: Stephen.Alerhand@gmail.com

Emerg Med Clin N Am 35 (2017) 825–845
http://dx.doi.org/10.1016/j.emc.2017.07.002

Box 1
Etiologies of spontaneous intracerebral hemorrhage

Hypertension

Amyloidopathy

Vascular malformation

Hemorrhagic brain tumor

Hemorrhagic conversion from prior ischemic stroke

Cerebral venous sinus thrombosis

in specific locations, including the deep structures of the basal ganglia and thalamus, as well as the pons, midbrain, and cerebellum.[8,9]

Complications from ICH occur in part owing to the limited space within the skull that is filled by brain tissue, blood, and cerebrospinal fluid. Increasing intracranial pressure (ICP) leads to decreased cerebral perfusion, as well as mechanical compression of brain contents that may ultimately lead to brain herniation. Blood may also leak into the cerebrospinal fluid drainage system and cause obstructive hydrocephalus.

CLINICAL PRESENTATION

Patients may present to the emergency department (ED) in a variety of ways, from those arriving on their own complaining of headache and vomiting, to those found obtunded and brought in by emergency medical services personnel. Even if focal neurologic deficits are not present immediately, a worsening level of alertness and potential loss of consciousness may develop quickly as the hematoma expands and causes compression of the surrounding brain parenchyma. The specific location of the ICH (ie, putamen, thalamus, caudate, lobes, cerebellum, pons) may correspond with particular neurologic signs and symptoms. For instance, thalamic hemorrhages may be associated with hallucinations or confusion, cortical hemorrhages with aphasia or neglect, and those in the posterior fossa with cerebellar or brainstem deficits. Early seizures in the first few days may also occur (14% incidence),[10] more commonly with lobar hemorrhages.

Box 2
Risk factors for spontaneous intracerebral hemorrhage

Hypertension

Cigarette smoking

Antithrombotic therapy

African American

Diabetes

Older age

Heavy alcohol intake

Chronic kidney disease

Male sex

Poor diet

DIAGNOSTIC CONSIDERATIONS

Clinical Assessment Scores

As part of the initial evaluation of patients with suspected ICH, the emergency physician should obtain a baseline severity score based on physical examination.[11] The National Institutes of Health Stroke Scale[11] may be used to achieve this purpose and is preferred over the Glasgow Coma Scale. The benefit of scoring systems lies in the ability to communicate effectively about a patient's dynamic medical condition over time to other medical providers. These providers, whether in the ED or an intensive care unit (ICU), can subsequently repeat the physical examination and identify changes.

Blood Testing

A rapid fingerstick glucose value should be obtained immediately in case the patient's condition is due to hypoglycemia. Intravenous access should also be obtained immediately upon the patient's arrival. The following markers should be ordered: complete blood count, basic metabolic panel including electrolytes and creatinine, troponin, prothrombin time, International Normalized Ratio (INR), partial thromboplastin time, and type and screen.

RADIOGRAPHIC STUDIES

Computed Tomography

The abrupt onset of focal neurologic symptoms should be presumed as an ischemic stroke until proven otherwise, because time-sensitive evidence-based treatments exist for this form of stroke. Rapid neuroimaging with noncontrast computed tomography (CT) scan or MRI should be obtained to distinguish ischemic stroke from ICH.[11] CT scan is the preferred imaging choice owing to its more rapid availability and lower cost. Hemorrhage appears as a high-density lesion. Its size and location can be visualized, as can the presence of intraventricular extension, edema, and/or brain herniation.

Computed Tomography Assessment

In a large retrospective study, ICH hematoma volumes greater than 32 mL supratentorially or 21 mL infratentorially were shown to be significant predictors of 30-day mortality.[12] To communicate hematoma size with neurosurgery and ICU consultants, this measurement can be calculated rapidly and easily using the ABC/2 method (**Fig. 1**).[13]

Additionally, the ICH score incorporates this volume to predict outcomes and assist with medical decision making. Higher scores are associated with increased risk of mortality and decreased likelihood of good functional outcome.[14] In the initial study of 152 patients with acute ICH, scores of 1, 2, 3, and 4 corresponded with 30-day mortality rates of 13%, 26%, 72%, and 97%, respectively (**Table 1**). Subsequent studies have supported this positive association with mortality.[15,16]

Location Corresponds with Etiology

Varying etiologies of spontaneous ICH may exert their effect within characteristic areas of the brain (**Figs. 2–5**). Accordingly, the location of the hemorrhage may help point to the underlying etiology. For instance, bleeding from hypertensive ICH occurs most commonly in the basal ganglia (40%–50%) and other deeper structures within the parenchyma (thalamus, cerebellum, pons). ICH owing to amyloid (almost exclusively in elderly patients) or arteriovenous malformation (AVM) tends to occur in the lobar regions. Those originating from mass lesions may demonstrate edema surrounding the tumor and be seen in the grey–white junctions. Hemorrhagic conversion of a prior ischemic stroke may show hypodensity and edema in the middle cerebral

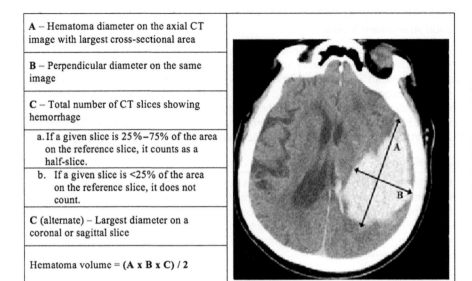

A – Hematoma diameter on the axial CT image with largest cross-sectional area	
B – Perpendicular diameter on the same image	
C – Total number of CT slices showing hemorrhage	
a. If a given slice is 25%–75% of the area on the reference slice, it counts as a half-slice.	
b. If a given slice is <25% of the area on the reference slice, it does not count.	
C (alternate) – Largest diameter on a coronal or sagittal slice	
Hematoma volume = **(A x B x C) / 2**	

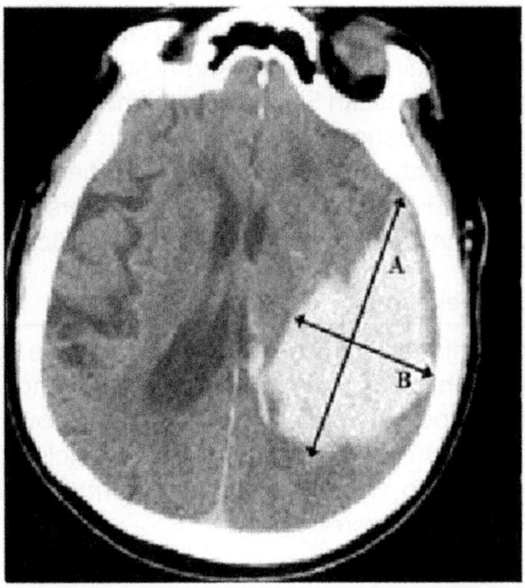

Fig. 1. The ABC/2 method for rapidly obtaining hematoma volume. CT, computed tomography. (*From* Morotti A, Goldstein JN. Diagnosis and management of acute intracerebral hemorrhage. Emerg Med Clin North Am 2016;34(4):883–99.)

Table 1
Obtaining the ICH score

Component	Points
GCS score	
3–4	2
5–12	1
13–15	0
ICH volume (cm^3)	
≥30	1
<30	0
Presence of IVH	
Yes	1
No	0
Infratentorial origin of ICH	
Yes	1
No	0
Age (y)	
≥80	1
<80	0
Total ICH score	0–6

Abbreviations: GCS, Glasgow Coma Scale; ICH, intracerebral hemorrhage; IVH, intraventricular hemorrhage.

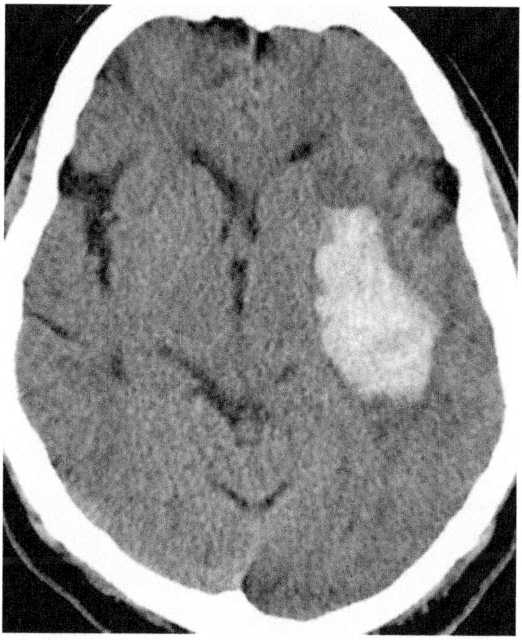

Fig. 2. Hypertensive hemorrhage. (*From* Fatterpekar GM, Naidich TP, Som PM. In: Silva IS, Muller NL, editors. The teaching files: chest: expert consult - online and print, 1e (teaching files in radiology). Philadelphia: Elsevier; 2012. p. 210–1.)

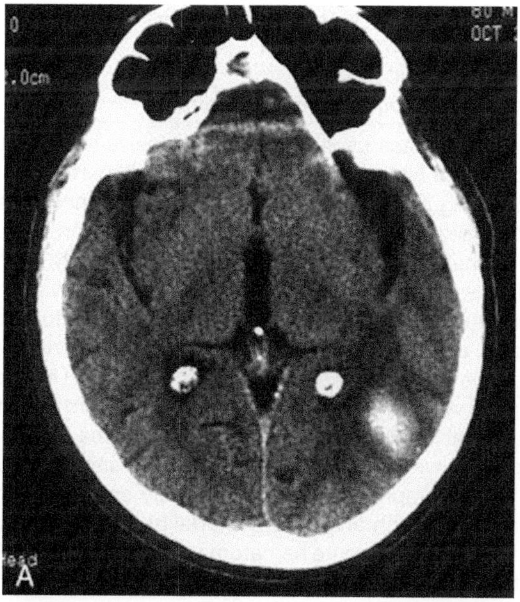

Fig. 3. Cerebral amyloid lobar hemorrhage. (*From* Kase CS, Shoamanesh A, Greenberg SM, et al. Intracerebral Hemorrhage. In: Grotta JC, Albers GW, Broderick JP, et al, editors. Stroke: pathophysiology, diagnosis, and management. vol. 28. Philadelphia: Elsevier; 2016. p. 466–515.e12.)

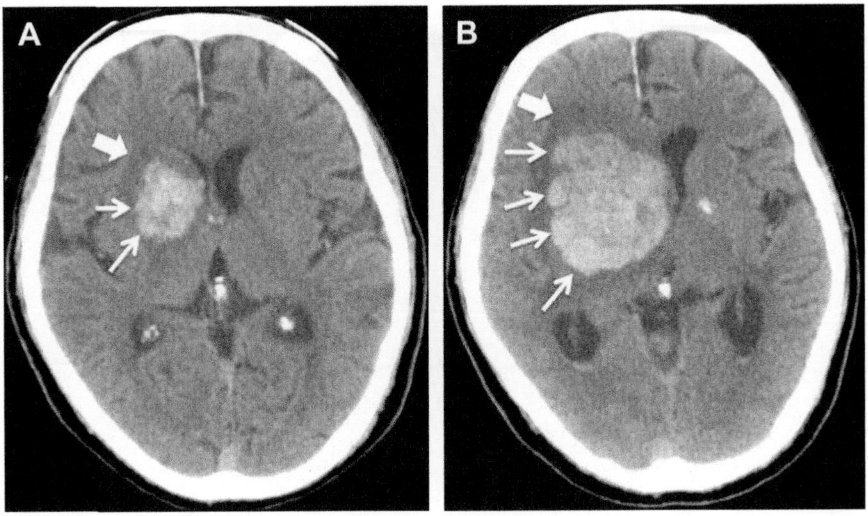

Fig. 4. Hemorrhagic brain metastasis. (*A*) The initial axial CT image at the level of the basal ganglia showed a hemorrhagic lesion with a slightly undulated or finger-in-glove appearance in the right lentiform nucleus (*thin arrows*) along with perifocal edema (*bold arrow*). (*B*) A subsequent axial CT image disclosed a growing hemorrhagic lesion with a remarkable finger-in-glove sign (*thin arrows*) and more pronounced perifocal edema (*bold arrow*). (*From* Juan YH, Hsuan HF, Cheung YC. Pointing to the diagnosis: hemorrhagic brain metastasis. Am J Med 2016;129(12):1268–9.)

artery territory with hemorrhage within it. ICH from a cerebral venous sinus thrombosis commonly appear at the sagittal and transverse sinuses.

ADVANCED IMAGING TECHNIQUES

Computed Tomography Angiography of the Brain

Follow-up brain imaging is less useful when hypertensive hemorrhage is suspected, such as in patients with a history of poorly controlled hypertension and a CT image showing a deep bleeding pattern. However, beyond the noncontrast CT scan, additional imaging modalities may provide important information about the underlying cause of an ICH. CT head angiography is performed routinely for patients in whom spontaneous ICH is suspected owing to secondary etiology, such as aneurysm, AVM, tumor, or cerebral venous thrombosis. Certain indicators for such bleeds include lobar ICH, young age, and absence of cardiovascular disease risk factors.[11] Suggestive radiologic evidence for vascular abnormalities causing ICH includes subarachnoid hemorrhage, enlarged vessels or calcifications along hemorrhage margins, hyperattenuation within a dural venous sinus, unusual hematoma shape and/or location, edema out of proportion with the presumed onset time, and the presence of a mass.

Furthermore, CT angiographic studies may identify contrast extravasation that is predictive of hematoma growth and 30-day mortality.[17–19] Extravasation is reflected by tiny enhancing foci within the acute hematoma called spot signs (**Fig. 6**). Spot signs are associated with intraoperative bleeding, postoperative bleeding, and larger residual ICH volumes during surgical evacuation.[20] Their number, diameter, and attenuation are used to calculate the Spot Sign Score, which has been shown to independently predict poor functional outcomes and in-hospital mortality.[21] This diagnostic marker does not have a clear role in determining management.

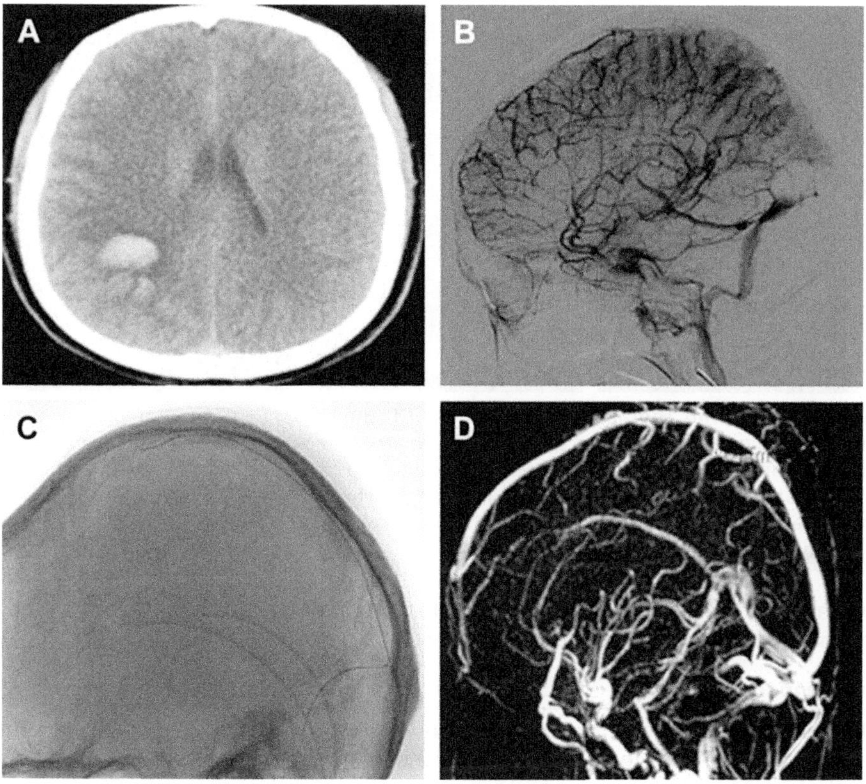

Fig. 5. Cerebral venous infarction owing to superior sagittal sinus thrombosis. A 32-year-old representative female presented with acute onset severe headache, vomiting and left hemiparesis. (*A*) CT scan revealed intracranial hemorrhage and infarct; (*B*) DSA revealed features of cerebral venous sinus thrombosis involving superior sagittal sinus, left transverse sinus; (*C*) microcatheter was advanced into the SSS; (*D*) MRV showed complete recanalization of superior sagittal sinus after 6-day local urokinase administration. She was asymptomatic at the time of discharge. (*From* Guo XB, Fu Z, Song LJ, et al. Local thrombolysis for patients of severe cerebral venous sinus thrombosis during puerperium. Eur J Radiol 2013;82(1):165–8.)

MRI

MRI takes longer to perform and is more expensive than CT imaging. Although much less frequently used, MRI may nevertheless be performed to evaluate for secondary causes of ICH, including hemorrhagic conversion of prior ischemic stroke.[22] With high diagnostic accuracy, it may also detect AVMs, tumors, and cerebral venous thrombosis.[23] MRI without contrast may be most useful in patients who are unable to receive intravenous (IV) contrast agents owing to allergy or renal disease.

EVALUATION AND MANAGEMENT

Initial Assessment

Even before the patient is taken for CT imaging, the initial evaluation for any patient with suspected ICH begins with assessment of airway, breathing, and circulation (ABCs). Given the varying etiologies of ICH, it is also important for the emergency physician to obtain a focused yet detailed history from the patient, family members, and/or emergency medical services personnel (**Table 2**). Although there is some

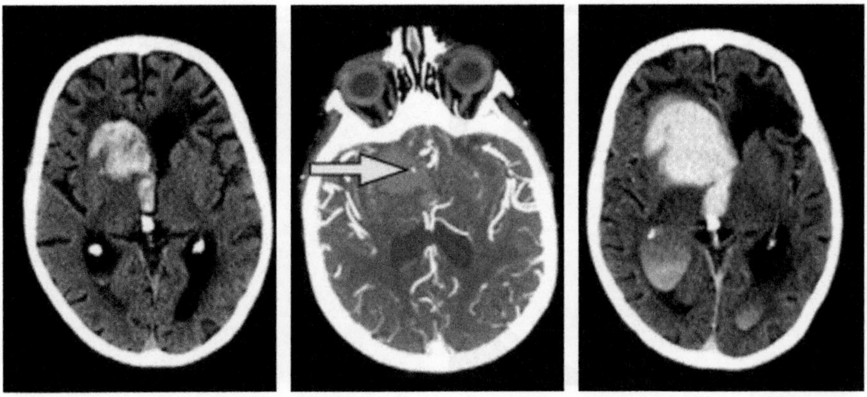

Fig. 6. A sign with spot-like appearance on CT angiography (CTA) in a patient with intracerebral haemorrhage. The spot sign (*green arrow*) measures 2·2 mm in maximal axial diameter, and has a density of 173 Hounsfield units. (*From* Demchuk AM et al. Prediction of haematoma growth and outcome in patients with intracerebral haemorrhage using the CT-angiography spot sign (PREDICT): a prospective observational study. Lancet Neurology 2012;11(4):307–14.)

overlap, the different etiologies call for certain focused management strategies, with the major difference being blood pressure control parameters.

Intervention Overview

Overall, treatment is generally supportive and aimed at preventing further injury to the brain by preventing the following complications: (1) hematoma expansion, (2) development of edema, (3) obstructive hydrocephalus, and (4) brain herniation. Some interventions must be taken immediately, whereas others may come secondarily (**Table 3**).

Rapid initiation of interventions may improve functional outcomes, because clinical deterioration may occur early. For instance, early hematoma expansion occurs in 18% to 38% of patients who receive repeat CT scan within 3 hours of onset.[24–26] This has been shown to carry an association with poor clinical outcomes including an increased mortality rate[24,26–31] of up to 30% to 55% at 30 days.[32,33] These sobering statistics highlight the importance of mitigating ICH growth in the ED.

REVERSAL OF ANTICOAGULATION

Antithrombotic Agents

Patients taking the vitamin K antagonist warfarin carry a 5- to 10-fold increased risk of suffering an ICH, and approximately 15% of cases are associated with its use.[34] Once the ICH occurs, prolonged bleeding causes 27% to 54% of patients to develop early hematoma expansion[35–37] that is associated with doubling of the mortality risk.[38]

Table 2
Focused yet detailed history taking

Components of Patient History to Obtain		
Patient age	Time of symptom onset	History of prior stroke
Antiplatelet agents and/or anticoagulation	Hypertension	Liver disease
Bleeding diathesis	Drug use	Alcohol use

Table 3
Interventions for spontaneous intracerebral hemorrhage

Primary Management			
Reversal of anticoagulation	Blood pressure control	ICP control	Surgery as needed
Secondary goals			
Seizure management	Glycemic control	Fever control	Intensive care disposition

These life-threatening risks are further exacerbated when coagulopathy is not corrected rapidly.[39]

Current guidelines recommend administration of IV vitamin K (5–10 mg) by slow push over 10 minutes.[40] Although long lasting, it takes 6 to 24 hours for vitamin K to achieve its reversal effects.

Fresh frozen plasma (FFP) contains factors I (fibrinogen), II, V, VII, IX, X, XI, XIII, and antithrombin. Relatively large volumes of FFP (10–15 mL/kg) are administered, which puts patients at risk for volume overload and pulmonary edema. Moreover, the INR of FFP itself is about 1.6, limiting the extent to which the coagulopathy can be reversed. Along with its required blood type matching, thawing time, and longer duration of administration, FFP takes several hours to achieve its INR reversal effects.[11]

Prothrombin complex concentrate (PCC) contains vitamin K–dependent coagulation factors II, VII, IX, and X. Compared with FFP, the vials contain a higher concentration of clotting factors within a smaller volume and take only minutes to fully administer. PCC can normalize the INR completely within 10 minutes,[11] although it brings a higher risk of disseminated intravascular coagulation.[39] The INR needs to be checked within 30 minutes and redosed as needed.

Research shows that PCC should be the first-line reversal agent for most patients with therapeutic warfarin levels (**Table 4**). Three randomized controlled trials comparing the two reversal agents found that PCC lowered the INR more rapidly than FFP and with no clear difference in thromboembolic risk.[41–43] In terms of outcomes research supporting PCC, one prospective observational study showed a lower risk of death or severe disability at 3 months,[44] whereas a retrospective study showed an increased 1-year survival.[45] Another study comparing the two treatments for Warfarin reversal showed that in patients whose INR was corrected within 2 hours, there was no difference in hematoma growth incidence or extent.[36] Even if it may not necessarily be the agent but rather the timing of coagulopathy reversal that imparts a greater effect, FFP takes longer than PCC to administer for the reasons mentioned.

Antiplatelet Agents

The use of antiplatelet drugs such as aspirin and clopidogrel is extremely common. In patients with ICH, they are associated with a greater baseline hematoma volume, hematoma growth, and increased mortality in patients with ICH.[46,47] Emergency

Table 4
PCC dosing recommendations

Pre-treatment INR	2–4	4–6	>6
4-Factor PCC dose (units of factor IX/kg)	25	35	50
Maximum dose (units of Factor IX)	2500	3500	5000

Abbreviations: INR, International Normalized Ratio; PCC, prothrombin complex concentrate.

physicians commonly administer platelets and desmopressin in the setting of ICH to reverse the effects of these drugs, with the intent of reducing hematoma growth. In patients with ICH taking antiplatelet drugs, however, there has not been any evidence that platelet transfusion improves outcomes.[11] Recently, in the PATCH trial (Platelet transfusion versus standard care after acute stroke due to spontaneous cerebral haemorrhage associated with antiplatelet therapy), platelet transfusion was compared with standard care in a randomized trial of patients with ICH taking antiplatelet drugs before hospital admission.[48] Platelet transfusion was associated with greater odds of death or dependence at 3 months, and a higher percentage of in-hospital adverse events and deaths. Based on this recent study, we recommend avoiding routine platelet transfusions for patients with ICH who are taking antiplatelet medications. Desmopressin helps to stop bleeding by stimulating von Willebrand's antigen release from the platelets and cells that line blood vessels. At this time, there are no randomized controlled data to guide its use in patients with ICH. Dosing is 0.3 μg/kg IV over 15 to 30 minutes.

Heparin

Protamine sulfate should be administered for those patients receiving IV heparin or low-molecular-weight heparin (LMWH). It is given slowly as 1 mg per 100 units of heparin, with a maximum dose of 50 mg.[11] For LMWH administered within 8 hours of hemorrhage, protamine sulfate is dosed at 1 mg for each mg of LMWH. For LMWH administered more than 8 hours before hemorrhage onset, 0.5 mg protamine sulfate per 1 mg of LMWH is advised.

Novel Oral Anticoagulants

There are no laboratory tests to assess for plasma levels of the newer factors Xa inhibitors (apixaban, rivaroxaban, and edoxaban) and direct thrombin inhibitor (dabigatran). These drugs generally have shorter half-lives than warfarin, so the time of most recent dosing and renal function should be taken into account.[49] For dabigatran, there is a reversal agent (idarucizumab) to which dabigatran binds with a higher affinity than to thrombin, thereby reversing the drug's coagulopathic effect.[50–55] There has been no evidence to show that it reduces hematoma expansion, but many centers have incorporated its use. For apixaban and rivaroxaban, there is an experimental reversal agent named andexanet alfa that binds the drugs and prevents their binding to factor Xa.[55,56] Clinical trials examining its effect on ICH progression associated with Xa inhibitors are not available at this early stage. In the absence of specific reversal agents for the novel oral anticoagulants, the optimal strategy for their reversal remains unclear, but many centers have used PCC as the reversal agent of choice based on early studies and expert recommendation.[57–61]

BLOOD PRESSURE MANAGEMENT

Elevated blood pressure in a patient with ICH can drive continued bleeding and hematoma expansion. It is very common for patients with acute ICH to have elevated blood pressure,[62] even in those without history of hypertension. This may occur secondary to pain, stress, or as a compensatory response to maintain perfusion in the setting of increased ICP. Hypertension in patients with ICH is independently associated with poor outcomes.[63,64] It is associated with hematoma expansion, neurologic deterioration, and death and dependency.[65–67]

Emergency providers routinely initiate immediate therapy to lower blood pressure, but the precise targets for blood pressure lowering have been controversial. The INTERACT1 trial (Intensive Blood Pressure Reduction in Acute Cerebral

Hemorrhage)[68] concluded that aggressive systolic blood pressure (SBP) reduction to less than 140 mm Hg was clinically feasible and that it seemed to reduce hematoma growth at 24 hours versus targeting to SBP of 180 mm Hg.[69] Based on this trial, the American Heart Association and American Stroke Association recommended that, for patients with ICH with a SBP between 150 to 220 mm Hg, acute lowering of SBP to 140 mm Hg is safe.[11]

The subsequent INTERACT2 study randomized patients to targeted goals of an SBP of less than 140 mm Hg versus an SBP of less than 180 mm Hg within the first 24 hours. It found no evidence of improved outcome at 90 days in the aggressive treatment group.[70] The ATACH2 trial (Antihypertensive Treatment of Acute Cerebral Hemorrhage) found that aiming for an SBP of 110 to 139 mm Hg did not result in a lower rate of death or disability at 3 months versus aiming for a target SBP of 140 to 179 mm Hg.[71] Furthermore, not only was there no difference in the proportion of patients who died, but the aggressive treatment group had a higher rate of adverse renal events within 7 days. Based on the most recent data (**Table 5**), we therefore recommend that, in hypertensive ICH, routinely lowering the SBP below 140 mm Hg should be avoided. Aiming for a target SBP of 140 to 160 mm Hg in these patients is reasonable.

Of note, in patients who have ICH associated with either a ruptured aneurysm or ruptured AVM, blood pressure goals are typically lower, as the risk of rebleeding in these patients with elevated blood pressure is higher.[72,73] At our center, SBP targeting between 120 and 140 mm Hg is typical in these patients.

The objective of intervention is to lower SBP as quickly as possible, as well as to maintain the proper parameters as previously discussed. This highlights the importance of using agents that are easily titratable. Labetalol has mixed alpha and beta adrenergic antagonism and is short acting. It is administered as 5 to 20 mg IV, with repeat boluses double the initial dose, without exceeding a maximum dose of 300 mg. Nicardipine is a calcium channel blocker of the dihydropyridine class that is more selective for coronary and cerebral vasculature. Common initial bolus dose is 5 mg/h by slow infusion (50 mL/h), titrated by 2.5 mg/h every 5 minutes as indicated, without exceeding 15 mg/h. Clevidipine is another calcium channel blocker that acts even more rapidly and can thus be titrated at smaller time intervals. Nitroprusside and hydralazine are contraindicated owing to the risk of venodilation and increased ICP.[74]

EMPIRIC INTRACRANIAL PRESSURE MANAGEMENT

In patients suspected to have increased ICP based on clinical (anisocoria, decreased level of consciousness, posturing) or radiographic signs (significant midline shift, cerebral edema, hydrocephalus, effacement of basal cisterns), blood pressure management should ideally be guided by the use of an ICP monitor. However, ICP monitors

Table 5
Summary of blood pressure management trials

Name of Study	Outcomes for SBP <140 mm Hg vs <180 mm Hg
INTERACT1	Reduction in hematoma growth at 24 h (not after adjusting for initial volume and onset-to-CT time). No change in adverse events at 90 d.
INTERACT2	No improvement in death or severe disability at 90 d.
ATACH2	No improvement in death or disability at 3 mo. Higher rate of renal adverse events within 7 d.

Abbreviations: CT, computed tomography; SBP, systolic blood pressure.

are rarely placed within the first few hours of ED management. Emergency physicians should therefore take measures to treat ICP empirically when elevation is suspected.

This may be achieved through several means. To begin with, the head of the bed should be elevated to 30°. The physician may also administer intravenous medications such as 20% mannitol at 0.5 to 1.5 g/kg over 30 to 60 minutes, which can be repeated at 0.25 to 0.5 g/kg as needed every 6 to 8 hours. Alternatively, in the setting of hypotension, 30 mL boluses of 23.4% hypertonic saline may be administered centrally, or 150 mL boluses of 3% hypertonic saline peripherally, with repeat bolusing as indicated. If the patient has been intubated, ventilator settings should initially be set to hyperventilate the patient to a P_{CO_2} of 30 to 35 mm Hg.

NEUROSURGICAL INTERVENTION

Just as hematoma expansion may occur early in the course of ICH, neurosurgical intervention may also achieve its most beneficial effect if performed early. It is important for ED physicians to recognize the indications for early neurosurgery and the techniques that may be applied.

Extraventricular Drain Placement

An extraventricular drain relieves elevated ICP using a catheter to drain blood and cerebrospinal fluid from the brain ventricles. It also provides the physician a way of monitoring ICP through its connection to a pressure transducer. It is recommended in patients with hydrocephalus and intraventricular extension,[11] which occurs in almost one-half of patients with ICH[75] and has been shown to predict poor outcomes.[76–78]

Craniotomy and Hematoma Evacuation for Supratentorial Hemorrhage

Craniotomy temporarily removes a part of the skull to evacuate the hematoma. This procedure aims to prevent brain herniation, reduce ICP, and decreased the cytotoxicity of blood products on the parenchyma. In the STICH study (Surgical Trial for Intracerebral Hemorrhage), early hematoma evacuation was compared with conservative (medical) management of ICH in terms of 6-month mortality and neurologic outcome, as determined by the Extended Glasgow Outcome Scale.[79] The study found no difference between the two groups overall. However, early surgery was more likely to produce a favorable outcome for patients having hematomas located within 1 cm of the cortical surface compared with those with deep hematomas. The subsequent STICH II trial sought to determine whether early hematoma evacuation would be beneficial in patients with superficial lobar hemorrhages of 10 to 100 mL without IVH.[80] Just as with STICH I, there was no difference in 6-month favorable outcome between the 2 groups as determined by the Extended Glasgow Outcome Scale. At this point, the benefit of early hematoma evacuation for patients with supratentorial ICH has not been established.

Craniotomy and Hematoma Evacuation for Posterior Fossa Hemorrhage

In contrast with supratentorial ICH, posterior fossa hemorrhage is a neurosurgical emergency for which there is agreement over the defined role for surgical decompression. Hemorrhage in this location may rapidly lead to obstructive hydrocephalus through compression of the fourth ventricle and subsequent downward herniation (**Fig. 7**). In addition, forward compression of the brainstem may itself lead to rapid death. Several studies have suggested that patients with cerebellar hemorrhage may achieve lower mortality rates and improved functional outcomes with surgical decompression.[81–84] It is recommended that patients with cerebellar hemorrhage

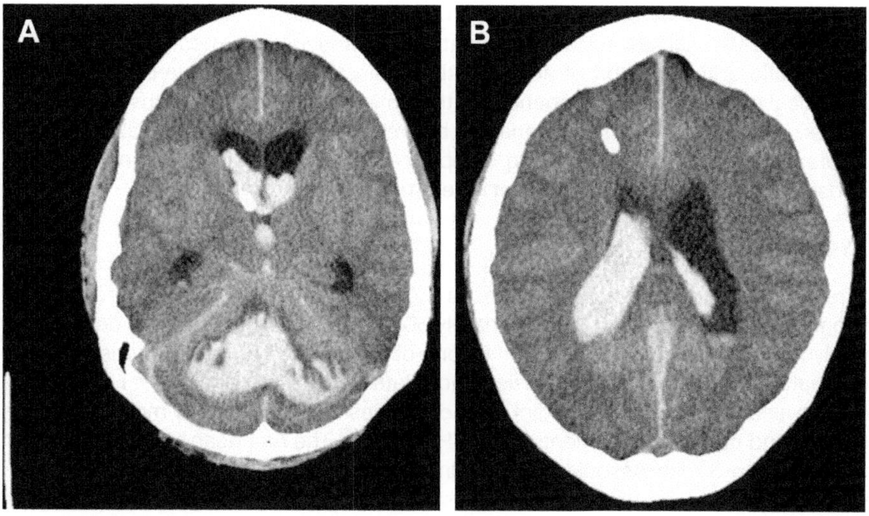

Fig. 7. Large cerebellar hemorrhage with intraventricular extension and hydrocephalus. (*Data from* Aoun SG, Bendok BR, Batjer HH. Acute management of ruptured arteriovenous malformations and dural arteriovenous fistulas. Large cerebellar hemorrhage with intraventricular extension and hydrocephalus. Neurosurg Clin N Am 2012;23(1):87–103.)

who are deteriorating neurologically or who have brainstem compression and/or hydrocephalus from ventricular obstruction undergo surgical hematoma evacuation as soon as possible.[11]

Hemicraniectomy

Neurosurgeons may perform hemicraniectomy as a last resort when other options are neither available nor feasible. This procedure entails removing a potentially large part of the skull without plans to replace it, to allow the brain to swell outward and prevent herniation. Some studies suggest that it may reduce midline shift and potentially improve functional outcomes based on modified Rankin Scale in certain patients with supratentorial hemorrhage.[85–88]

Specifically, this procedure may be considered in patients with coma, large hematomas with significant midline shift, or elevated ICP refractory to medical management.[11] However, owing to the risk of poor neurologic outcome, hemicraniectomy remains a controversial procedure and thus warrants discussion with family members and health proxies regarding expected prognoses and goals of care.

SEIZURE MANAGEMENT

Damage to brain tissue may lead to seizure activity in patients with ICH. The precise mechanism remains unclear, but it may result from sudden development of the space-occupying lesion with mass effect, focal ischemia, and blood breakdown products. Approximately 14% of patients with spontaneous ICH develop seizures within 7 days.[10] About 50% to 70% of seizures occur in the first 24 hours and 90% within the first 3 days.[10,89–93] The most important risk factor for early seizures is cortical involvement of the hemorrhage.[90,94] Both prospective and population-based studies, however, have not shown an association between clinical seizures and neurologic outcome or mortality.[89,90,95–97]

The American Heart Association and American Stroke Association guidelines recommend that clinical seizures be treated with antiepileptic medications, but that prophylactic administration of antiepileptic medications not be given.[11] The choice of medication to administer depends on the patient's other medications and comorbidities. Acute seizures should generally be treated with an IV benzodiazepine such as lorazepam at 0.05 to 0.1 mg/kg, supplemented by a loading dose of phenytoin or fosphenytoin at 20 mg/kg, or levetiracetam at 50 mg/kg.

GLYCEMIC CONTROL

Increased blood glucose that develops in the setting of ICH may arise from the condition's associated stress.[98] Approximately 60% of patients with ICH may develop hyperglycemia, even without a prior history of diabetes.[99] It has demonstrated an association with hematoma expansion and relative edema expansion.[100] Hyperglycemia has also been shown to predict poor outcomes including 30-day mortality in both diabetic and nondiabetic patients with ICH.[98,101–103] The American Heart Association and American Stroke Association guidelines recommend avoiding both hyperglycemia and hypoglycemia without offering a specific target range.[11] For safety purposes, we suggest maintaining glucose levels between 140 and 180 mg/dL.

THERMOREGULATION

Patients with ICH commonly develop fevers, which are associated with poor outcomes.[94,104] In those who survive beyond the first 72 hours after admission, fever duration seems to be an unfavorable independent prognostic factor.[105] Fevers should thus be treated aggressively with acetaminophen and cooling blankets.

DISPOSITION

All patients diagnosed with ICH must be admitted to an ICU or dedicated stroke unit.[11] This disposition is strongly recommended for at least the first 24 hours of inpatient care, because the risk of neurologic deterioration is highest within this period.[106] Care of patients with ICH in a dedicated neurosurgical ICU is associated with a lower mortality rate and better functional outcome.[107,108]

PROGNOSIS

The 30-day mortality rate for ICH ranges between 30% and 55%, with one-half of mortalities occurring within the first 48 hours.[32,33] The clinical deterioration and poor outcomes of ICH are in large part determined by its major complications, as discussed, including perihematoma edema, intraventricular extension, hydrocephalus, seizures, fever, and infections.[109] A large systematic review found that fewer than one-half of patients with ICH survived 1 year, and fewer than one-third survived 5 years.[110]

SUMMARY

Although most commonly arising from poorly controlled hypertension, spontaneous ICH may occur secondary to several other etiologies as well. Clinical presentation to the ED ranges on a wide spectrum from headache with vomiting to coma. In addition to managing the ABCs, the crux of emergency management lies in stopping hematoma expansion and other complications to prevent clinical deterioration. This may be achieved primarily through anticoagulation reversal, blood pressure and empiric ICP management, and early neurosurgical consultation most commonly for posterior fossa hemorrhage. Patients must be admitted to an ICU. Nevertheless, the effects of ICH are potentially devastating with very poor prognoses for functional outcome and mortality.

REFERENCES

1. Broderick JP, Brott T, Tomsick T, et al. Intracerebral hemorrhage more than twice as common as subarachnoid hemorrhage. J Neurosurg 1993;78(2):188–91.
2. O'Donnell MJ, Xavier D, Liu L, et al. Risk factors for ischaemic and intracerebral haemorrhagic stroke in 22 countries (the INTERSTROKE study): a case-control study. Lancet 2010;376(9735):112–23.
3. Feldmann E, Broderick JP, Kernan WN, et al. Major risk factors for intracerebral hemorrhage in the young are modifiable. Stroke 2005;36(9):1881–5.
4. Ariesen MJ, Claus SP, Rinkel GJ, et al. Risk factors for intracerebral hemorrhage in the general population: a systematic review. Stroke 2003;34(8):2060–5.
5. Sturgeon JD, Folsom AR, Longstreth WT Jr, et al. Risk factors for intracerebral hemorrhage in a pooled prospective study. Stroke 2007;38(10):2718–25.
6. Woo D, Haverbusch M, Sekar P, et al. Effect of untreated hypertension on hemorrhagic stroke. Stroke 2004;35(7):1703–8.
7. Zia E, Hedblad B, Pessah-Rasmussen H, et al. Blood pressure in relation to the incidence of cerebral infarction and intracerebral hemorrhage. Hypertensive hemorrhage: debated nomenclature is still relevant. Stroke 2007;38(10):2681–5.
8. Martini SR, Flaherty ML, Brown WM, et al. Risk factors for intracerebral hemorrhage differ according to hemorrhage location. Neurology 2012;79(23): 2275–82.
9. Jackson CA, Sudlow CL. Is hypertension a more frequent risk factor for deep than for lobar supratentorial intracerebral haemorrhage? J Neurol Neurosurg Psychiatry 2006;77(11):1244–52.
10. De Herdt V, Dumont F, Henon H, et al. Early seizures in intracerebral hemorrhage: incidence, associated factors, and outcome. Neurology 2011;77(20): 1794–800.
11. Hemphill JC 3rd, Greenberg SM, Anderson CS, et al. Guidelines for the management of spontaneous intracerebral hemorrhage: a guideline for healthcare professionals from the American Heart Association/American Stroke Association. Stroke 2015;46(7):2032–60.
12. Safatli DA, Gunther A, Schlattmann P, et al. Predictors of 30-day mortality in patients with spontaneous primary intracerebral hemorrhage. Surg Neurol Int 2016;7(Suppl 18):S510–7.
13. Kothari RU, Brott T, Broderick JP, et al. The ABCs of measuring intracerebral hemorrhage volumes. Stroke 1996;27(8):1304–5.
14. Hemphill JC 3rd, Bonovich DC, Besmertis L, et al. The ICH score: a simple, reliable grading scale for intracerebral hemorrhage. Stroke 2001;32(4):891–7.
15. Meyer DM, Begtrup K, Grotta JC. Recombinant activated factor VIIIHTI. Is the ICH score a valid predictor of mortality in intracerebral hemorrhage? J Am Assoc Nurse Pract 2015;27(7):351–5.
16. Wang CW, Liu YJ, Lee YH, et al. Hematoma shape, hematoma size, Glasgow Coma Scale score and ICH score: which predicts the 30-day mortality better for intracerebral hematoma? PLoS One 2014;9(7):e102326.
17. Goldstein JN, Fazen LE, Snider R, et al. Contrast extravasation on CT angiography predicts hematoma expansion in intracerebral hemorrhage. Neurology 2007;68(12):889–94.

18. Wada R, Aviv RI, Fox AJ, et al. CT angiography "spot sign" predicts hematoma expansion in acute intracerebral hemorrhage. Stroke 2007;38(4):1257–62.
19. Kim J, Smith A, Hemphill JC 3rd, et al. Contrast extravasation on CT predicts mortality in primary intracerebral hemorrhage. AJNR Am J Neuroradiol 2008; 29(3):520–5.
20. Brouwers HB, Raffeld MR, van Nieuwenhuizen KM, et al. CT angiography spot sign in intracerebral hemorrhage predicts active bleeding during surgery. Neurology 2014;83(10):883–9.
21. Delgado Almandoz JE, Yoo AJ, Stone MJ, et al. The spot sign score in primary intracerebral hemorrhage identifies patients at highest risk of in-hospital mortality and poor outcome among survivors. Stroke 2010;41(1):54–60.
22. Macellari F, Paciaroni M, Agnelli G, et al. Neuroimaging in intracerebral hemorrhage. Stroke 2014;45(3):903–8.
23. Kamel H, Navi BB, Hemphill JC 3rd. A rule to identify patients who require magnetic resonance imaging after intracerebral hemorrhage. Neurocrit Care 2013; 18(1):59–63.
24. Fujii Y, Takeuchi S, Sasaki O, et al. Multivariate analysis of predictors of hematoma enlargement in spontaneous intracerebral hemorrhage. Stroke 1998; 29(6):1160–6.
25. Brott T, Broderick J, Kothari R, et al. Early hemorrhage growth in patients with intracerebral hemorrhage. Stroke 1997;28(1):1–5.
26. Fujitsu K, Muramoto M, Ikeda Y, et al. Indications for surgical treatment of putaminal hemorrhage. Comparative study based on serial CT and time-course analysis. J Neurosurg 1990;73(4):518–25.
27. Delcourt C, Huang Y, Arima H, et al. Hematoma growth and outcomes in intracerebral hemorrhage: the INTERACT1 study. Neurology 2012;79(4):314–9.
28. Davis SM, Broderick J, Hennerici M, et al. Hematoma growth is a determinant of mortality and poor outcome after intracerebral hemorrhage. Neurology 2006; 66(8):1175–81.
29. Leira R, Davalos A, Silva Y, et al. Early neurologic deterioration in intracerebral hemorrhage: predictors and associated factors. Neurology 2004;63(3):461–7.
30. Kazui S, Naritomi H, Yamamoto H, et al. Enlargement of spontaneous intracerebral hemorrhage. Incidence and time course. Stroke 1996;27(10):1783–7.
31. Fujii Y, Tanaka R, Takeuchi S, et al. Hematoma enlargement in spontaneous intracerebral hemorrhage. J Neurosurg 1994;80(1):51–7.
32. van Asch CJ, Luitse MJ, Rinkel GJ, et al. Incidence, case fatality, and functional outcome of intracerebral haemorrhage over time, according to age, sex, and ethnic origin: a systematic review and meta-analysis. Lancet Neurol 2010;9(2): 167–76.
33. Naidech AM, Jovanovic B, Liebling S, et al. Reduced platelet activity is associated with early clot growth and worse 3-month outcome after intracerebral hemorrhage. Stroke 2009;40(7):2398–401.
34. Wintzen AR, de Jonge H, Loeliger EA, et al. The risk of intracerebral hemorrhage during oral anticoagulant treatment: a population study. Ann Neurol 1984;16(5): 553–8.
35. Cucchiara B, Messe S, Sansing L, et al. Hematoma growth in oral anticoagulant related intracerebral hemorrhage. Stroke 2008;39(11):2993–6.
36. Huttner HB, Schellinger PD, Hartmann M, et al. Hematoma growth and outcome in treated neurocritical care patients with intracerebral hemorrhage related to oral anticoagulant therapy: comparison of acute treatment strategies using

vitamin K, fresh frozen plasma, and prothrombin complex concentrates. Stroke 2006;37(6):1465–70.
37. Flibotte JJ, Hagan N, O'Donnell J, et al. Warfarin, hematoma expansion, and outcome of intracerebral hemorrhage. Neurology 2004;63(6):1059–64.
38. Hart RG, Boop BS, Anderson DC. Oral anticoagulants and intracranial hemorrhage. Facts and hypotheses. Stroke 1995;26(8):1471–7.
39. Fredriksson K, Norrving B, Stromblad LG. Emergency reversal of anticoagulation after intracerebral hemorrhage. Stroke 1992;23(7):972–7.
40. Ansell J, Hirsh J, Poller L, et al. The pharmacology and management of the vitamin K antagonists: the Seventh ACCP Conference on Antithrombotic and Thrombolytic Therapy. Chest 2004;126(3 Suppl):204S–33S.
41. Milling TJ Jr, Refaai MA, Goldstein JN, et al. Thromboembolic events after vitamin K antagonist reversal with 4-factor prothrombin complex concentrate: exploratory analyses of two randomized, plasma-controlled studies. Ann Emerg Med 2016;67(1):96–105.e5.
42. Steiner T, Poli S, Griebe M, et al. Fresh frozen plasma versus prothrombin complex concentrate in patients with intracranial haemorrhage related to vitamin K antagonists (INCH): a randomised trial. Lancet Neurol 2016;15(6):566–73.
43. Goldstein JN, Refaai MA, Milling TJ Jr, et al. Four-factor prothrombin complex concentrate versus plasma for rapid vitamin K antagonist reversal in patients needing urgent surgical or invasive interventions: a phase 3b, open-label, non-inferiority, randomised trial. Lancet 2015;385(9982):2077–87.
44. Frontera JA, Gordon E, Zach V, et al. Reversal of coagulopathy using prothrombin complex concentrates is associated with improved outcome compared to fresh frozen plasma in warfarin-associated intracranial hemorrhage. Neurocrit Care 2014;21(3):397–406.
45. Huhtakangas J, Tetri S, Juvela S, et al. Improved survival of patients with warfarin-associated intracerebral haemorrhage: a retrospective longitudinal population-based study. Int J Stroke 2015;10(6):876–81.
46. Camps-Renom P, Alejaldre-Monforte A, Delgado-Mederos R, et al. Does prior antiplatelet therapy influence hematoma volume and hematoma growth following intracerebral hemorrhage? Results from a prospective study and a meta-analysis. Eur J Neurol 2017;24(2):302–8.
47. Thompson BB, Bejot Y, Caso V, et al. Prior antiplatelet therapy and outcome following intracerebral hemorrhage: a systematic review. Neurology 2010; 75(15):1333–42.
48. Baharoglu MI, Cordonnier C, Al-Shahi Salman R, et al. Platelet transfusion versus standard care after acute stroke due to spontaneous cerebral haemorrhage associated with antiplatelet therapy (PATCH): a randomised, open-label, phase 3 trial. Lancet 2016;387(10038):2605–13.
49. Miller MP, Trujillo TC, Nordenholz KE. Practical considerations in emergency management of bleeding in the setting of target-specific oral anticoagulants. Am J Emerg Med 2014;32(4):375–82.
50. Pollack CV Jr, Reilly PA, Eikelboom J, et al. Idarucizumab for dabigatran reversal. N Engl J Med 2015;373(6):511–20.
51. Glund S, Stangier J, Schmohl M, et al. Safety, tolerability, and efficacy of idarucizumab for the reversal of the anticoagulant effect of dabigatran in healthy male volunteers: a randomised, placebo-controlled, double-blind phase 1 trial. Lancet 2015;386(9994):680–90.

52. Reilly PA, van Ryn J, Grottke O, et al. Idarucizumab, a specific reversal agent for dabigatran: mode of action, pharmacokinetics and pharmacodynamics, and safety and efficacy in phase 1 subjects. Am J Emerg Med 2016;34(11S):26–32.
53. Thibault N, Morrill AM, Willett KC. Idarucizumab for reversing dabigatran-induced anticoagulation: a systematic review. Am J Ther 2016. [Epub ahead of print].
54. Schiele F, van Ryn J, Canada K, et al. A specific antidote for dabigatran: functional and structural characterization. Blood 2013;121(18):3554–62.
55. Dalal J, Bhave A, Chaudhry G, et al. Reversal agents for NOACs: connecting the dots. Indian Heart J 2016;68(4):559–63.
56. Balla S, Koerber S, Flaker G. Management of bleeding in patients receiving non-vitamin K antagonists. Postgrad Med J 2017;93(1098):221–5.
57. Eerenberg ES, Kamphuisen PW, Sijpkens MK, et al. Reversal of rivaroxaban and dabigatran by prothrombin complex concentrate: a randomized, placebo-controlled, crossover study in healthy subjects. Circulation 2011;124(14): 1573–9.
58. Levi M, Moore KT, Castillejos CF, et al. Comparison of three-factor and four-factor prothrombin complex concentrates regarding reversal of the anticoagulant effects of rivaroxaban in healthy volunteers. J Thromb Haemost 2014; 12(9):1428–36.
59. Baumann Kreuziger LM, Keenan JC, Morton CT, et al. Management of the bleeding patient receiving new oral anticoagulants: a role for prothrombin complex concentrates. Biomed Res Int 2014;2014:583794.
60. Steiner T, Bohm M, Dichgans M, et al. Recommendations for the emergency management of complications associated with the new direct oral anticoagulants (DOACs), apixaban, dabigatran and rivaroxaban. Clin Res Cardiol 2013; 102(6):399–412.
61. Kaatz S, Kouides PA, Garcia DA, et al. Guidance on the emergent reversal of oral thrombin and factor Xa inhibitors. Am J Hematol 2012;87(Suppl 1):S141–5.
62. Qureshi AI, Ezzeddine MA, Nasar A, et al. Prevalence of elevated blood pressure in 563,704 adult patients with stroke presenting to the ED in the United States. Am J Emerg Med 2007;25(1):32–8.
63. Willmot M, Leonardi-Bee J, Bath PM. High blood pressure in acute stroke and subsequent outcome: a systematic review. Hypertension 2004;43(1):18–24.
64. Qureshi AI. Acute hypertensive response in patients with stroke: pathophysiology and management. Circulation 2008;118(2):176–87.
65. Rodriguez-Luna D, Pineiro S, Rubiera M, et al. Impact of blood pressure changes and course on hematoma growth in acute intracerebral hemorrhage. Eur J Neurol 2013;20(9):1277–83.
66. Sakamoto Y, Koga M, Yamagami H, et al. Systolic blood pressure after intravenous antihypertensive treatment and clinical outcomes in hyperacute intracerebral hemorrhage: the stroke acute management with urgent risk-factor assessment and improvement-intracerebral hemorrhage study. Stroke 2013; 44(7):1846–51.
67. Qureshi AI, Mendelow AD, Hanley DF. Intracerebral haemorrhage. Lancet 2009; 373(9675):1632–44.
68. Anderson CS, Huang Y, Wang JG, et al. Intensive blood pressure reduction in acute cerebral haemorrhage trial (INTERACT): a randomised pilot trial. Lancet Neurol 2008;7(5):391–9.

69. Arima H, Anderson CS, Wang JG, et al. Lower treatment blood pressure is associated with greatest reduction in hematoma growth after acute intracerebral hemorrhage. Hypertension 2010;56(5):852–8.
70. Anderson CS, Heeley E, Huang Y, et al. Rapid blood-pressure lowering in patients with acute intracerebral hemorrhage. N Engl J Med 2013;368(25): 2355–65.
71. Qureshi AI, Palesch YY, Barsan WG, et al. Intensive blood-pressure lowering in patients with acute cerebral hemorrhage. N Engl J Med 2016;375(11):1033–43.
72. Alfotih GT, Li F, Xu X, et al. Risk factors for re-bleeding of aneurysmal subarachnoid hemorrhage: meta-analysis of observational studies. Neurol Neurochir Pol 2014;48(5):346–55.
73. Tang C, Zhang TS, Zhou LF. Risk factors for rebleeding of aneurysmal subarachnoid hemorrhage: a meta-analysis. PLoS One 2014;9(6):e99536.
74. Qureshi AI, Palesch YY, Martin R, et al. Interpretation and implementation of intensive blood pressure reduction in acute cerebral hemorrhage trial (INTERACT II). J Vasc Interv Neurol 2014;7(2):34–40.
75. Hallevi H, Albright KC, Aronowski J, et al. Intraventricular hemorrhage: anatomic relationships and clinical implications. Neurology 2008;70(11):848–52.
76. Suthar NN, Patel KL, Saparia C, et al. Study of clinical and radiological profile and outcome in patients of intracranial hemorrhage. Ann Afr Med 2016;15(2): 69–77.
77. Bhattathiri PS, Gregson B, Prasad KS, et al. Intraventricular hemorrhage and hydrocephalus after spontaneous intracerebral hemorrhage: results from the STICH trial. Acta Neurochir Suppl 2006;96:65–8.
78. Hallevy C, Ifergane G, Kordysh E, et al. Spontaneous supratentorial intracerebral hemorrhage. Criteria for short-term functional outcome prediction. J Neurol 2002;249(12):1704–9.
79. Mendelow AD, Gregson BA, Fernandes HM, et al. Early surgery versus initial conservative treatment in patients with spontaneous supratentorial intracerebral haematomas in the International Surgical Trial in Intracerebral Haemorrhage (STICH): a randomised trial. Lancet 2005;365(9457):387–97.
80. Mendelow AD, Gregson BA, Rowan EN, et al. Early surgery versus initial conservative treatment in patients with spontaneous supratentorial lobar intracerebral haematomas (STICH II): a randomised trial. Lancet 2013;382(9890):397–408.
81. Han J, Lee HK, Cho TG, et al. Management and outcome of spontaneous cerebellar hemorrhage. J Cerebrovasc Endovasc Neurosurg 2015;17(3):185–93.
82. Dahdaleh NS, Dlouhy BJ, Viljoen SV, et al. Clinical and radiographic predictors of neurological outcome following posterior fossa decompression for spontaneous cerebellar hemorrhage. J Clin Neurosci 2012;19(9):1236–41.
83. Kirollos RW, Tyagi AK, Ross SA, et al. Management of spontaneous cerebellar hematomas: a prospective treatment protocol. Neurosurgery 2001;49(6): 1378–86 [discussion: 1386–7].
84. van Loon J, Van Calenbergh F, Goffin J, et al. Controversies in the management of spontaneous cerebellar haemorrhage. A consecutive series of 49 cases and review of the literature. Acta Neurochir (Wien) 1993;122(3–4):187–93.
85. Esquenazi Y, Savitz SI, El Khoury R, et al. Decompressive hemicraniectomy with or without clot evacuation for large spontaneous supratentorial intracerebral hemorrhages. Clin Neurol Neurosurg 2015;128:117–22.
86. Takeuchi S, Wada K, Nagatani K, et al. Decompressive hemicraniectomy for spontaneous intracerebral hemorrhage. Neurosurg Focus 2013;34(5):E5.

87. Fung C, Murek M, Z'Graggen WJ, et al. Decompressive hemicraniectomy in patients with supratentorial intracerebral hemorrhage. Stroke 2012;43(12): 3207–11.
88. Hayes SB, Benveniste RJ, Morcos JJ, et al. Retrospective comparison of craniotomy and decompressive craniectomy for surgical evacuation of nontraumatic, supratentorial intracerebral hemorrhage. Neurosurg Focus 2013;34(5):E3.
89. Beghi E, D'Alessandro R, Beretta S, et al. Incidence and predictors of acute symptomatic seizures after stroke. Neurology 2011;77(20):1785–93.
90. Bladin CF, Alexandrov AV, Bellavance A, et al. Seizures after stroke: a prospective multicenter study. Arch Neurol 2000;57(11):1617–22.
91. Claassen J, Jette N, Chum F, et al. Electrographic seizures and periodic discharges after intracerebral hemorrhage. Neurology 2007;69(13):1356–65.
92. Vespa PM, O'Phelan K, Shah M, et al. Acute seizures after intracerebral hemorrhage: a factor in progressive midline shift and outcome. Neurology 2003;60(9): 1441–6.
93. Faught E, Peters D, Bartolucci A, et al. Seizures after primary intracerebral hemorrhage. Neurology 1989;39(8):1089–93.
94. Passero S, Rocchi R, Rossi S, et al. Seizures after spontaneous supratentorial intracerebral hemorrhage. Epilepsia 2002;43(10):1175–80.
95. Mullen MT, Kasner SE, Messe SR. Seizures do not increase in-hospital mortality after intracerebral hemorrhage in the nationwide inpatient sample. Neurocrit Care 2013;19(1):19–24.
96. Andaluz N, Zuccarello M. Recent trends in the treatment of spontaneous intracerebral hemorrhage: analysis of a nationwide inpatient database. J Neurosurg 2009;110(3):403–10.
97. Szaflarski JP, Rackley AY, Kleindorfer DO, et al. Incidence of seizures in the acute phase of stroke: a population-based study. Epilepsia 2008;49(6):974–81.
98. Fogelholm R, Murros K, Rissanen A, et al. Admission blood glucose and short term survival in primary intracerebral haemorrhage: a population based study. J Neurol Neurosurg Psychiatry 2005;76(3):349–53.
99. Godoy DA, Pinero GR, Svampa S, et al. Hyperglycemia and short-term outcome in patients with spontaneous intracerebral hemorrhage. Neurocrit Care 2008; 9(2):217–29.
100. Qureshi AI, Palesch YY, Martin R, et al. Association of serum glucose concentrations during acute hospitalization with hematoma expansion, perihematomal edema, and three month outcome among patients with intracerebral hemorrhage. Neurocrit Care 2011;15(3):428–35.
101. Stead LG, Jain A, Bellolio MF, et al. Emergency department hyperglycemia as a predictor of early mortality and worse functional outcome after intracerebral hemorrhage. Neurocrit Care 2010;13(1):67–74.
102. Kimura K, Iguchi Y, Inoue T, et al. Hyperglycemia independently increases the risk of early death in acute spontaneous intracerebral hemorrhage. J Neurol Sci 2007;255(1–2):90–4.
103. Passero S, Ciacci G, Ulivelli M. The influence of diabetes and hyperglycemia on clinical course after intracerebral hemorrhage. Neurology 2003;61(10):1351–6.
104. Middleton S, McElduff P, Ward J, et al. Implementation of evidence-based treatment protocols to manage fever, hyperglycaemia, and swallowing dysfunction in acute stroke (QASC): a cluster randomised controlled trial. Lancet 2011; 378(9804):1699–706.
105. Schwarz S, Hafner K, Aschoff A, et al. Incidence and prognostic significance of fever following intracerebral hemorrhage. Neurology 2000;54(2):354–61.

106. Mayer SA, Sacco RL, Shi T, et al. Neurologic deterioration in noncomatose patients with supratentorial intracerebral hemorrhage. Neurology 1994;44(8): 1379–84.
107. Langhorne P, Fearon P, Ronning OM, et al. Stroke unit care benefits patients with intracerebral hemorrhage: systematic review and meta-analysis. Stroke 2013; 44(11):3044–9.
108. Diringer MN, Edwards DF. Admission to a neurologic/neurosurgical intensive care unit is associated with reduced mortality rate after intracerebral hemorrhage. Crit Care Med 2001;29(3):635–40.
109. Lord AS, Gilmore E, Choi HA, et al, Collaboration V-I. Time course and predictors of neurological deterioration after intracerebral hemorrhage. Stroke 2015; 46(3):647–52.
110. Poon MT, Fonville AF, Al-Shahi Salman R. Long-term prognosis after intracerebral haemorrhage: systematic review and meta-analysis. J Neurol Neurosurg Psychiatry 2014;85(6):660–7.

Abdominal Aortic Emergencies

Christie Lech, MD*, Anand Swaminathan, MD, MPH

KEYWORDS

- Abdominal aorta • Dissection • Aneurysm • Aortic rupture • Acute aortic syndrome

KEY POINTS

- Acute aortic syndrome is a group of diagnoses, including aortic dissection, intramural hematoma, and penetrating atherosclerotic ulcer. These have similar risk factors, including hypertension and dyslipidemia, as well as comparable presentations.
- Aortic aneurysm can be a precursor to dissection and rupture. Close surveillance and risk factor modification are key to prevention of aneurysm progression.
- Aortic endoleak and aortoenteric fistula can be either primary processes or, more commonly, a postoperative complication after aortic repair. Although some endoleaks can be managed conservatively, aortoenteric fistulas are surgical emergencies.

INTRODUCTION

The abdominal aorta is the continuation of the descending thoracic aorta. It begins at the aortic hiatus of the diaphragm at the level of the twelfth thoracic vertebrae and ends on the body of the fourth lumbar vertebrae where it divides into the 2 common iliac arteries. The abdominal aorta is broadly subdivided into suprarenal and infrarenal segments at the level of the renal arteries. The wall of the aorta is composed of 3 layers (tunicae): the intima, media, and adventitia. Advanced age, as well as degenerative processes (and those factors that accelerate them), such as atherosclerosis, fibrosis, and calcification of the aortic wall, impair its elasticity.[1]

ACUTE AORTIC SYNDROME

Acute aortic syndrome (AAS) encompasses a constellation of conditions that have a similar presentation. These pathologic conditions include aortic dissection (AD), intramural hematoma (IMH), and penetrating atherosclerotic ulcer (PAU).

Each of these diseases is described in detail in the following sections. Common features of these conditions are discussed, including risk factors and classification systems used to categorize them.

Financial Disclosures: The authors have nothing to disclose.
Department of Emergency Medicine, New York University Medical Center, Bellevue Hospital Center, 462 First Avenue, Room 345A, New York, NY 10016, USA
* Corresponding author.
E-mail address: christie.lech@nyumc.org

Emerg Med Clin N Am 35 (2017) 847–867
http://dx.doi.org/10.1016/j.emc.2017.07.003
emed.theclinics.com

Definition

Abdominal aortic dissection

AD occurs when there is a tear in the aortic intima, leading to separation of the media and the intima. (See aortic dissection at: https://radiopaedia.org/cases/aortic-dissection.) This is often preceded by medial degeneration or cystic medial necrosis. There are 2 theories that describe the pathogenesis of AD. The first theory is that there is a primary tear in the intimal layer and, during a subsequent hypertensive attack, blood enters the media at the location of the intimal tear and dissects into the media. The second theory is that the catalyst to dissection is rupture of the vasa vasorum with the development of an IMH, and that the intimal tear occurs as a result of increased wall stress.[1]

AD can propagate in both an anterograde and retrograde manner. As an AD propagates in an anterograde fashion, it can spread to the iliac bifurcation. This usually occurs along the convexity of the aorta, which preferentially involves the left side of the aorta and can lead to occlusion of branching arteries (renal and brachiocephalic), leading to end-organ ischemia and necrosis.[1]

Dissection can be classified as hyperacute (<24 hours), acute (2–7 days), subacute (8–30 days), and chronic (>30 days). Of the 3 conditions that define AAS, abdominal AD is the most common.[2]

Intramural hematoma

IMH is defined as hemorrhage from the vasa vasorum into the media layer of the aortic wall in the absence of a demonstrable 2-lumen flow and primary intimal tear. IMHs comprise approximately 5% to 15% of AASs.[2] Whereas classic AD more commonly affects the ascending aorta, IMH more commonly involves the descending aorta.[3] Approximately two-thirds of IMHs degenerate into aneurysm or dissection, and IMH is often thought of as a precursor to AD.[2] IMH can lead to AD in 28% to 47% of patients and aortic rupture in 21% to 47% of patients.[1] Approximately one-third of IMHs resolve spontaneously.[2]

Of the conditions of AAS, the risk of aortic rupture is higher in patients with IMH and PAU than in those with AD.[1]

Penetrating atherosclerotic ulcer

PAU is defined as ulceration of an atherosclerotic plaque in the intimal layer of the aorta that extends into the media with rupture of the internal elastic lamina. Alternatively, PAU can be thought of as a localized dissection that is limited by extensive calcification associated with progressive atherothrombosis.[3] PAU makes up approximately 2% to 7% of AAS.[3] PAU is most commonly seen in patients with extensive atherosclerotic disease who are often 70 years or older. Complications of PAU include false aneurysm, aortoenteric fistula, AD, and aortic rupture. Ulcers with an initial diameter greater than 20 mm and a depth of greater than 10 mm are associated with a high risk of ulcer progression.[4]

Of the conditions of AAS, the risk of aortic rupture is higher in IMH and PAU patients than in those with AD.[1]

Causes and Risk Factors

Abdominal aortic dissection

One of the major risk factors for dissection is hypertension (prevalence ~70%), especially in patients with poorly controlled blood pressure despite multidrug therapy.[2] Chronic hypertension leads to intimal thickening, fibrosis, calcification, and extracellular fatty acid deposition, in addition to extracellular matrix degradation, elastolysis, and apoptosis.[1] This leads to intimal disruption and thickening. This cascade leads to necrosis of smooth muscle cells and fibrosis of elastic structures in the aortic wall, which can lead to both aneurysm and dissection.[1]

A history of connective tissue disease (Marfan syndrome, Ehlers-Danlos syndrome, Turner syndrome, Loeys-Dietz syndrome) is also a risk factor for dissection. Approximately 20% of cases of dissection are associated with a genetic disorder that affects the connective tissues.[5] Moreover, those with connective tissue disorders can present at a younger age with AD compared with those with dissection without history of a connective tissue disorder.[2]

There is a male predominance in AD; approximately 60% of patients with dissection are men.[5] However, this predominance may equalize with time because research has shown that for patients older than 75 years, there is similar incidence of dissection for men and women.[2] Additional risk factors include history of atherosclerosis; cigarette use; illicit drug use, in particular cocaine or amphetamine use; dyslipidemia; history of blunt trauma; recent aortic manipulation; or family history of aortic disease. Patients with inflammatory disorders, including autoimmune (eg, Behçet syndrome, polyarteritis nodosa) and infectious (eg, tuberculosis, syphilis), are at increased risk for development of AD, as well as rupture. AD has been reported in pregnancy, most commonly in the third trimester or early puerperium; however, many of these woman are hypothesized or known to have an underlying connective tissue disorder.[2]

Intramural hematoma

Risk factors for the development of IMH include hypertension, vascular disorders, arteriosclerosis, trauma, and iatrogenic causes.[4] Unlike in AD, patients with IMH are typically older in age, and IMH rarely occurs in those with Marfan syndrome.[3] There is a greater prevalence of IMH in patients of Chinese, Korean, and Japanese descent compared with European and American patients.[3]

Penetrating atherosclerotic ulcer

Age (>70 year old), atherosclerotic disease, coronary artery disease, hypertension, hyperlipidemia, history of cigarette use, and renal disease are all risk factors for development of a penetrating aortic ulcer.[3] Moreover, compared with patients with AD, those with PAU are typically a decade older and have more extensive atherothrombotic degeneration their vessels.[1]

Clinical Presentation

AD, IMH, and PAU can have similar clinical presentations and, as such, they are discussed together. There is a particular emphasis on AD because it makes up almost all AASs.

AD is the great mimicker because it can present with myriad of signs and symptoms that can be subtle and nonspecific. Studies have demonstrated that the diagnosis of dissection can be missed up to 40% of the time at symptom onset.[1]

The most common presentation (~90% of patients) is sudden onset and severe pain located in the chest, abdomen, flank, or back. Abruptness of pain symptoms for AD, as well as other aortic emergencies, is highly sensitive and is present in approximately 90% of affected patients.[1] That being said, in about 5% of cases dissections may be painless.[6] Although classic features of AD (ie, abrupt onset of severe chest or abdominal pain that is tearing or ripping in nature and radiates to the back) often increase the clinician's suspicion for dissection. Those who present with painless dissections are often subject to delays in diagnosis and potentially worse outcomes.

Other presenting symptoms, which can be nonspecific in isolation, include neurologic symptoms such as paresis, paraplegia, or syncope. Syncope, which occurs in approximately 13% of patients, can signal evidence of cardiac tamponade or stroke.[2]

Neurologic deficits (eg, paresis, paraplegia) occur more commonly with type A dissections and can be found in approximately 17% of patients with AD.[2]

On physical examination, a pulse deficit, which is associated with increased in-hospital mortality, may also be noted. Pulse deficits occur in 19% to 30% of patients with type A dissection and 9% to 21% of patients with type B dissection. The commonly noted pulse deficits include decreased or absent right brachial pulse, right femoral pulse (15%), left femoral pulse (14%), left brachial pulse (12%), and left common carotid pulse.[1]

One highly specific, although less sensitive, finding of dissection is auscultation of the murmur of aortic insufficiency. This murmur was appreciated in 12% of patients with type B AD and 44% of patients with type A dissection in the study population of the International Registry of Acute Aortic Dissection (IRAD) study. It was more common than other examination findings, including pulse deficit, cerebrovascular accident, or congestive heart failure.[6] Less commonly on examination, patients may demonstrate gastrointestinal bleeding or hematuria or anuria.[2] Ominous signs indicating evolution of the dissection include myocardial ischemia, cardiac tamponade, cardiogenic shock, acute aortic regurgitation, and mesenteric ischemia.[2]

Hypertension is noted in over 60% of patients.[6,7] Older patients ($\geq$70 years) are more likely to be hypertensive at presentation.[1] Conversely, younger patients (<40 years) more often present without hypertension.[1] Approximately 34% of patients with AD are normotensive, defined as a systolic blood pressure (SBP) between 100 to 149 mm Hg, and approximately 8% of patients with dissection present with shock, defined as an SBP less than or equal to 80.[6]

IMH and PAU can present as abrupt onset of chest, back, abdominal, and/or flank pain, mimicking AD. Pain is a more common presenting symptom in IMH compared with AD,[3] although the pain quality of IMH and PAU is usually clinically indistinguishable.

Classification

The initial management of patients with AD always includes medical management and may include surgical intervention. The classification schemes (see later discussion) can help with clinical decision-making for clinical management.

The DeBakey classification system describes the site of the origin of the intimal tear and the extent of the dissection (**Table 1**).

The Stanford classification system is used for AD, IMH, and PAU, and it describes the absence or presence of ascending aorta involvement (**Table 2**).

The Working Group on Aortic Diseases of the DEFINE project created a novel classification system for AD: the DISSECT mnemonic. The purpose of this new system is to provide a way to describe multiple characteristics of a dissection that are important in the decision-making pathway for dissection management. The group makes it clear that this new system supplements, rather than replaces, the traditional DeBakey and Stanford systems.[8]

DISSECT mnemonic

D: dissection less than 2 weeks, 2 weeks to 3 months, or greater than 3 months from initial symptoms
I: intimal tear location (ascending aorta, arch, descending, abdominal, or unknown)
S: size of the aorta
SE: segmental extent
C: clinical complications; that is, cardiac tamponade, aortic valve compromise, rupture, or branch malperfusion
T: thrombosis and extent of the false lumen.

Table 1
DeBakey system

Category	Description
I	Tear in the ascending aorta propagating distally to include at least the aortic arch and typically the descending aorta
II	Tear only in the ascending aorta
III	Tear in the descending aorta most often propagating distally
IIIa	Tear only in the descending thoracic aorta
IIIb	Tear extending below the diaphragm

Diagnosis

The evaluation of a patient with suspected AAS should include a focused history and physical examination, particularly looking for risk factors, signs, or symptoms, as previously described.

Computed tomography with angiography

Computed tomography (CT) with angiography (CT-A) is the imaging modality of choice for the diagnosis and follow-up of aortic disease because it has a sensitivity and specificity of almost 100%.[4] CT-A allows for the examination of the entire thoracic and abdominal aorta and their branches and evaluates nonaortic diseases.

Abdominal aortic dissection CT scans can be useful to evaluate the location of the intimal flap to guide surgical intervention. In addition, CT scanning can identify involvement of branch vessels and other nonaortic diseases. Also, CT scanning can assist in the differentiation between the false and the true lumen. The false lumen usually is rounded and biconvex in shape. Additionally, the false lumen may demonstrate the presence of a thrombus or other radiographic sign, such as the cobwebs sign (strands of media that appear as filling defects because they cross the false lumen) and the beak sign (a wedge of hematoma that permits propagation of the false lumen)[4] (**Fig. 1**).

Intramural hematoma An IMH appears as a circular or crescentic hyperdensity (thickening >5 mm) of the aortic wall in the absence of detectable blood flow in the vessel wall.[4] In addition, the aortic wall can be observed to be thickened, and there is no communication with the lumen or contrast flow into the aortic wall (**Fig. 2**).[4]

Penetrating atherosclerotic ulcer On contrast-enhanced images, PAU appears as a localized, crater-like, contrast-filled out-pouching of the aorta through the intimal layer (**Fig. 3**). Noncontrast CT scan imaging of a PAU appears as displacement of intimal calcifications.[1]

Ultrasonography

This modality can be performed at the bedside, which is useful for the unstable patient. Additional benefits of ultrasound are that it is noninvasive, safe, accurate, and does not involve the use of radiation or potentially nephrotoxic contrast material. In the

Table 2
Stanford system

Type	Description
A	Dissection involving the ascending aorta irrespective of the site of tear
B	Dissection that does not involve the ascending aorta

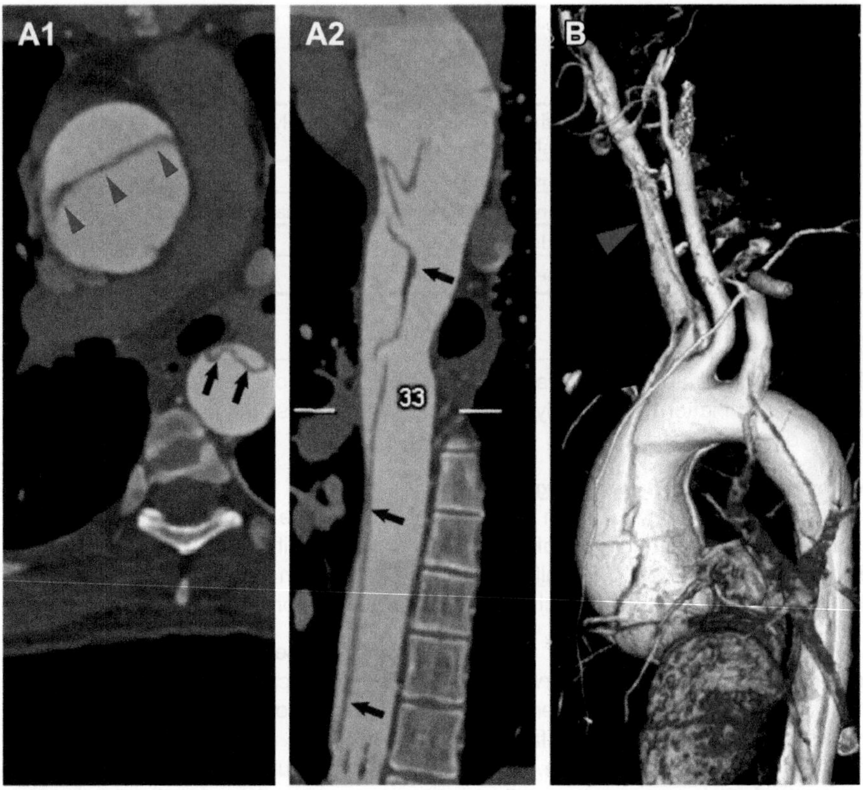

Fig. 1. AD, computed tomography. CT scan of the thorax and neck. (*A1*) Type A AD with dissecting membrane in the aneurysmatic ascending (*red arrowheads*) and descending aorta (*black arrows*). Red arrowheads are located in the true lumen, black arrows in the false lumen. (*A2*) Sagittal view of the descending aorta showing dissecting membrane (*black arrows*). The white horizontal line indicates the plane of the axial view shown in A1. (*B*) Reconstruction of the aortic arch and supra-aortic branches: dissecting membrane extending into the right common carotid artery (CCA) (*red arrowhead*) and the outflow of the left CCA. (*From* Witsch T, Stephan A, Hederer P, et al. Aortic dissection presenting as "Hysteria". J Emerg Med 2015;49(5):627–9.)

emergency department, the use of transabdominal ultrasound to evaluate the aorta has a sensitivity of 70% to 80% and a specificity of 100%.[9]

Limitations of ultrasonography include that it provides a restricted field of view and that its accuracy is operator-dependent. It is also affected by patient characteristics, including body habitus.

MRI and magnetic resonance angiography

MRI is a sensitive imaging modality for the detection of AD.[10] Other benefits of MRI or magnetic resonance angiography (MRA) are lack of ionizing radiation and that use of iodinated contrast medium is not needed. MRI is superior to CT scan with regard to ability to characterize tissue and fluid components, which is particularly important in the evaluation of inflammation-related edema and hematoma age. However, because MRI or MRA requires that the patient to be hemodynamically stable, and necessitates a longer amount of time to obtain as well as interpret, this modality is often not feasible.

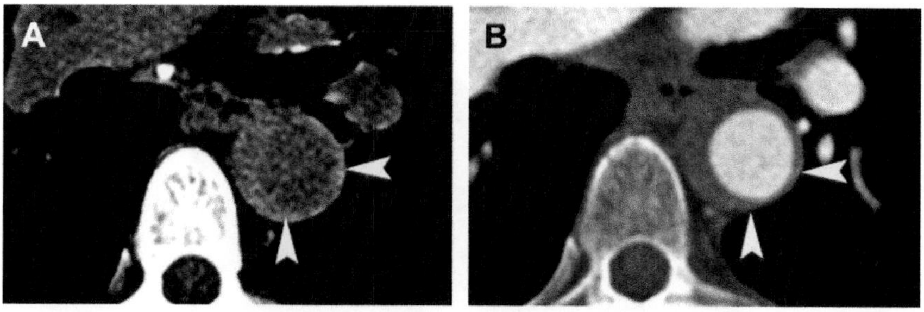

Fig. 2. IMH. (*A*) Noncontrast CT demonstrates a high-attenuation hemorrhage (*arrowheads*) in the wall of the descending thoracic aorta that indicates IMH. (*B*) Postcontrast CT obscures the high attenuation of an acute IMH (*arrowheads*). (*From* Brant WE. Peritoneal cavity, vessels, nodes, and abdominal wall. In: Webb WR, Brant WE, Major NM, et al, editors. Fundamentals of body CT. 4th edition. Philadelphia: Elsevier; 2015. p. 158–74.)

Abdominal aortic dissection MRI or MRA also provides detail regarding the location and extent of the area of dissection (**Fig. 4**).

Intramural hematoma On MRI, an IMH appears as a crescent-shaped area of eccentric thickening and has intermediate signal intensity in the acute setting.[4] MRI is superior to CT scan with regard to ability to characterize tissue and fluid components, which is particularly important in the evaluation of inflammation-related edema and hematoma age.

Penetrating atherosclerotic ulcer On MRI imaging, PAU appears as high intensity in the aortic wall in both T1-weighted and T2-weighted images. MRI is superior to CT scan with regard to the ability to characterize tissue and fluid components, which is particularly important in the evaluation of inflammation-related edema and hematoma age. However, due to the time needed to obtain and interpret the study, this modality is often not feasible.

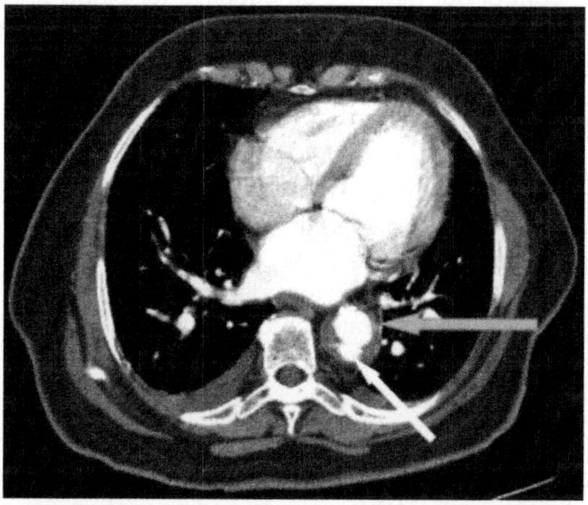

Fig. 3. PAU. CT scan of the chest that shows a localized plaque, seen as a crater-like, contrast-filled protrusion of contrast material outside the aortic lumen without surrounding stranding (*white arrow*). There is absence of a dissection flap or false lumen. There is also an intimal calcification or atheromatous ulcer (*gray arrow*). (*From* Roldan CJ. Penetrating atherosclerotic ulcerative disease of the aorta: do emergency physicians need to worry? J Emerg Med 2012;43(1):196–203.)

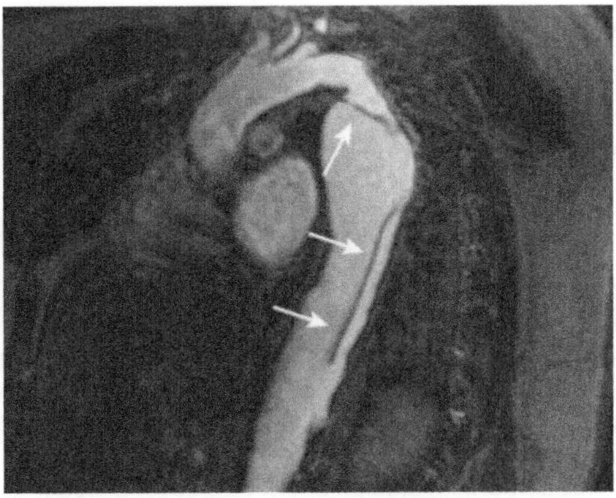

Fig. 4. MRI demonstrating AD. The dissection flaps (*arrows*) are clearly delineated. (*Courtesy of* Dr Lars Grenacher; and *From* Cardiac magnetic resonance imaging. In: Levine GN, editor. Cardiology secrets. Philadelphia: Elsevier; 2018. p. 86.)

Treatment

Patients who are diagnosed with AAS may require aggressive resuscitation to stabilize them for potential surgical intervention, as well as emergent cardiothoracic and vascular surgery consultation. In addition, medical treatment focused on anti-impulse therapy should be initiated. All patients diagnosed with AAS should be first treated medically in parallel with emergent surgical consultation for surgical intervention.

Medications used to treat AAS are aimed at anti-impulse therapy: controlling heart rate, blood pressure, and rate of increase of blood pressure dP/dT. Medical treatment involves administration of intravenous beta-blockade as the first-line treatment. Beta-blockers are used to lower heart rate and blood pressure. Esmolol is a short-acting beta-blocker medication that can be titrated to goal vital signs. Esmolol can be used for heart rate control but may not be effective for blood pressure control and thus often necessitates the use of a calcium channel blocker. Labetalol may also be used. Labetalol provides both beta-blockade and alpha-blockade, lowering blood pressure and reducing the change in pressure over time.

If the patient cannot tolerate beta-blockers, nondihydropyridine calcium channel blockers can be used. Caution is advised regarding the use of calcium channel blockers in patients who are hemodynamically unstable or have acute severe aortic regurgitation on examination.[2] Opiate medications provide analgesia and also mitigate sympathetic release of catecholamines.

The goal SBP is 100 to 120 mm Hg, and the goal heart rate is 60 to 80 beats per minute, though no studies definitively demonstrate improved outcome with these targets (**Table 3**).

Abdominal aortic dissection

Type A ADs are a surgical emergency. Dissection that is confined to the descending aorta may also require surgical intervention if the following complications are present: uncontrolled hypertension, intractable pain, impeding rupture (ie, extra-aortic blood collection), early false lumen expansion, organ or extremity malperfusion, or progressive dissection. These are known as complicated type B dissections. Surgical repair most often occurs through endovascular repair rather than open repair.

The mortality rate for untreated AD is 1% to 2% per hour over the first 24 hours.[2] In addition, the 30 day mortality for patients with dissection is greater than 50%.[2]

Table 3
Antihypertensive agents

Antihypertensive Agent	Preferred Use	Starting Dose	Side Effects & Contraindications
Nicardipine	Hypertensive encephalopathy, myocardial infarction, congestive heart failure, cerebral infarction or hemorrhage, AAS	5 mg/h IV GTT, increasing by 2.5 mg/h IV every 5 min to a max of 30 mg/h IV GTT	Hypotension Contraindicated in severe aortic stenosis Reflex tachycardia
Labetalol	Hypertensive encephalopathy, myocardial infarction, preeclampsia or eclampsia, cerebral infarction or hemorrhage, AAS	20–80 mg IV bolus every 10 min, 0.5–2 mg/min IV GTT	Hypotension Contraindicated in acute asthma, COPD, acute CHF, heart block and sympathomimetic intoxication (eg, cocaine)
Esmolol	Hypertensive encephalopathy, myocardial infarction, eclampsia, cerebral infarction or hemorrhage, AAS	Loading dose 500 mcg/kg IV over 1 min, 25–50 mcg/kg/min IV GTT titrate every 10–20 min	See labetalol

Abbreviations: CHF, congestive heart failure; COPD, chronic obstructive pulmonary disease; GTT, glucose tolerance test; IV, intravenous.

Intramural hematoma

Type A IMH is a high risk for both early complications and death; as such, surgical intervention is usually indicated. High-risk features of type B IMH include patient age older than 70 years, initial aortic diameter greater than 45 mm, mean aortic diameter growth greater than or equal to 5 mm per year, wall thickness of involved segment greater than or equal to 10 mm, the presence of pleural effusion and/or aortic ulcer, and the presence of an ulcer-like projection.[11] As such, type B IMH patients who are stable can be managed with conservative medical therapy, whereas complicated cases or hemodynamically unstable patients require surgical or endovascular treatment.[4] Without treatment, the mortality for IMH is more than 35%.[1]

Penetrating atherosclerotic ulcer

If the PAU is uncomplicated in the hemodynamically stable patient, follow-up with a vascular or cardiothoracic surgeon is warranted, along with medical treatment. If the ulcer is complicated, that is, persistently symptomatic despite medical treatment, asymptomatic patients with large pleural effusion, presence of IMH, and initial ulcer depth greater than 10 mm and diameter greater than 20 mm, endovascular aortic repair or surgical therapy should be pursued.[4] In addition, type A PAU is almost always treated surgically given its propensity for rupture even in asymptomatic, stable patients.[3,11] Without treatment, the mortality for PAU is approximately 42%.[1]

ABDOMINAL AORTIC ANEURYSM

Definition

A true aortic aneurysm is defined as dilation of all the layers (intima, media, and adventitia) of the aortic wall. False aneurysms, also known as pseudoaneurysms, occur when the intima is disrupted and blood is contained by the adventitia and periadventitial tissues. This section focuses exclusively on true aneurysms.

Abdominal aortic aneurysms (AAAs) are classified based on their location: supraceliac, juxtarenal, infrarenal, and aortoiliac. In addition, these aneurysms can be categorized based on cause: degenerative, inflammatory, or mycotic. Aneurysms secondary to degeneration occur because of breakdown of elastin and collagen fibers that make up the media layer. Degenerative aneurysms can be linked to arterial hypertension and atherosclerotic disease, as well a combination of other factors: anatomic, inflammatory, infectious, and so forth. Inflammatory aortic aneurysms involve chronic inflammation in the intima, media, and adventitia. Most mycotic aneurysms are secondary to bacterial infections; fungal infections are less likely. *Salmonella* species are the most frequently found bacteria, followed by *Streptococcus* and *Staphylococcus* species.[12] Infection can be spread both from direct inoculation from adjacent infections (renal, lumbar spine osteomyelitis, psoas muscle abscess) or from hematogenous spread (gastroenteritis, pneumonia).[12] Mycotic aneurysms are more likely to rupture than aneurysms that occur secondary to atherosclerosis.[12]

Aortic aneurysms are described as either fusiform (75%) or saccular (25%). A fusiform aneurysm involves symmetric dilation of the full circumference of the aortic wall. With regard to the abdominal aorta, fusiform aneurysms are typically of atherosclerotic origin.[1] Saccular aneurysms demonstrate localized dilatation.[1]

When the aortic diameter exceeds 3 cm, it becomes significant. Studies have postulated that in patients with aneurysms less than 3.5 cm, annual screening of aortic size should occur. For those with aneurysms greater that 3.5 cm, evaluation for change in size should occur every 6 months.[13] In addition, those patients who have a rapid increase in aneurysm size, defined as increase in size of greater than 0.5 cm in 6 months, should be subject to closer surveillance.[13] AAAs that are greater than 5.5 cm expand at a rate of approximately 10% per year, with risk of rupture increasing exponentially.[9]

Causes and Risk Factors

Certain syndromes can predispose individuals to aneurysm formation. These include connective tissues disorders: Marfan, Turner, and Loeys-Dietz syndromes, as well as bicuspid aortic valve and a family history of aortic aneurysms.

Patients with AAAs often have a history of hypertension, dyslipidemia, atherosclerosis, cigarette use, or AD. With regard to cigarette use, the growth rate of AAA is 0.16 cm per year, which is significantly greater than nonsmokers at 0.09 cm per year.[1] In addition, cigarette use is associated with increased mortality attributable to abdominal aortic aneursyms.[1]

Both male gender and age older than 65 years are associated with increased risk of aneurysm. The incidence of AAA in all patients older than 65 years is 5% to 10%.[4] Given these data, the US Preventative Services Task Force recommends that men between the ages of 65 and 75 years with a history of cigarette use be screened for AAA.

Aneurysms greater than 5.5 cm expand at a rate of approximately 10% per year, and the associated risk of rupture increases exponentially.[9] Moreover, the risk of rupture almost doubles with each 1 cm increase in aneurysmal diameter.[1]

Clinical Presentation

Patients may report a history of gradually worsening abdominal and/or flank and/or back pain. The pain may radiate to the groin or scrotum. AAAs may be painless and are often incidentally found on imaging performed for other clinical concerns. Aneurysms are more likely to be asymptomatic in patients with connective tissue disorders, with studies indicating that only approximately 5% of patients are symptomatic before an acute event occurs.[1]

They may also present with evidence of gastrointestinal bleeding. This bleeding can be secondary to duodenal erosion.[1] Similarly, an AAA can cause compression of the porta hepatis, leading to jaundice.[1]

On physical examination, a pulsatile mass may be present. A palpable abdominal mass has a wide range of sensitivity of 29% to 76%.[14] Despite this, patients with AAA are often asymptomatic until a complication, such as rupture, occurs. Approximately 75% of AAAs are asymptomatic.[13] For those with asymptomatic AAAs, the sensitivity of abdominal palpation of the aneurysm can range from 65% to 100%.[15] Urologic symptoms (eg, typical pain presentation of renal colic) can be present in up to 10% of patients with AAA.[16] Approximately 5% of symptomatic AAAs present with neurologic findings such as syncope.[16]

Diagnosis

The evaluation of a patient with suspected aortic aneurysm should include a focused history and physical examination, particularly looking for risk factors, signs, or symptoms as previously described.

Ultrasound

This modality can be performed at the bedside, which is useful for the unstable patient. Additional benefits of ultrasound are that it is noninvasive, safe, accurate, and does not involve the use of radiation or potentially nephrotoxic contrast material.[1]

Sensitivity and specificity is nearly 100% for the detection of AAAs. This modality can be used to rapidly detect peritoneal rupture; however, it is less sensitive than CT scan in the detection of intra-abdominal free fluid and rupture.[4]

Limitations of ultrasonography include that it provides a restricted field of view and that its accuracy is operator-dependent also affected by the patient characteristics.[1]

Computed tomography with angiography

CT-A is the imaging modality of choice for the diagnosis and follow-up of aortic disease. CT-A is useful in determining the size of an AAA in the stable patient.

Inflammatory aneurysms demonstrate a thickened aortic wall and, on noncontrast enhanced images, the wall of this type of aneurysm tends to depict soft tissue attenuation.[12] Mycotic aneurysms appear as saccular, eccentric aneurysms with irregular contour and often gas in the periaortic fat of the retroperitoneum.[12]

Extravasation of intravenous contrast indicates rupture. CT scan results are useful for surgeons because it can guide surgical approach (open vs endovascular repair).

MRI and magnetic resonance angiography

When compared with CT-A scans, the benefits of MRI or MRA are lack of ionizing radiation and that use of iodinated contrast medium is not needed. Like CT scan, this imaging modality is useful in determining the size of an AAA. MRI is superior to CT scan with regard to the ability to characterize tissue and fluid components, which is particularly important in the evaluation of inflammation-related edema and hematoma age.[1] However, due to the time needed to obtain and interpret the study, this modality is often not feasible.

Treatment

If the AAA is symptomatic, surgical intervention is required. Also, if an asymptomatic aneurysm is greater than 5 cm, operative repair is usually recommended. Patients with intact, asymptomatic AAAs less than 5 cm may be discharged from the emergency department with follow-up with a cardiothoracic or vascular surgeon and strict return precautions. In addition, these patients should be counseled regarding smoking cessation if they are tobacco users, as well as be started on a beta-blocker medication.

ABDOMINAL AORTIC ANEURYSM RUPTURE

Definition

Abdominal aortic rupture occurs when there is a tear in all 3 layers of the wall of the aorta. This leads to massive internal bleeding. Most AAAs rupture into the retroperitoneal space (88%), a few rupture into the intraperitoneal cavity (12%), and rarely rupture can occur into the duodenum or inferior vena cava.[17] Approximately 98% of ruptures occur infrarenally. The media layer of the aorta, where the strength of the aortic structure lies, contains elastic lamellae (which make up lamellar units). The number of elastic lamellae progressively decreases in the abdominal aorta.[1] Hemorrhage from aortic rupture may be limited secondary to factors such as clot formation, retroperitoneal tamponade, increased abdominal muscle tone, and hypotension.[17]

Causes and Risk Factors

Risk factors for a ruptured abdominal aorta include age older than 60 years, male sex, history of tobacco use, hypertension, history of heart or peripheral vascular disease, and family history of AAA. One study showed that aortic rupture occurred in 72% of subjects with AAA who had diastolic hypertension, and other studies have similarly supported a link between hypertension and risk of aortic rupture.[1] Similarly, another study looked at actuarial data of factors related to abdominal aortic rupture and found that diastolic blood pressure, initial aneurysm size, and degree of obstructive pulmonary disease were independently predictive of aortic rupture.[18]

Clinical Presentation

Patients with a ruptured AAA can present with severe abdominal and/or flank and/or back pain. The pain of a ruptured aortic aneurysm may mimic that of renal colic; therefore, in patient populations with risk factors for aortic disease, there should remain a high clinical suspicion of this devastating diagnosis. Impending rupture of an aortic aneurysm may be heralded by pain that remits and then recurs.[1]

In addition to pain symptoms, patients also may present with syncope or near syncope. Aortic rupture can also cause urologic symptoms either via direct compression or irritation of the ureter.[16]

These patients can exhibit hypotension or shock, which can occur secondary to different mechanisms. One way in which this occurs is frank internal hemorrhage. In addition, hypotension can be secondary to retrograde rupture into the pericardium (leading to tamponade), impaired left ventricular function, myocardial ischemia, or severe aortic regurgitation.[9]

These patients commonly have abdominal tenderness on physical examination. In addition, a pulsating mass may be noted. A palpable abdominal mass has a wide range of sensitivity of 29% to 76%.[14] The classic triad of abdominal pain, hypotension, and pulsatile mass of patients with a ruptured aortic aneurysm is not always found. Studies estimate this to be present in between 30% to 50% of patients.[16] Up to 30% of patients with a ruptured AAA may be misdiagnosed if they present with 1 of the 3 aforementioned signs or symptoms.[12]

Diagnosis

The evaluation of a patient with suspected aortic rupture should include a focused history and physical examination, particularly looking for risk factors, signs, or symptoms as previously described.

Computed tomography with angiography

CT-A is the gold standard of imaging for both impending and acute aortic rupture in the hemodynamically stable patient. The presence of contrast extravasation indicates active bleeding and rupture. From a radiographic perspective, high risk for impending rupture is defined as an increased in aneurysm size (>7 cm diameter or >10 mm increase per year) and irregularity in aortic wall calcifications.[4] Classic findings of a ruptured AAA on CT scan include retroperitoneal hematoma, point discontinuity in circumferential calcification, and frank contrast medium extravasation[12] (**Fig. 5**). If there is marked blood loss, the volume of blood can displace kidneys anteriorly or laterally.[12] The draped aorta sign signifies contained rupture in the posterior wall of the aorta as an indistinct posterior aortic wall that lays over the lumbar vertebra. The crescent sign is another radiographic finding that is predictive of rupture. It is defined as a crescent-shaped area of hyperattenuation within a thrombus.[4]

Ultrasound

This modality can be performed at the bedside, which is useful for the unstable patient. Additional benefits of ultrasound are that it is noninvasive, safe, accurate, and does not involve the use of radiation or potentially nephrotoxic contrast material.[1]

Ultrasound is very sensitive for evaluation of the size of an aortic aneurysm; however, it is less sensitive than CT scan in determining rupture. If clinical examination and history suggest aortic rupture, and ultrasound evaluation demonstrates intraperitoneal free fluid, this can confirm a diagnosis of rupture. Despite this, approximately 80% of ruptures occur in the retroperitoneum[6] and, therefore, this fluid is not visible on ultrasound.

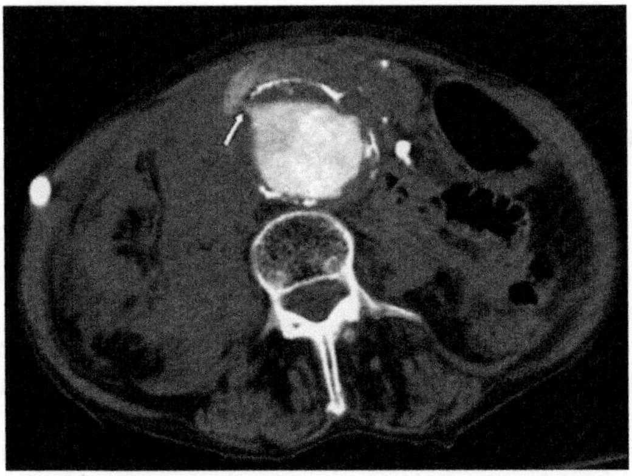

Fig. 5. Active rupture of an AAA: CT findings. Contrast (*arrow*) is actively extravasating from the right anterolateral aspect of the aorta. (*From* Gore RM, Levine MS. High-yield imaging: gastrointestinal. Philadelphia: Elsevier; 2010.)

MRI and magnetic resonance angiography

When compared with CT-A scans, the benefits of MRI or MRA are lack of ionizing radiation and that use of iodinated contrast medium is not needed. MRI is superior to CT scan with regard to ability to characterize tissue and fluid components, which is particularly important in the evaluation of inflammation-related edema and hematoma age.[1] However, due to the time needed to obtain and interpret the study, this modality is often not feasible.

Treatment

These patients require emergent resuscitation. Multiple large-bore intravenous access should be obtained. Large-volume resuscitation, ideally with blood products, should occur if the patient demonstrates evidence of poor perfusion or is hypotensive (mean arterial pressure <60–65 mm Hg).[14] At the same time, over-resuscitation should also be avoided because it can lead to clot disruption. Providers must also ascertain if the patient with aortic rupture is currently taking anticoagulants and ensure reversal of the anticoagulation with the appropriate medications or blood products. In parallel to the resuscitation, vascular or cardiothoracic surgery teams should be consulted. If they are not present at the institution, arrangements for rapid transfer should occur.

A ruptured aortic aneurysm has an overall mortality of approximately 90% and a 5-year survival of less than 20%.[4]

ABDOMINAL AORTIC ANEURYSMAL ENDOLEAK

Definition

Aortic aneurysm endoleak is related to the acute expansion of aneurysm secondary to vessel dilatation and subsequent increased vessel wall tension. Although the purpose of endovascular repair of an aortic aneurysm is to prevent rupture and subsequent mortality, at least 1% of patients experience aortic rupture postrepair annually.[19] It has been hypothesized that this risk of subsequent rupture is related to the complexities of the prior aortic aneurysm, as well as endoleaks and endotension.[19] Leakage is the most frequent complication after endovascular repair of an AAA, with the prevalence of endoleaks on postoperative follow-up found to be approximately 20%.[19] Endoleaks can cause an increase in aneurysm sac size, as well as intraluminal pressure, which could lead to aortic rupture.

Causes and Risk Factors

Risk factors for occurrence of endoleak include size of aneurysm (aneurysm diameter) as well as age (>75 years), hypertension, and history of cigarette use.[20–22] Similarly, another study found that preoperative aneurysm size, angulation of the infrarenal neck, patency of the IMA, and the magnitude of sac thrombus were associated with an increased risk of endoleak occurrence.[19]

Clinical Presentation

Endoleaks are often asymptomatic and may be found incidentally on routine follow-up. As the endoleak continues to expand, patients may experience abdominal or flank pain because the aorta is at increased risk of rupture.

Classification

Endoleaks are classified according to their cause, specifically, the source of the blood flow.[23]

Type	Description
I	Occurs secondary to a failure to create an adequate circumferential seal Ia: involves the proximal attachment site Ib: involves the distal attachment site Ic: involves the common iliac artery
II	Occurs secondary to backflow from collateral arteries IIa: simple to-and-from leak, 1 patent branch IIb: complex leak, $\geq$2 patent branches
III	Occurs secondary to structural failure of the endograft. IIIa: component disconnection IIIb: stent fabric disturbance IIIc: other causes
IV	Occurs secondary to an issue with the graft fabric porosity
V	High intrasac pressure following endovascular aneurysm repair without evidence of aneurysm sac perfusion Va: with no endoleak Vb: with sealed endoleak Vc: with type I or III endoleak Vd: with type II endoleak

Data from Brown A, Saggu GK, Bown MJ, et al. Type II endoleaks: challenges and solutions. Vasc Health Risk Manag 2016;12:53–63; and Carrafiello G, Recaldini C, Laganà D, et al. Endoleak detection and classification after endovascular treatment of abdominal aortic aneurysm: value of CEUS over CTA. Abdom Imaging 2008;33:357–62.

Diagnosis

The evaluation of a patient with suspected aortic endoleak should include a focused history and physical examination, particularly looking for risk factors, signs, or symptoms as previously described.

Computed tomography with angiography

CT-A is the imaging modality of choice for the diagnosis and follow-up of aortic disease. As such, CT-A is the gold standard imaging for assessment of endoleaks and has high sensitivity. On CT-A scan, endoleaks appear as a contrast-enhanced area within the aneurysm sac and outside the stent graft.[1] More specifically, type I endoleak appears as persistent blood flow communicating with 1 of the graft attachment sites, type II endoleak appears as contrast leakage in the periphery of the aneurysm sac, and type III endoleak appears as a contrast collection inside the aneurysm sac.[1]

Ultrasound

Ultrasound may be used to detect endoleak, but it has lower sensitivity and specificity for endoleak than CT-A. Limitations of ultrasonography include that it provides a restricted field of view, its accuracy is operator-dependent, and it is affected by patient characteristics.[1]

MRI and magnetic resonance angiography

MRA has high accuracy in the diagnosis and classification of endoleaks because it provides excellent resolution and tissue differentiation.[1] Compared with CT-A scans, the benefits of MRI or MRA are lack of ionizing radiation and that use of iodinated contrast medium is not needed. MRI is superior to CT scan with regard to the ability to characterize tissue and fluid components, which is particularly important in the evaluation of inflammation-related edema and hematoma age.[1] However, due to the time needed to obtain and interpret the study, this modality is often not feasible.

Treatment

For stable patients, conservative management may be used for endoleaks. However, embolization or embolotherapy, or endoscopic or open surgical intervention may be indicated.

Type I and III endoleaks require immediate angiographic evaluation and surgical intervention.[1] Type II endoleaks may or may not require immediate surgical intervention, with the decision resting on multiple factors.

ACUTE ABDOMINAL AORTIC OCCLUSION

Definition

Acute aortic occlusion occurs through 3 mechanisms: (1) saddle embolus to the distal infrarenal aorta, (2) in situ thrombosis of the abdominal aorta, or (3) thrombosis of the infrarenal AAA.[24] Other types of emboli are rare causes of acute aortic occlusion, and these include emboli from infections such as echinococcus.[12]

Approximately 85% of these emboli are cardiac in origin (ie, secondary to ventricular wall motion abnormalities in acute coronary syndrome, atrial fibrillation, or valvular disease).[9]

Causes and Risk Factors

Common risk factors for aortic occlusion include hypertension, atherosclerotic disease, history of cigarette use, diabetes mellitus, dyslipidemia, history of hypercoagulable state, or history of aortic aneurysm or dissection. In addition, states that put a patient at increased risk for emboli formation, including atrial fibrillation, myocardial infarction, rheumatic valvular heart disease, also increase risk for acute aortic occlusion.[25]

Clinical Presentation

Patients can present with abdominal pain, as well as neurovascular findings in their lower extremities. Typically, these symptoms include bilateral lower extremity ischemia or sudden worsening of pre-existing ischemia.[25]

Physical examination can demonstrate either diminished or absent distal lower extremity pulses, which can mimic symptoms of peripheral arterial occlusion. In addition, patients can present with extremity pain and/or weakness or paresthesias. The patient may experience pain in their lower back and buttocks.[25] Mottling of the lower extremities, usually up to the level of the umbilicus, occurs in approximately 60% of patients.[26] Pain and pallor can be early signs of ischemia, with preservation of light touch indicating tissue viability. Complete loss of movement or lack of sensation can indicate irreversible ischemia.

Unlike chronic aortic occlusion, in acute aortic occlusion, collateral circulation is not present; therefore, mortality is greater than 75%.[12]

Classification

The Rutherford and Fontaine scoring systems, which are used to evaluate peripheral arterial disease, can also be applied to aortoiliac disease.[27]

Fontaine stages

Stage	Clinical Features
Claudication	
I	Asymptomatic
IIa	Mild claudication
IIb	Moderate to severe claudication
Critical limb ischemia	
III	Ischemic rest pain
IV	Ulceration or gangrene

Rutherford categories

Grade	Category	Clinical
0	0	Asymptomatic
I	1	Mild claudication
I	2	Moderate claudication
I	3	Severe claudication
II	4	Ischemic rest pain
III	5	Minor tissue loss
III	6	Major tissue loss

Diagnosis

The evaluation of a patient with suspected aortic occlusion should include a focused history and physical examination, particularly looking for risk factors, signs, or symptoms as previously described.

Computed tomography with angiography

CT-A is the standard imaging modality of choice for the diagnosis and follow-up of aortic disease. As such, CT-A is the preferred imaging modality for the diagnosis of acute aortic occlusion. CT findings include lack of blood flow in the abdominal aorta and absence of defined collateral vessels.[12]

MRI and magnetic resonance angiography

Contrast-enhanced MRI can also be used to diagnose acute aortic occlusion. MRI is superior to CT scan with regard to the ability to characterize tissue and fluid components, which is particularly important in the evaluation of inflammation-related edema and hematoma age. However, due to the time needed to obtain and interpret the study, this modality is often not feasible.

Treatment

Without treatment, studies have demonstrated that irreversible ischemia of the distal tissue begins within 6 hours of the occlusion. Acute aortoiliac occlusion is a surgical emergency and, as such, a vascular surgeon should be consulted, along with interventional radiology as appropriate. Surgical interventions include embolectomy, thrombectomy, or bypass. Heparin can be given to minimize clot propagation. If treated only conservatively, mortality rates approach 75%.[25]

AORTOENTERIC FISTULA

Definition

An aortoenteric fistula is an erosion of a portion of the aorta that is adjacent to a portion of the gastrointestinal tract. This can be either a primary event related to an AAA or a secondary event postoperatively after aortic repair, which is more common. Primary aortoenteric fistula typically arises from an atherosclerotic aneurysm but can also originate from gastric ulcers, gastrointestinal foreign bodies, intestinal carcinoma, gallstones, or diverticulitis.[12] The postoperative fistula occurs between the vascular graft and an adjacent portion of the gastrointestinal tract. Infection of the graft is the most common cause of postoperative aortoenteric fistula.[28] The most common location in the gastrointestinal tract of an aortoenteric fistula is the duodenum because the third part of the duodenum is located between the superior mesenteric artery and the abdominal aorta.[28] The median time between aortic graft placement and the formation of an aortoenteric fistula is 6 years.[14]

Causes and Risk Factors

Risk factors for primary aortoenteric fistula formation include atherosclerosis, infection (tuberculosis and syphilis), and mechanical stress (ulcer, radiation, biliary calculi). Similarly, risk factors for secondary aortoenteric fistula formation include aortic pulsations that cause pseudoaneurysm formation, as well as graft infection.

Clinical Presentation

An aortoenteric fistula can present as a gastrointestinal bleed of varying severity (18%–100%).[28] Herald bleeding, defined as a transient episode of hemorrhage, can precede significant gastrointestinal hemorrhage.[28] Patients may also present with hematemesis and melena (64%), abdominal pain (32%), and palpation of an abdominal pulsating mass (25%).[29] Secondary aortoenteric fistulas may also present with infectious signs and symptoms, including fever, malaise, and evidence of local wound infection (30%–87%).[28] The classic triad of abdominal pain, gastrointestinal bleed, and abdominal mass may be present.[28]

Diagnosis

This diagnosis should be suspected in all patients with gastrointestinal bleeding who have a known AAA repair.

The evaluation of a patient with suspected aortoenteric fistula should include a focused history and physical examination, particularly looking for risk factors, signs, or symptoms as previously described.

Computed tomography with angiography

CT-A is the standard imaging modality of choice for the diagnosis and follow-up of aortic disease. CT-A is the gold standard of imaging for the diagnosis of aortoenteric fistula in the hemodynamically stable patient. Despite this, studies have shown that CT scan confirms the diagnosis of aortoenteric fistula in 33% to 80% of cases and, at times, surgical exploration of the aorta.[30]

CT scan of an aortoenteric fistula demonstrates intra-aortic or ectopic gas, as well as bowel wall thickening, leakage of contrast into the bowel lumen, swelling or hematoma around the graft, loss of calcifications around or tear in the aortic wall, and obliteration of fat planes around the aorta.[4] CT scan is also useful in demonstrating if abscess or other infection is present.

Esophagogastroduodenoscopy

Unlike a CT scan, an esophagogastroduodenoscopy can be performed on an unstable patient and can elucidate alternative causes of gastrointestinal bleeding. Despite this, endoscopy can be time-consuming and require resources not present at every hospital, which may further delay definitive intervention. Also, although endoscopy can locate the hemorrhage source, it may be negative in up to 5% of cases. In these instances, use of CT scan can be useful to exclude the diagnosis of aortoenteric fistula.[12] Other studies have shown that the sensitivity of endoscopy to detect aortoenteric fistula was less than 25%.[29]

Treatment

These patients require emergent resuscitation. Multiple large-bore intravenous access should be obtained. Large-volume resuscitation, ideally with blood products, should occur if the patient demonstrates evidence of poor perfusion or is hypotensive. Aortoenteric fistula is an emergency that ultimately requires surgical intervention. In addition, patients with aortoenteric fistulas should receive broad-spectrum antibiotic treatment because infection is often present.[28]

SUMMARY

Diseases of the abdominal aorta represent a category of pathologic conditions that can have catastrophic consequences for the patient. These are high-risk diagnoses and are often difficult diagnoses to make given that they can present with nonspecific and vague symptoms. By understanding common risk factors and features of each of these abdominal aortic diseases, the emergency medicine provider will develop an appropriate level of clinical suspicion for these diagnoses. With consideration of aortic disease on the differential diagnosis, the correct imaging modalities for diagnosis arms the provider with the correct steps for emergent resuscitation, management, and patient disposition. This set of knowledge and skills allows the clinician to provide earlier diagnoses, decreases time to definitive intervention, and potentially decreases patient morbidity and mortality.

REFERENCES

1. Chiesa R, Melissano G, Zangrillo A, editors. Thoraco-abdominal aorta: surgical and anesthetic management. New York: Springer Links Books Medicine; 2011.

2. Bonaca MP, O'Gara PT. Diagnosis and management of acute aortic syndromes: dissection, intramural hematoma, and penetrating aortic ulcer. Curr Cardiol Rep 2014;16(10):536.
3. Corvera JS. Acute aortic syndrome. Ann Cardiothorac Surg 2016;5(3):188–93.
4. Missiroli C, Singh AK. Nontraumatic emergencies of abdominal aorta. Semin Ultrasound CT MR 2008;29(5):369–77.
5. Nienaber CA, Clough RE. Management of acute aortic dissection. Lancet 2015; 382:800–11.
6. Hagan PG, Nienaber CA, Isselbacher EM, et al. The International Registry of Acute Aortic Dissection (IRAD) new insights into an old disease. JAMA 2000; 283(7):897–903.
7. Wittels K. Aortic emergencies. Emerg Med Clin North Am 2011;29(4):789–800.
8. Dake MD, Thompson M, van Sambeek M, et al. DISSECT: a new mnemonic-based approach to the categorization of aortic dissection. Eur J Vasc Endovasc Surg 2013;46(2):175–90.
9. Knaut AL, Cleveland JC. Aortic emergencies. Emerg Med Clin North Am 2003;21: 817–45.
10. Litmanovich D, Bankier AA, Cantin L, et al. CT and MRI in diseases of the aorta. J Vasc Interv Radiol 2009;193:928–40.
11. Evangelista A, Czerny M, Nienaber C, et al. Interdisciplinary expert consensus on management of type B intramural haematoma and penetrating aortic ulcer. Eur J Cardiothorac Surg 2015;47(2):209–17.
12. Bhalla S, Menias CO, Heiken JP. CT of acute abdominal aortic disorders. Radiol Clin North Am 2003;41(6):1153–69.
13. Santilli JD, Santilli SM. Diagnosis and treatment of abdominal aortic aneurysms. Am Fam Physician 1997;56(4):1081–90.
14. White A, Broder J. Acute aortic emergencies – part 1: aortic aneurysms. Adv Emerg Nurs 2012;34(3):216–29.
15. Lederle FA, Simel DL. Does this patient have abdominal aortic aneurysm? JAMA 1999;281(1):77–82.
16. Rogers RL, McCormack R. Aortic disasters. Emerg Med Clin North Am 2004; 22(4):887–908.
17. Brimacombe J, Berry A. Haemodynamic management in ruptured abdominal aortic aneurysm. Postgrad Med J 1994;70(822):252–6.
18. Cronenwett JL, Murphy TF, Zelenock GB, et al. Actuarial analysis of variables associated with rupture of small abdominal aortic aneurysms. Surgery 1985; 98(3):472–83.
19. van Marrewijk C, Buth J, Harris PL, et al. Significance of endoleaks after endovascular repair of abdominal aortic aneurysm: the EUROSTAR experience. J Vasc Surg 2002;35(3):461–73.
20. Brown A, Saggu GK, Bown MJ, et al. Type II endoleaks: challenges and solutions. Vasc Health Risk Manag 2016;12:53–63.
21. Frego M, Lumachi F, Bianchera G, et al. Risk factors of endoleak following endovascular repair of abdominal aortic aneurysm. A multicentric retrospective study. In Vivo 2007;21:1099–102.
22. Mohan IV, Lajeij RJF, Harris PL. Risk factor for endoleak and the evidence for stent-graft oversizing in patients undergoing endovascular aneurysm repair. Eur J Vasc Endovasc Surg 2001;21:344–9.
23. Carrafiello G, Recaldini C, Laganà D, et al. Endoleak detection and classification after endovascular treatment of abdominal aortic aneurysm: value of CEUS over CTA. Abdom Imaging 2008;33:357–62.

24. Robinson WP, Patel RK, Columbo JA, et al. Contemporary management of acute aortic occlusion has evolved but outcomes have not significantly improved. Ann Vasc Surg 2016;34:178–86.
25. Surowiec SM, Isiklar H, Sreeram S, et al. Acute occlusion of the abdominal aorta. Am J Surg 1998;176:193–7.
26. Johnston RB, Cohn E, Cotlar AM. Acute embolic occlusion of the distal aorta. Curr Surg 2003;60(2):191–2.
27. Neisen MJ. Endovascular management of aortoiliac occlusive disease. Semin Intervent Radiol 2009;26:296–302.
28. Malik MU, Ucbilek E, Sherwal AS. Critical gastrointestinal bleed due to secondary aortoenteric fistula. J Community Hosp Intern Med Perspect 2015;5(6):1–7.
29. Varetto G, Gibello L, Castagno C, et al. Use of contrast-enhanced ultrasound in carotid atherosclerotic disease: limits and perspectives. Biomed Res Int 2015; 2015:293163.
30. Chenu C, Marchiex B, Barcelo C, et al. Aorto-enteric fistula after endovascular abdominal aortic aneurysm repair: case report and review. Eur J Vasc Endovasc Surg 2009;37:401–6.

Cerebral Venous Thrombosis

A Challenging Neurologic Diagnosis

Brit Long, MD[a,*], Alex Koyfman, MD[b,1],
Michael S. Runyon, MD, MPH[c,1]

KEYWORDS

• Cerebral venous thrombosis • Stroke • Seizure • Focal neurologic deficit
• Anticoagulation

KEY POINTS

- Cerebral venous thrombosis (CVT) is a rare and difficult diagnosis owing to a wide variety of signs and symptoms, commonly occurring in patients under 50 years of age.
- Scenarios warranting CVT investigation include atypical headache, stroke without risk factors or with seizure, unexplained intracranial hypertension, multiple hemorrhagic infarcts, hemorrhagic infarcts not in a specific arterial distribution, or objective neurologic examination findings.
- Laboratory examination, such as D-dimer testing and lumbar puncture, is not reliable for diagnosis.
- Imaging is required, including computed tomography with venography or magnetic resonance (MR) imaging/MR venography
- Treatment includes immediate stabilization, anticoagulation (even with hemorrhage present), and managing complications.

INTRODUCTION

Many conditions emergency physicians evaluate are simple and straightforward; however, emergency physicians train to recognize conditions that can be life threatening. Most patients with headaches will have benign etiologies, although some may be suffering a condition with high morbidity and mortality. Emergency physicians must

Disclosure Statement: This review does not reflect the views or opinions of the U.S. government, Department of Defense, SAUSHEC EM Program, or U.S. Air Force.

[a] Department of Emergency Medicine, San Antonio Military Medical Center, 3841 Roger Brooke Drive, Fort Sam Houston, TX 78234, USA; [b] Department of Emergency Medicine, The University of Texas Southwestern Medical Center, 5323 Harry Hines Boulevard, Dallas, TX 75390, USA; [c] Department of Emergency Medicine, Carolinas HealthCare System, Medical Education Bldg., Third floor, 1000 Blythe Blvd, Charlotte, NC 28203, USA
[1] Present address: 3841 Roger Brooke Drive, Fort Sam Houston, TX 78234.
* Corresponding author. 3841 Roger Brooke Drive, Fort Sam Houston, TX 78234.
E-mail address: Brit.long@yahoo.com

Emerg Med Clin N Am 35 (2017) 869–878
http://dx.doi.org/10.1016/j.emc.2017.07.004
0733-8627/17/Published by Elsevier Inc.

expertly evaluate each patient for "red flags" that signify potential risk for morbidity and mortality. Cerebral venous thrombosis (CVT) is one such disorder.

CVT is a rare, accounting for approximately 0.5% to 1.0% of strokes, with an annual incidence of 1.32 cases per 100,000 population in the Netherlands and 0.22 cases per 100,000 population in Portugal.[1–6] The disease includes thrombosis of the cerebral veins and major dural sinuses. CVT is more common in patients with a history of thrombophilia, women on oral contraceptives, and during pregnancy.[1–4,7] It is 3 times more common in women.[7] The diagnosis is often delayed, approximately 4 to 7 days after symptoms onset.[8–10] The majority of patients present under the age of 50 years (80%), with a mean age of 39 years.[1,2,8] Less than 10% of patients present over the age of 60 years.[3,7,8]

DISCUSSION

Disease Presentation

Owing to the variety of signs and symptoms, CVT can be a challenging diagnosis. CVT should be suspected in several clinical scenarios (**Box 1**). The signs and symptoms are highly variable, as is the onset, which may be acute, subacute, or chronic.[1–3] The wide variety of symptoms and signs, combined with the rarity of the disease, make CVT an easy diagnosis to overlook. For example, a young female on oral contraceptive pills with a persistent headache is more likely to be experiencing a tension or migraine headache, and certainly neuroimaging is not appropriate in all such patients. However, the emergency physician must closely evaluate for other features of the presentation that are concerning for CVT, especially objective neurologic findings.

Symptoms may vary with thrombus location.[3,4,7,8] However, thrombus location does not reliably predict the actual clinical presentation, and patients may experience bilateral symptoms owing to venous sinus anatomy. Cortical vein thrombosis frequently presents with motor and sensory deficits, as well as seizure. Sagittal sinus thrombosis may present with motor deficits, sometimes bilateral, and seizures. Lateral sinus thrombosis may present with intracranial hypertension and headache alone. Thrombosis of the left transverse sinus can present as aphasia, whereas thrombosis of the deep venous sinus can cause behavioral symptoms owing to thalamic involvement. Cavernous sinus thrombosis, a different entity, is associated with eye pain, chemosis, proptosis, and oculomotor palsies.[3,4] This condition is often associated with sinus infection; thus, treatment usually requires antibiotics in addition to the other standard treatments for CVT.[4,7,8]

Four major CVT syndromes have been described in the literature: isolated intracranial hypertension (which is the most common), focal neurologic abnormality, seizure, and encephalopathy. The patient may present with one or more of the following syndromes.[2–4]

Box 1
Scenarios warranting cerebral venous thrombosis investigation

- Headache in a patient with risk factors and focal neurologic findings.
- Stroke without typical risk factors or in the setting of seizure.
- Unexplained intracranial hypertension.
- Multiple hemorrhagic infarcts, or hemorrhagic infarcts not in a specific arterial distribution.
- Objective neurologic deficits in a patient with risk factors for cerebral venous thrombosis.

Data from Refs.[1–4]

1. For intracranial hypertension, the most frequent symptom is a localized, persistent headache, which is seen in up to 90% of patients presenting acutely. This means that 10% of patients will not have a headache during their course, often accounting for a delay in diagnosis.[9–11] Headache may be sudden in onset and severe, mimicking subarachnoid hemorrhage, or it may be persistent and gradually worsening. Visual symptoms may occur in association with the headache.[2] The intensity of pain often increases with coughing, Valsalva maneuver, or bending over owing to increased intracranial pressure (ICP).[11,12]
2. Focal neurologic deficits are found in 37% to 44% of patients, with motor weakness the most common focal symptom.[9,11] Motor weakness may include monoparesis, hemiparesis, or bilateral involvement.[2,8,9] Fluent aphasia may also be seen, although sensory deficits are not common.[1,2]
3. Seizures, including focal, generalized, and status epilepticus, are seen in 30% to 40% of patients.[9,11,13] Because seizures are rare in strokes, CVT should be considered in any patient with a focal neurologic deficit and seizure.[1,2]
4. The final syndrome is encephalitis, which can be found in patients with thrombosis of the straight sinus or with severe cases, including extensive hemorrhage, edema, and large venous infarcts leading to herniation.[1,2,4] Elderly patients more commonly present with altered mental status and confusion.[14]

Pathophysiology

Two major pathophysiologic mechanisms are associated with CVT, both leading to increased ICP, vasogenic and cytotoxic edema, and hemorrhage.[3,4,9,11] The first mechanism includes thrombosis of cerebral veins and sinuses with increasing venular and capillary pressures. As local venous pressure increases, cerebral perfusion decreases causing ischemic injury and cytotoxic edema. Vasogenic edema occurs owing to disruption of the blood–brain barrier. This may lead to parenchymal hemorrhage if pressures continue to increase.[15,16] The second mechanism includes decreased absorption of cerebrospinal fluid owing to obstruction of the cerebral sinuses. This blockage also leads to increased pressures, cytotoxic and vasogenic edema, and parenchymal hemorrhage.[15,16]

Risk Factors

At least 1 risk factor is present in 85% of patients with CVT, although many of these risk factors are not identified until the diagnosis is made and further testing for thrombophilic conditions is completed. CVT is often multifactorial with several risk factors present, such as infection in a patient with an underlying thrombophilia.[3,4,9] In fact, multiple risk factors are found in 50% of cases.[1,17] A thrombophilia, such as deficiencies of antithrombin, protein C, and protein S, or the factor V Leiden mutation, is present in 34% of patients.[1–4,7–9] Pregnancy, the postpartum state, and hormonal contraceptives are frequent risk factors in women. Local infections, including osteitis, mastoiditis, sinusitis, and meningitis, are associated with CVT. Chronic inflammatory states, such vasculitis, inflammatory bowel disease, malignancy, nephrotic syndrome, and hematologic disorders such as polycythemia and essential thrombocytosis, may also be contributory. Other risk factors include head trauma, local injury to the cerebral sinuses, and neurosurgical procedures (**Box 2**).[1,2,4]

Diagnosis

Delays in diagnosis are common owing to the wide variety of presentations. This disease must be considered in patients under 50 years of age with acute, subacute, or chronic headaches with atypical features, including focal neurologic deficit(s) (often

Box 2
Cerebral venous thrombosis risk factors

- Thrombophilic state
- Oral contraceptive use
- The puerperium
- Central nervous system infection
- Systemic inflammatory states such as lupus or inflammatory bowel disease
- Cancer
- Hematologic disorders
- Neighboring site infection, such as sinusitis

Data from Refs.[1–9,17]

not fitting a specific anatomic distribution or involving multiple vascular territories), seizures, signs of intracranial hypertension, or hemorrhagic infarction.[1–4] Papilledema may be present on funduscopic examination, but this is neither sensitive nor specific.[1–5] Patients may improve with pain medication; however, if focal deficit or seizure is present, further evaluation for CVT should be considered. Emergency physicians are masters of considering and evaluating for the subtle nuances of common complaints. This clinical acumen plays a large role in selecting the subset of patients with headache or neurologic symptoms for whom neuroimaging for possible CVT is appropriate.

Laboratory examination including complete blood cell count, metabolic panel, and a coagulation panel should be obtained. An elevated D-dimer may be found in patients with CVT.[4,9,11,18,19] However, a D-dimer test cannot rule out the condition, especially in patients with risk factors. One study found a false-negative rate of 24% and false-positive rate of 9% in a cohort of 239 patients. Other studies have found a false-negative rate approaching 40% in patients with CVT presenting with isolated headache.[11,18,19] Unfortunately, emergency physicians cannot rely on a normal D-dimer to rule out CVT, and a positive test does little to increase the likelihood of the diagnosis.

A lumbar puncture may be considered to evaluate for other causes of headache, such as meningitis or subarachnoid hemorrhage. Notably, in patients with CVT the lumbar puncture often reveals nonspecific findings such as increased protein, increased red blood cells, and lymphocytosis that may mimic other disease processes, including viral meningitis.[8,9,11] These are present in 30% to 50% of cases. Increased ICP may occur in 25% of patients.[9,11] If concern for CVT remains after obtaining lumbar puncture, neuroimaging should be strongly considered.[1,2,4,8,9,11]

Neuroimaging is ultimately required for diagnosis. The American Heart Association and American Stroke Association guidelines recommend imaging of the cerebral venous system for patients with lobar intracerebral hemorrhage of unclear origin or with infarction in multiple arterial territories.[4,7,8] Imaging should also be obtained in patients with idiopathic intracranial hypertension and headache with atypical features.[4,8]

1. Head computed tomography (CT) is the most common imaging modality in many neurologic situations, including patients with a new headache, focal neurologic deficit, seizure, or altered mental status. The American College of Emergency Physicians 2008 clinical policy provides a level B recommendation for obtaining head CT in any patient with headache and new abnormal neurologic finding(s).[20] A noncontrast head CT is normal in 30% of CVTs, with the majority of scans demonstrating

nonspecific abnormalities.[1–4,9,11] As such, a negative noncontrast head CT cannot be used to rule out the disease. One-third of noncontrast head CTs demonstrate signs of CVT.[1–4] Head CT noncontrast followed by administration of intravenous contrast may demonstrate direct signs, such as dense triangle sign (hyperdensity with triangular shape in posterior superior sagittal sinus), empty delta sign (triangular pattern of contrast enhancement surrounding a central area with no enhancement), and the cord sign (curvilinear density over the cerebral cortex).[3,4,8,21–23] Indirect signs of CVT are more common and include contrast enhancement over the falx and tentorium, dilated venous structures, small ventricles, and parenchymal abnormalities (seen in 80%, including hemorrhagic and nonhemorrhagic lesions).[21–23] As discussed and as shown in **Box 1**, multiple infarctions or infarctions in several arterial distributions warrant further testing.[1–4] **Fig. 1** and the following images (https://radiopaedia.org/cases/cerebral-venous-thrombosis-ct-only and https://radiopaedia.org/cases/cerebral-venous-thrombosis-5) demonstrate CT findings of CVT.

2. Intravenous contrast-enhanced CT combined with venous phase imaging is rapid and reliable, detecting the heterogeneous density of the thrombus. It can be used in patients with MRI contraindications, such as those with a pacemaker. CT venography has an overall sensitivity of 95% and is helpful for patients with subacute or chronic presentations.[1–4,8,24] The associated radiation exposure potential complications from the intravenous contrast material must be considered. Although these risks are real and reinforce the importance of carefully selecting patients who require neuroimaging, in cases of suspected CVT the benefits of rapid diagnosis and treatment far exceed the risks. Owing to availability, CT is often the most feasible test in the emergency department setting.

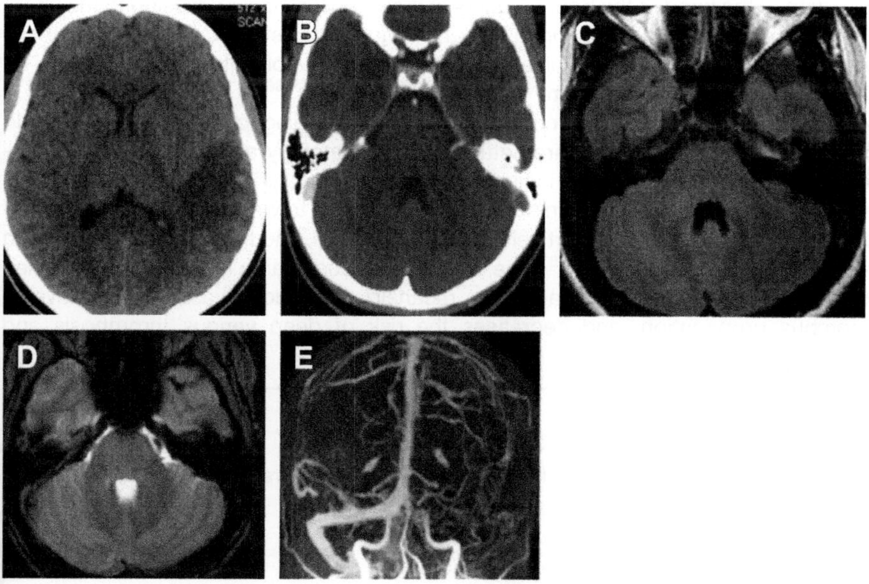

Fig. 1. Imaging of cerebral venous thrombosis. (*A*) Unenhanced computed tomography (CT) scan. (*B*) Axial slice of a CT angiography. (*C*) Axial fluid-attenuated inversion recovery image. (*D*) Axial T2*. (*E*) venous MRA with contrast. The CT scan shows a typical left superficial temporal venous infarction. Note the occasional foci of subcortical hemorrhage within this large area of vasogenic edema of the white matter. (*From* Bonneville F. Imaging of cerebral venous thrombosis. Diagn Interv Imaging 2014;95(12):1145–50.)

3. MRI with T2-weighted imaging and MR venography are the most sensitive imaging modalities for diagnosis in all phases and can be used to avoid exposure to radiation.[1–4,8,9,11] MRI findings depend on the thrombus age. Acute thrombosis appears isointense to brain on T1-weighted imaging, but hypointense on T2-weighted imaging. Subacute thrombus is hyperintense on T1-weighted and T2-weighted imaging. In chronic presentations, the thrombus may be heterogeneous and of variable intensity. MR is better than CT at diagnosing and evaluating parenchymal lesions associated with CVT, such as hemorrhage.[1,3,8,24–30] If the diagnosis is based on a lack of blood flow only, the test may be falsely positive.[3,4,24,31] Contrast enhancement with venous phase imaging improves detection, because MRI alone will not identify thrombus and lack of blood flow.[1,4,8] (See https://radiopaedia.org/cases/cerebral-venous-thrombosis-1 and **Fig. 1** for images displaying MRIs of CVT.)
4. Cerebral angiography with venous phase imaging may be used if CT and MRI modalities do not reveal the diagnosis but the diagnosis is still under consideration.[3,8,32,33] This test is best for cortical vein thrombosis or if endovascular treatment is available.[2–4,7,8]

Management

Management focuses on first addressing life-threatening complications, including respiratory compromise, seizures, or increased ICP. These procedures are followed by specific therapy, supportive care, and treatment of underlying causes and complications.[1–4,8] Treatment goals are outlined in **Box 3**.

For patients with signs or symptoms concerning for increased ICP (posturing, change in breathing pattern, decreased mental status, lateralizing neurologic findings, or hypertension with bradycardia), immediate treatment is warranted to reduce ICP. Elevation of the head of the bed, mannitol or hypertonic saline, admission to the intensive care unit, and ICP monitoring may be required for stabilization.[3,4,8,34] If these measures are ineffective at initial ICP management, consulting neurosurgery for decompressive hemicraniectomy may be indicated.[1,2,34–36]

Owing to the risk of rapid decompensation, patients diagnosed with a CVT should be admitted to an intensive care setting, with hematology and neurology consultations.[1,2,9,11] Specific therapy includes initial anticoagulation with low-molecular-weight or unfractionated heparin, followed by transition to warfarin once clinically stable.[1–3,8,37] The literature supports either type of heparin, and this should be discussed with the admitting service.[1–3,8,37] The new oral anticoagulants have not been studied for use in this disease. Anticoagulation recanalizes occluded vasculature, prevents thrombus propagation, and decreases the risk of deep venous thrombosis and

Box 3
Goals of management

- Evaluate and stabilize the immediate condition – increased intracranial pressure, seizure, or respiratory compromise
- Anticoagulation for recanalization of venous thrombosis
- Thrombolytic use in selected patients
- Use of antiepileptic agents in patients with seizures or intracerebral lesion
- Treat underlying condition such as infection and address risk factors such as oral contraceptive pill use or thrombophilia

Data from Refs.[1–4,8]

pulmonary embolism. In the past, anticoagulation has been controversial, because approximately 50% of patients will experience hemorrhagic transformation.[2,37,38] However, this risk is not a contraindication for anticoagulation. The available evidence suggests that patients with hemorrhage present before treatment do not experience increased bleeding with anticoagulation.[2–4,38] Thus, anticoagulation is usually warranted, even when associated intracranial hemorrhage is present.[1–4,7,8] The duration of anticoagulation is 3 to 6 months if provoked and 6 to 12 months if unprovoked, with a target International Normalized Ratio goal of 2.0 to 3.0.[3,8] If a thrombophilic condition is discovered, anticoagulation may be lifelong. Thrombolysis, either systemic or catheter directed, may be indicated in the setting of large and extensive thrombus or if anticoagulation fails, but imposes a risk of new or worsening hemorrhage. Surgical thrombectomy is used in the setting of clinical deterioration despite maximal medical treatment.[1,2,36,39,40]

Supportive care includes addressing risk factors, such as discontinuing hormonal contraceptives and seeking and treating associated infections. Antiepileptic therapy is warranted with levetiracetam, phenytoin, fosphenytoin, or valproic acid if the patient experiences a seizure or has an intracerebral lesion with edema, hemorrhage, or infarction on imaging. Seizure prophylaxis otherwise is not required.[1,2,11,13,41] Further testing for an underlying etiology, including thrombophilia, is recommended.[1–4,8] Currently, little literature is present concerning evaluation for underlying malignancy, which is present in 7.4% of cases, but the American Heart Association makes few recommendations for evaluating for malignancy in patients with new CVT and no prior cancer.[8,9] With evaluation for an underlying condition, follow-up imaging including computed tomography venography or magnetic resonance venography at 3 to 6 months is required to assess for recanalization of the affected area.[1–4,7,8] Failure to recanalize the affected vessel requires further anticoagulation.[8,9,11]

Prognosis

The mortality from CVT is 4.3% to 5.6% within 30 days of the acute event and hospitalization. This is most commonly owing to herniation or status epilepticus.[1–3,8] Death most commonly occurs with intracranial lesions due to increased ICP and herniation.[1–3,15] Overall mortality and dependency rates approach 15%.[7,44] Approximately 88% of patients experience complete recovery or experience only mild residual deficits.[1–4,42] Unfortunately, one-half of patients have ongoing headaches that occur intermittently.[1,2,12,42] A second CVT may occur, with 3% to 5% of patients experiencing recurrence.[42,43] Two-thirds of patients achieve recanalization of the vasculature with treatment.[3,8,44,45] However, patients with CVT are at higher risk than the general population for venous thrombosis of a different organ system, such as deep venous thrombosis.[2,8,9] Markers for worse long-term prognosis include malignancy or infection as the instigating event, associated intracranial hemorrhage, altered mental status on admission (particularly a Glasgow Coma Score of <9), male gender, age greater than 37 years, and deep venous system involvement.[1–3,8,9,46]

SUMMARY

Although CVT is a rare condition, accounting for 1% of strokes, it may impart significant morbidity and mortality. Owing to a wide variety of presentations, the diagnosis is often delayed. Although headache is a common presentation to the emergency department, the emergency physician must consider CVT in the differential diagnosis in several clinical scenarios: a headache in a pregnant patient, a headache in a young female on oral contraceptive pills, or a headache that is atypical and persistent. CVT should also be considered in the following cases: stroke without typical risk factors or when accompanied by a seizure, unexplained intracranial hypertension, multiple hemorrhagic infarcts or hemorrhagic infarcts that are not attributable to a specific arterial distribution, and with neurologic deficits in a patient with risk factors for CVT. Diagnosis requires imaging, most commonly contrast-enhanced CT of the head with venous phase imaging. Treatment includes initial stabilization, anticoagulation, managing complications, and addressing risk factors. With an understanding of the risk factors and various scenarios warranting investigation, emergency physicians can expertly diagnose and manage this potentially deadly condition.

REFERENCES

1. Piazza G. Cerebral venous thrombosis. Circulation 2012;125:1704–9.
2. Thorell SE, Parry-Jones AR, Punter M, et al. Cerebral venous thrombosis – A primer for the haematologist. Blood Rev 2015;29:45–50.
3. Bousser MG, Ferro JM. Cerebral venous thrombosis: an update. Lancet Neurol 2007;6:162–70.
4. Stam J. Thrombosis of the cerebral veins and sinuses. N Engl J Med 2005;352: 1791–8.
5. Ferro JM, Correia M, Pontes C, et al. Cerebral vein and dural sinus thrombosis in Portugal: 1980-1998. Cerebrovasc Dis 2001;11:177.
6. Coutinho JM, Zuurbier SM, Aramideh M, et al. The incidence of cerebral venous thrombosis: a cross-sectional study. Stroke 2012;43:3375.
7. Coutinho JM, Ferro JM, Canhao P, et al. Cerebral venous and sinus thrombosis in women. Stroke 2009;40:2356–61.
8. Saposnik G, Barinagarrementeria F, Brown RD Jr, et al. Diagnosis and management of cerebral venous thrombosis: a statement for healthcare professionals from the American Heart Association/American Stroke Association. Stroke 2011;42:1158–92.
9. Ferro JM, Canhao P, Stam J, et al. Prognosis of cerebral vein and dural sinus thrombosis: results of the International Study on Cerebral Vein and Dural Sinus Thrombosis (ISCVT). Stroke 2004;35:664–70.
10. Ferro JM, Canhao P, Stam J, et al. Delay in the diagnosis of cerebral vein and dural sinus thrombosis: influence on outcome. Stroke 2009;40:3133–8.
11. Tanislav C, Siekmann R, Sieweke N, et al. Cerebral vein thrombosis: clinical manifestation and diagnosis. BMC Neurol 2011;11:69.
12. Agostoni E. Headache in cerebral venous thrombosis. Neurol Sci 2004;25(Suppl 3):S206–10.
13. Ferro JM, Canhao P, Bousser MG, et al. Early seizures in cerebral vein and dural sinus thrombosis: risk factors and role of antiepileptics. Stroke 2008;39:1152–8.
14. Ferro JM, Canhao P, Bousser MG, et al. Cerebral vein and dural sinus thrombosis in elderly patients. Stroke 2005;36:1927–32.
15. Schaller B, Graf R. Cerebral venous infarction: the pathophysiological concept. Cerebrovasc Dis 2004;18:179.
16. Gotoh M, Ohmoto T, Kuyama H. Experimental study of venous circulatory disturbance by dural sinus occlusion. Acta Neurochir (Wien) 1993;124:120.
17. Canhao P, Ferro JM, Lindgren AG, et al. Causes and predictors of death in cerebral venous thrombosis. Stroke 2005;36:1720–5.

18. Crassard I, Soria C, Tzourio C, et al. A negative D-dimer assay does not rule out cerebral venous thrombosis: a series of seventy-three patients. Stroke 2005;36: 1716–9.
19. Kosinski CM, Mull M, Schwarz M, et al. Do normal D-dimer levels reliably exclude cerebral sinus thrombosis? Stroke 2004;35:2820–5.
20. Edlow JA, Panagos PD, Godwin SA, et al. Clinical policy: critical issues in the evaluation and management of adult patients presenting to the Emergency Department with acute headache. Ann Emerg Med 2008;52(4):407–30.
21. Virapongse C, Cazenave C, Quisling R, et al. The empty delta sign: frequency and significance in 76 cases of dural sinus thrombosis. Radiology 1987;162:779.
22. Lee EJ. The empty delta sign. Radiology 2002;224:788.
23. Boukobza M, Crassard I, Bousser MG. When the "dense triangle" in dural sinus thrombosis is round. Neurology 2007;69:808.
24. Khandelwal N, Agarwal A, Kochhar R, et al. Comparison of CT venography with MR venography in cerebral sinovenous thrombosis. AJR Am J Roentgenol 2006; 187:1637–43.
25. Chu K, Kang DW, Yoon BW, et al. Diffusion-weighted magnetic resonance in cerebral venous thrombosis. Arch Neurol 2001;58:1569–76.
26. Dormont D, Anxionnat R, Evrard S, et al. MRI in cerebral venous thrombosis. J Neuroradiol 1994;21:81–99.
27. Lafitte F, Boukobza M, Guichard JP, et al. MRI and MRA for diagnosis and follow-up of cerebral venous thrombosis (CVT). Clin Radiol 1997;52:672–9.
28. Selim M, Fink J, Linfante I, et al. Diagnosis of cerebral venous thrombosis with echo-planar T2-weighted magnetic resonance imaging. Arch Neurol 2002;59: 1021–6.
29. Leach JL, Fortuna RB, Jones BV, et al. Imaging of cerebral venous thrombosis: current techniques, spectrum of findings, and diagnostic pitfalls. Radiographics 2006;26(Suppl. 1):S19–41 [discussion: S42–3].
30. Meckel S, Reisinger C, Bremerich J, et al. Cerebral venous thrombosis: diagnostic accuracy of combined, dynamic and static, contrast-enhanced 4D MR venography. AJNR Am J Neuroradiol 2010;31:527–35.
31. Linn J, Ertl-Wagner B, Seelos KC, et al. Diagnostic value of multidetector-row CT angiography in the evaluation of thrombosis of the cerebral venous sinuses. AJNR Am J Neuroradiol 2007;28:946–52.
32. Ayanzen RH, Bird CR, Keller PJ, et al. Cerebral MR venography: normal anatomy and potential diagnostic pitfalls. AJNR Am J Neuroradiol 2000;21:74–8.
33. Zouaoui A, Hidden G. Cerebral venous sinuses: anatomical variants or thrombosis? Acta Anat 1988;133:318–24.
34. Carney N, Totten AM, O'Reilly C, et al. Guidelines for the Management of Severe Traumatic Brain Injury, Fourth Edition. Neurosurgery 2016. Available at: https://braintrauma.org/uploads/07/04/Guidelines_for_the_Management_of_Severe_Traumatic.97250__2_.pdf.
35. Stefini R, Latronico N, Cornali C, et al. Emergent decompressive craniectomy in patients with fixed dilated pupils due to cerebral venous and dural sinus thrombosis: report of three cases. Neurosurgery 1999;45(3):626–9.
36. Ferro JM, Crassard I, Coutinho JM, et al. Decompressive surgery in cerebrovenous thrombosis: a multicenter registry and a systematic review of individual patient data. Stroke 2011;42:2825–31.
37. Stam J, De Bruijn SF, DeVeber G. Anticoagulation for cerebral sinus thrombosis. Cochrane Database Syst Rev 2002;(4):CD002005.

38. Tait C, Baglin T, Watson H, et al. Guidelines on the investigation and management of venous thrombosis at unusual sites. Br J Haematol 2012;159:28–38.
39. Canhao P, Falcao F, Ferro JM. Thrombolytics for cerebral sinus thrombosis: a systematic review. Cerebrovasc Dis 2003;15:159–66.
40. Dentali F, Squizzato A, Gianni M, et al. Safety of thrombolysis in cerebral venous thrombosis: a systematic review of the literature. Thromb Haemost 2010;104: 1055–62.
41. Masuhr F, Busch M, Amberger N, et al. Risk and predictors of early epileptic seizures in acute cerebral venous and sinus thrombosis. Eur J Neurol 2006;13: 852–6.
42. Dentali F, Gianni M, Crowther MA, et al. Natural history of cerebral vein thrombosis: a systematic review. Blood 2006;108:1129–34.
43. Martinelli I, Bucciarelli P, Passamonti SM, et al. Long-term evaluation of the risk of recurrence after cerebral sinus-venous thrombosis. Circulation 2010;121:2740.
44. Baumgartner RW, Studer A, Arnold M, et al. Recanalisation of cerebral venous thrombosis. J Neurol Neurosurg Psychiatry 2003;74:459.
45. Arauz A, Vargas-González JC, Arguelles-Morales N, et al. Time to recanalisation in patients with cerebral venous thrombosis under anticoagulation therapy. J Neurol Neurosurg Psychiatry 2016;87:247.
46. Ferro J, Canhao P, Crassard I. External validation of a prognostic model of cerebral vein and dural sinus thrombosis. Cerebrovasc Dis 2005;19(Suppl. 2):154.

Mesenteric Ischemia

A Deadly Miss

Manpreet Singh, MD[a,*], Brit Long, MD[b], Alex Koyfman, MD[c]

KEYWORDS

- Mesenteric ischemia • Pain out of proportion • Time is bowel • Acute arterial emboli • Acute arterial thrombosis • Mesenteric venous thrombosis • Nonocclusive

KEY POINTS

- Mesenteric ischemia has a variety of etiologies, each with its own historical clues to assist in diagnosis.
- Early computed tomography angiography without waiting for administration of oral contrast should be pursued in suspected cases of mesenteric ischemia.
- Laboratory findings do not have sufficient sensitivity and specificity for ruling out or in the disease.
- Treatment requires surgery and interventional radiology consultation, intravenous antibiotics and fluids, and anticoagulation.

INTRODUCTION

Mesenteric ischemia is one of a few vascular abdominal catastrophes where rapid diagnosis and initiation of treatment are imperative to reduce long-term morbidity and prevent mortality. There are 4 major etiologies of acute mesenteric ischemia, namely, arterial embolus, arterial thrombosis, venous thrombosis, and nonocclusive, which are discussed in detail. The presentation of patients with mesenteric ischemia is usually nonspecific with a "benign" objective abdominal examination, which can provide a false sense of security because the late findings of this disease process (ie, absent bowel sounds, positive fecal occult blood test, focal or generalized peritonitis from visceral ischemia, elevated lactate, hypotension, fever) have not revealed

Disclosure Statement: The authors have no financial relationships to disclose. This review does not reflect the views or opinions of the US government, Department of Defense, US Air Force, or SAUSHEC EM Residency Program.
[a] Department of Emergency Medicine, Harbor-UCLA Medical Center, David Geffen School of Medicine at UCLA, Torrance, 1000 W. Carson Street, Box 21, Torrance, CA 90502, USA; [b] Department of Emergency Medicine, San Antonio Military Medical Center, 3841 Roger Brooke Drive, Fort Sam Houston, TX 78234, USA; [c] Department of Emergency Medicine, The University of Texas Southwestern Medical Center, 5323 Harry Hines Boulevard, Dallas, TX 75390, USA
* Corresponding author.
E-mail address: ManpreetS2006@gmail.com

Emerg Med Clin N Am 35 (2017) 879–888
http://dx.doi.org/10.1016/j.emc.2017.07.005 **emed.theclinics.com**

themselves. In general, a high degree of clinical suspicion should be based on the combination of history, examination, laboratory results, and imaging studies to arrive to this diagnosis.

EPIDEMIOLOGY

Although a rare case of abdominal pain with an annual incidence of 0.09% to 0.2% per year and approximately 1% of acute abdomen hospitalizations,[1,2] this is offset with a 60% to 80% mortality within the first 24 hours.[3] With the ever-expanding geriatric population, this disease is expected to increase.

ANATOMY

The abdominal aorta gives off 3 major branches to the intestines, which are the celiac artery (CA), superior mesenteric artery (SMA), and inferior mesenteric artery.[4] The CA perfuses the foregut (distal esophagus to second portion of duodenum). Acute mesenteric ischemia of the foregut is very rare, because the CA is a short, wide artery with good collateral flow. The SMA perfuses the midgut (duodenum to distal transverse colon), which encompasses nearly the entire small bowel and two-thirds of the large bowel. This is the most common embolic site of mesenteric ischemia owing to a favorable take-off angle (approximately 45°) from the aorta. The inferior mesenteric artery perfuses the hindgut (transverse colon to rectum) and is rarely the sole vessel involved in mesenteric ischemia. Collateral circulation from the CA or inferior mesenteric artery generally allows sufficient perfusion in reduced SMA flow states, such as nonocclusive or thrombotic mesenteric ischemia.

PATHOPHYSIOLOGY

Beside the abdominal aortic anatomy, it is important to understand how the bowel layers are affected by mesenteric ischemia starting from the inner to most outer layer (mucosa, submucosa, muscularis, and serosa). With mesenteric ischemia early on, the furthest layer (mucosa) from the blood supply is the first to become ischemic and is the reason for extreme, visceral pain. However, because the outer structures (musclaris and serosa) have not become ischemic, there is minimal irritation of the parietal peritoneum when the examiner indents down against the serosa and the external layers of the bowel. Hence, there is pain "out of proportion" to examination early in the disease process, where there is no focal localization or peritonitis. Eventually, the muscularis and serosal layers become ischemic and infarct, leading to peritoneal irritation and guarding with rigidity. At this point, the pain is "in proportion" to the examination with development of peritonitis. It is also important to consider that, between the early and late presentations mentioned, there may be a deceptive pain-free interval of 3 to 6 hours caused by a decline in intramural pain receptors from hypoperfusion.

THE CLASSIC TYPES

Mesenteric ischemia can be classified as acute versus chronic or occlusive versus nonocclusive. The following are the major 4 etiologies of acute mesenteric ischemia[5]: Acute arterial emboli, acute arterial thrombosis, mesenteric venous thrombosis, and nonocclusive.

Acute Arterial Emboli

In the most frequent cause of mesenteric ischemia, accounting for 40% to 50% of cases, the embolus lodges in the SMA.[3] The proximal branches of the SMA (jejunal and middle colic arteries) are usually preserved, because generally the embolus lodges 3 to 10 cm distally from the SMA takeoff, where the artery tapers. This is just after the first major branch of the SMA (the middle colic artery). As a result, the proximal small and large bowels are usually spared.[6] Owing to poorly developed collateral circulation, the onset of symptoms in cases of embolus is usually severe and dramatic pain.[4] When the bowel becomes ischemic, it has a propensity to empty itself, leading to vomiting or diarrhea, so-called gut emptying. This is one reason mesenteric ischemia is often misdiagnosed as gastroenteritis. Common predisposing factors include atrial fibrillation, cardiomyopathy, recent angiography, and valvular disorders, such as rheumatic valve disease.[5]

Acute Arterial Thrombosis

Patients with long-standing atherosclerosis may experience plaque development at the origin of the SMA, a site of turbulent blood flow. This subsequent stenosis may lead to long-standing postprandial pain ("intestinal angina") and "food fear" with resultant weight loss. These symptoms of chronic mesenteric ischemia can be seen in up to 80% of patients who develop arterial thrombosis. If the plaque ruptures acutely or the stenosis reaches a critical level, patients may present with acute pain, similar to those with arterial emboli.[3,6,7]

Mesenteric Venous Thrombosis

This form of mesenteric ischemia is generally found in patients with an underlying hypercoagulable state, and mesenteric venous thrombosis accounts for 10% to 15% of the total cases. Patients typically present with less severe and more insidious pain than those with arterial occlusion.[5] Patients may demonstrate weight loss, depending on the duration of symptoms. Most patients present after more than 24 hours of symptoms. In 1 study, the mean symptom duration was 5 to 14 days, with many patients experiencing pain for 1 month before diagnosis.[8] Predisposing risk factors include malignancy, sepsis, liver disease or portal hypertension, sickle cell disease, and pancreatitis.[3,7] Many patients have heritable hematologic disorders including protein C and S deficiency, antithrombin III deficiency, and factor V Leiden mutation. One-half of patients with mesenteric venous thrombosis have a personal or family history of venous thromboembolism.[9,10]

Nonocclusive

This form of mesenterial ischemia occurs in 20% of patients owing to failure of autoregulation in low-flow states such as hypovolemia, potent vasopressor use, heart failure, or sepsis.[3,6] The underlying ischemia from splanchnic vasoconstriction can further lead to hypotension from endogenous substances, perpetuating a vicious cycle.[4,5] This accounts for the extremely high mortality rate, usually owing to the poor health of the affected population with multiple comorbidities, combined with the difficulty in treating the primary cause of diminished intestinal blood flow.

FEATURES AND PRESENTATION

Mesenteric ischemia is often described in 3 progressive phases when the pathophysiology is considered: the hyperactive phase, paralytic phase, and shock phase.

Hyperactive Phase

Severe abdominal pain out of proportion is the usual presenting symptom. Other early symptoms including emesis, diarrhea, and bloody stools are common, but not always present. Early emesis and diarrhea are due to ischemia of the innermost bowel layers leading to gut emptying and eventual bloody stools. Several studies have demonstrated that abnormal mental status may be associated with early presentation, but can also be indicative of late phase.[1]

Paralytic Phase

As ischemia progresses, the abdominal pain becomes in proportion to the examination leading to focal, localized tenderness. Bowel motility decreases, leading to abdominal distention and absent bowel sounds. However, bowel sounds are not helpful in ruling in or out the disease.[11,12]

Shock Phase

Eventual necrosis leads to leaking of fluid through the bowel wall, resulting in diffuse peritonitis. However, peritonitis is only reported in 16% of patients with necrotic bowel.[13] Sepsis with metabolic acidosis, dehydration, hypotension, tachycardia, and confusion often occurs. The typical patient is usually elderly (median age, 74 years) with multiple risk factors presenting with sudden onset of severe abdominal pain that is out of proportion to the examination (ie, pain out of proportion), meaning intense subjective pain with no objective tenderness on palpation. Risk factors including peripheral arterial disease (27%), coronary artery disease (46%), diabetes, dialysis, venous thromboembolism, and hypertension are common, but not always present. Pain is the most consistent presenting symptom, beginning as crampy, vague periumbilical abdominal pain that evolves over time to focal, localized tenderness and peritonitis owing to transmural infarction of all bowel layers, as discussed in the Pathophysiology section.

It is important to understand that presentation varies based on the etiology and type of mesenteric ischemia.[1,3,5] The presentation of mesenteric ischemia is typically acute severe abdominal pain with a paucity of physical examination findings. History and physical examination findings, such as acute abdominal pain, pain out of proportion, peritoneal signs, guaiac-positive stool, acute abdominal pain, heart failure, and atrial fibrillation, have a wide range of sensitivities and are frequently absent.[14,15] The presentation and examination are challenging; 1 study demonstrates the disease is suspected in only 22% of patients.[1] Therefore, clinicians should be vigilant in considering mesenteric ischemia in the differential of abdominal pain of unclear etiology. Assessing the patient's pretest probability for disease, actively searching for known risk factors, and adding in clues based on the patient's history and physical examination findings are important factors in the diagnostic process for wary clinicians.

DIAGNOSIS

Laboratory Tests

- White blood cell count
- Lactate
- D-Dimer
- Urine intestinal fatty acid binding protein

Diagnostic biomarkers are tools designed to improve clinical decision making, especially in mesenteric ischemia, where early symptoms are nonspecific, and mortality increases with delayed or missed diagnosis. Numerous laboratory abnormalities have been described in mesenteric ischemia, including elevated amylase, lactate dehydrogenase, large base deficit, hemoconcentration, leukocytosis, and high anion gap metabolic acidosis with elevated lactate (specifically D-lactate). None of these findings are sensitive or specific for mesenteric ischemia and are often late findings. Troponin I levels may be elevated, but this finding is not specific for mesenteric ischemia and has been shown to lead to delays in definitive care of these patients with inappropriate cardiology consultations.[16]

Laboratory tests include white blood cell count, pH from venous blood gas, D-dimer, lactate, and urine intestinal fatty acid binding protein. A summary of laboratory test sensitivity and specificity is provided in **Table 1**. Many physicians rely on these tests to enhance decision making and diagnosis, but this is a potential pitfall. Approximately 75% of patients will have a white blood cell count of greater than 15,000 cells/mm.[3,13] However, this does not differentiate mesenteric ischemia from other diagnoses, where 25% of cases do not have an increase. Metabolic acidosis is not always present, and metabolic alkalosis can present early if vomiting is a predominant symptom.[2] D-Dimer is 96% sensitive, but it is not specific.[17] Physicians should not rely on lactate for diagnosis, because this test is not always increased.[18] Early in the disease process, lactate is normal as it travels through the portal venous system to the liver, where it is converted into glucose via the Cori cycle. As gut ischemia increases, the liver is unable to keep up with converting lactate into glucose, and lactate spills over into the systemic circulation, where it eventually increases in late stages of disease.[1,3,19] A newer test is the urine intestinal fatty acid binding protein, and this test has demonstrated a sensitivity of 90% and specificity of 89% in 1 study.[20] However, these findings have not been validated, and the vast majority of emergency departments do not have access to this test.[2,21]

Imaging

- Abdominal plain films
- Ultrasound imaging
- Computed tomography (CT) angiography of the abdomen and pelvis
- Angiography
- Laparoscopy

Various imaging methods have been studied and used in the diagnosis of mesenteric ischemia, including lower gastrointestinal system endoscopy, radionuclide imaging, peritoneal fluid analysis, MRI, and peritoneoscopy.[16] Imaging that is insensitive or low yield should be avoided, and any imaging that is performed should be obtained as quickly as possible, given the time-sensitive nature of the disease. It has been shown that a multidisciplinary approach to suspected cases of mesenteric ischemia with streamlined protocols and early involvement of consultants can impact overall mortality.[22] The following are common diagnostic modalities often described: plain radiographs, ultrasound imaging, CT angiography of the abdomen and pelvis, angiography, and laparoscopy.

Table 1
Laboratory findings in mesenteric ischemia

Laboratory Test	Sensitivity (%)	Specificity (%)
White blood cells	80	50
Lactate	86	44
D-Dimer	96	40
Urine intestinal fatty acid binding protein	90	89

Plain Radiographs

The findings on a plain abdominal radiograph are usually nonspecific (ie, small bowel distention with air–fluid levels or ileus), and 25% of patients may have normal findings.[3] Patients with normal plain radiographs have a lower mortality rate, presumably because the findings that are visible on plain radiographs are late findings seen in more advanced disease.[23–25] Characteristic findings, such as thumbprinting or thickening of bowel loops, occur in fewer than 40% of patients.[3] Later findings, such as air in the bowel wall (pneumatosis intestinalis) and portal venous system, are ominous signs portending a poor prognosis.

Ultrasound imaging

Using ultrasound imaging to detect significant stenosis (>50%) in mesenteric vessels has been shown, and it has a role in chronic mesenteric ischemia. However, the role of ultrasound in diagnosing acute ischemia is less well-established.[26,27] This likely is due to limited operator experience in mesenteric ischemia and the abnormality in patient bowel gas patterns that often accompanies mesenteric ischemia, which make visualization of the mesenteric vessels difficult.[28]

Computed Tomography Angiography

This modality is the most commonly used diagnostic tool. With older technologies the initial sensitivity was 64%, which has improved to 93% with the use of dynamic contrast-enhanced CT.[29,30] With the addition of multidetector technology to CT scans, this has further improved results with reported sensitivity, specificity, positive predictive value, and negative predictive value of 93% to 95%, 92% to 100%, 90% to 100%, and 94% to 98%, respectively.[31–33] Because a delay in diagnosis can lead to significant morbidity and mortality, avoiding oral contrast in suspected cases to expedite the scan is key.[33] **Fig. 1**A–D demonstrates CT findings.

Angiography

Once the gold diagnostic standard in evaluation owing to its high accuracy and therapeutic role, today angiography is used primarily as a confirmatory tool when noninvasive radiologic studies do not produce conclusive results.[33,34] Catheter-based therapy and vasodilation still play a large role in management, especially in patients deemed too risky for open surgical techniques.

Laparoscopy

Depending on the institution, the availability of experienced radiologists to interpret CT angiograms and endovascular specialists to perform diagnostic and therapeutic angiography may be limited. In addition, acute renal failure from mesenteric ischemia or those with known contrast allergy may prohibit obtaining a contrast study.[35,36] Furthermore, a CT scan may not demonstrate vascular or intestinal pathologies in patients with a high pretest probability of mesenteric ischemia early in the disease course.[37] Thus, diagnostic laparoscopy can fill this diagnostic gap. Patients who have undergone successful revascularization (with or without developing short bowel syndrome) had a shorter mean time between admission and diagnostic laparoscopy.[30,37]

MANAGEMENT

Treatment of mesenteric ischemia should be initiated while the diagnostic evaluation is commencing. Aggressive fluid resuscitation should be started to correct fluid deficits

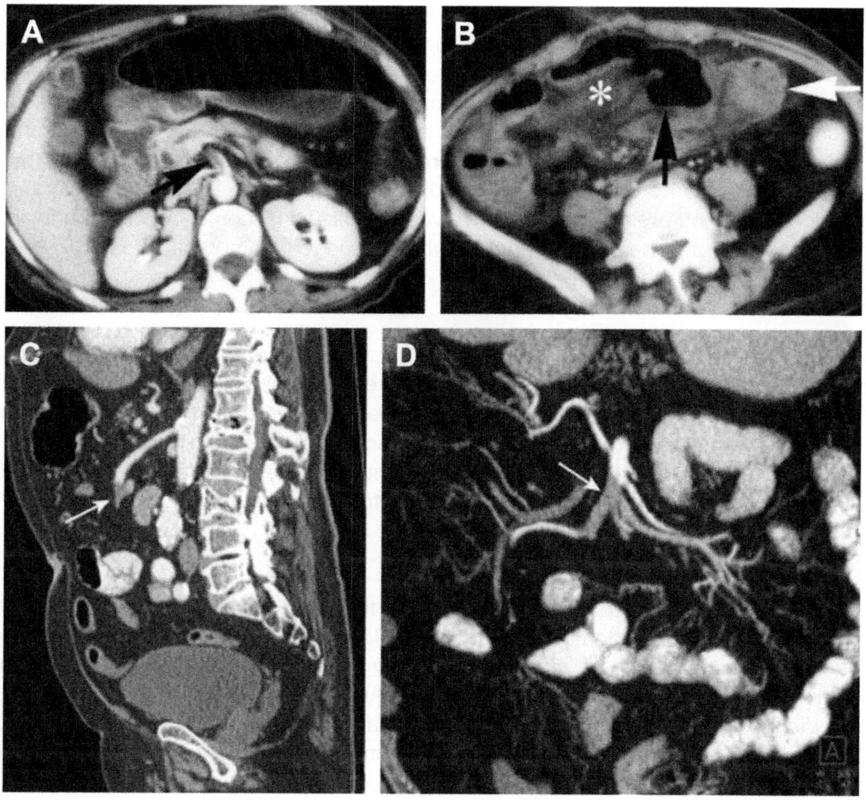

Fig. 1. (*A, B*) – Acute mesenteric ischemia with small intestinal infarction in a 65-year-old woman who complained of severe, acute abdominal pain. (*A, B*) Intravenous contrast-enhanced computed tomography scan shows hypoattenuating thrombus occluding the origin of the superior mesenteric artery (*arrow, A*), mesenteric edema (*asterisk, B*), mural thickening (*white arrow, B*) and dilatation (*black arrow, B*) of the small intestine. (*C, D*) An 80-year-old man with acute abdominal pain. A sagittal multiplanar reconstruction (*C*) and coronal maximum intensity projection (*D*) show a large thrombus in the middle of the superior mesenteric artery (*arrow*); this was embolic, presumably from a cardiogenic source. Surgical embolectomy was performed. (*From* [*A, B*] Levy AD. Mesenteric ischemia. Radiol Clin North Am 2007;45(3):593–9, x; and [*C, D*] Horton KM, Fishman EK. CT angiography of the mesenteric circulation. Radiol Clin North Am 2010;48:331–45, viii.)

often 8–20 L) and metabolic derangements, because there may be extensive capillary leak and third spacing of fluid. Broad-spectrum antibiotics are generally given to cover intestinal flora, such as ceftriaxone and metronidazole, or piperacillin and tazobactam.[38] Anticoagulation with a heparin drip should be started, in consultation with the treating surgeon.[39] Early surgical consultation is warranted, even before definitive testing is performed, especially in cases with a high pretest probability.[40] The presence of peritoneal signs is usually an indicator of late stages of the disease requiring emergency laparotomy and may obviate the need for any confirmatory imaging.[40,41]

Once the diagnosis is established, surgical management should be performed immediately.[3,40,41] Three guiding principles should be followed in the surgical management of thromboembolic mesenteric ischemia: revascularization, assessment of intestinal viability, and resection of necrotic bowel. Revascularization is often performed via open versus endovascular repair (ie, embolectomy, thrombectomy, endarterectomy, or bypass).

An important part of the postoperative care involves reducing the profound vasospasm that accompanies acute mesenteric ischemia.[11,42] This is typically accomplished through intraarterial papaverine infusion via an indwelling catheter in the SMA, but can also be performed by vasodilator prostaglandin E_1 via an intravenous line.[38,43] A growing area of research involves minimizing ischemia–reperfusion injury from these sort of ischemic pathologies, which leads to high complications.

OUTCOMES

Mortality was as high as 80% in 1999, but true mortality varies based on the underlying cause.[1,44,45] Early recognition can save lives. One study has shown a 70% mortality if time to diagnosis was more than 24 hours compared with a 14% mortality if less than 12 hours.[18,37] With a high likelihood of complications including respiratory failure, multiorgan system failure, sepsis, and short gut syndrome affecting 35% to 79% of patients after treatment, close intensive care monitoring is required.[18,36]

SUMMARY

Mesenteric ischemia is a vascular emergency that all emergency physicians must consider early in their abdominal pain differential. As highlighted in this review, it continues to remain a diagnostic challenge, and any delay in diagnosis can contribute to the increases in the already high mortality rate. Although the underlying cause varies, early diagnosis and prompt effective treatment can lead to improved clinical outcome. Delay in diagnosis can lead to significant morbidity and mortality, and a high suspicion for mesenteric ischemia warrants rapid surgery consultation and evaluation for mesenteric ischemia.

REFERENCES

1. Cudnik MT, Darbha J, Jones J, et al. The diagnosis of acute mesenteric ischemia: a systematic review and meta-analysis. Acad Emerg Med 2013;20(11):1087–100.
2. van den Heijkant TC, Aerts BA, Teijink JA, et al. Diagnosis of mesenteric ischemia. World J Gastroenterol 2013;19(9):1338–41.
3. Lewiss RE, Egan DJ, Shreves A. Vascular abdominal emergencies. Emerg Med Clin North Am 2011;29:253–72.
4. Oldenburg WA, Lau LL, Rodenberg TJ, et al. Acute mesenteric ischemia: a clinical review. Arch Intern Med 2004;164(10):1054–62.
5. Martinez JP, Hogan GJ. Mesenteric ischemia. Emerg Med Clin North Am 2004;22(4):909–28.
6. Lotterman S. Mesenteric ischemia: a power review. Available at: http://www.emdocs.net/mesenteric-ischemia-power-review/. Accessed May 29, 2016.
7. McKinsey JF, Gewertz BL. Acute mesenteric ischemia. Surg Clin North Am 1997;77:307–18.
8. Rhee RY, Gloviczki P, Mendonca CT, et al. Mesenteric venous thrombosis: still a lethal disease in the 1990s. J Vasc Surg 1994;20:688–97.
9. Boley SJ, Sprayregen S, Siegelman SJ, et al. Initial results from an aggressive roentgenologic and surgical approach to acute mesenteric ischemia. Surgery 1977;82:848.

10. Clark RA, Gallant TE. Acute mesenteric ischemia: angiographic spectrum. AJR Am J Roentgenol 1984;142:555.
11. Bobadilla JL. Mesenteric ischemia. Surg Clin North Am 2013;93:925–40, ix.
12. Wyers MC. Acute mesenteric ischemia: diagnostic approach and surgical treatment. Semin Vasc Surg 2010;23:9–20.
13. Acosta S, Block T, Bjornsson S, et al. Diagnostic pitfalls at admission in patients with acute superior mesenteric artery occlusion. J Emerg Med 2012;42(6): 635–41.
14. Park WM, Gloviczki P, Cherry KJ, et al. Contemporary management of acute mesenteric ischemia: factors associated with survival. J Vasc Surg 2002;35(3): 445–52.
15. Levy PJ, Krausz MM, Manny J. Acute mesenteric ischemia: improved results–a retrospective analysis of ninety-two patients. Surgery 1990;107(4):372–80.
16. Gagné DJ, Malay MB, Hogle NJ, et al. Bedside diagnostic minilaparoscopy in the intensive care patient. Surgery 2002;131(5):491–6.
17. Chiu YH, Huang MK, How CK, et al. D-Dimer in patients with suspected acute mesenteric ischemia. Am J Emerg Med 2009;27(8):975–9.
18. Dahlke MH, Asshoff L, Popp FC, et al. Mesenteric ischemia–outcome after surgical therapy in 83 patients. Dig Surg 2008;25:213–9.
19. Cohn B. Does this patient have acute mesenteric ischemia? Ann Emerg Med 2014;64(5):533–4.
20. Sun DL, Cen YY, Li SM, et al. Accuracy of the serum intestinal fatty-acid-binding protein for diagnosis of acute intestinal ischemia: a meta-analysis. Sci Rep 2016; 6:34371.
21. Thuijls G, van Wijck K, Grootjans J, et al. Early diagnosis of intestinal ischemia using urinary and plasma fatty acid binding proteins. Ann Surg 2011;253:303–8.
22. Bradbury AW, Brittenden J, McBride K, et al. Mesenteric ischaemia: a multidisciplinary approach. Br J Surg 1995;82(11):1446–59.
23. Smerud MJ, Johnson CD, Stephens DH. Diagnosis of bowel infarction: a comparison of plain films and CT scans in 23 cases. AJR Am J Roentgenol 1990;154: 99–103.
24. Duran M, Pohl E, Grabitz K, et al. The importance of open emergency surgery in the treatment of acute mesenteric ischemia. World J Emerg Surg 2015;10(1):45.
25. Sack J, Aldrete JS. Primary mesenteric venous thrombosis. Surg Gynecol Obstet 1982;154:205.
26. Zwolak RM. Can duplex ultrasound replace arteriography in screening for mesenteric ischemia? Semin Vasc Surg 1999;12(4):252–60.
27. Sartini S, Calosi G, Granai C, et al. Duplex ultrasound in the early diagnosis of acute mesenteric ischemia: a longitudinal cohort multicentric study. Eur J Emerg Med 2016. [Epub ahead of print].
28. Oliva IB, Davarpanah AH, Rybicki FJ, et al. ACR Appropriateness Criteria® imaging of mesenteric ischemia. Abdom Imaging 2013;38(4):714–9.
29. Menke J. Diagnostic accuracy of multidetector CT in acute mesenteric ischemia: systematic review and meta-analysis. Radiology 2010;256:93–101.
30. Kirkpatrick ID, Kroeker MA, Greenberg HM. Biphasic CT with mesenteric CT angiography in the evaluation of acute mesenteric ischemia: initial experience. Radiology 2003;229:91–8.
31. Klar E, Rahmanian PB, Bucker A, et al. Acute mesenteric ischemia: a vascular emergency. Dtsch Arztebl Int 2012;109:249–56.
32. Horton KM, Fishman EK. CT angiography of the mesenteric circulation. Radiol Clin North Am 2010;48:331–45.

33. Aschoff AJ, Stuber G, Becker BW, et al. Evaluation of acute mesenteric ischemia: accuracy of biphasic mesenteric multidetector CT angiography. Abdom Imaging 2009;34(3):345–57.
34. Ofer A, Abadi S, Nitecki S, et al. Multidetector CT angiography in the evaluation of acute mesenteric ischemia. Eur Radiol 2009;19:24–30.
35. Gupta PK, Natarajan B, Gupta H, et al. Morbidity and mortality after bowel resection for acute mesenteric ischemia. Surgery 2011;150:779–87.
36. Kougias P, Lau D, El Sayed HF, et al. Determinants of mortality and treatment outcome following surgical interventions for acute mesenteric ischemia. J Vasc Surg 2007;46:467–74.
37. Gonenc M, Dural CA, Kocatas A, et al. The impact of early diagnostic laparoscopy on the prognosis of patients with suspected acute mesenteric ischemia. Eur J Trauma Emerg Surg 2013;39(2):185–9.
38. Kozuch PL, Brandt LJ. Review article: diagnosis and management of mesenteric ischaemia with an emphasis on pharmacotherapy. Aliment Pharmacol Ther 2005; 21:201–15.
39. Frishman WH, Novak S, Brandt LJ, et al. Pharmacologic management of mesenteric occlusive disease. Cardiol Rev 2008;16:59–68.
40. Eltarawy IG, Etman YM, Zenati M, et al. Acute mesenteric ischemia: the importance of early surgical consultation. Am Surg 2009;75:212–9.
41. Ryer EJ, Kalra M, Oderich GS, et al. Revascularization for acute mesenteric ischemia. J Vasc Surg 2012;55:1682–9.
42. Sise MJ. Acute mesenteric ischemia. Surg Clin North Am 2014;94(1):165–81.
43. Mitsuyoshi A, Obama K, Shinkura N, et al. Survival in nonocclusive mesenteric ischemia: early diagnosis by multidetector row computed tomography and early treatment with continuous intravenous high-dose prostaglandin E(1). Ann Surg 2007;246:229–35.
44. Schoots IG, Koffeman GI, Legemate DA, et al. Systematic review of survival after acute mesenteric ischaemia according to disease aetiology. Br J Surg 2004;91: 17–27.
45. Beaulieu RJ, Arnaoutakis KD, Abularrage CJ, et al. Comparison of open and endovascular treatment of acute mesenteric ischemia. J Vasc Surg 2014;59: 159–64.

Acute Limb Ischemia

An Emergency Medicine Approach

Jamie R. Santistevan, MD[a,b,*]

KEYWORDS

• Acute limb ischemia • Peripheral arterial disease • Arterial thromboembolism • Arterial thrombosis • Compartment syndrome • Reperfusion injury

KEY POINTS

- Acute limb ischemia (ALI) occurs when there is sudden decrease in limb perfusion that threatens limb viability and requires urgent diagnosis and management to prevent loss of life and limb.
- If ALI is suspected based on history and physical examination, intravenous (IV) heparin should be initiated immediately and vascular surgery consulted.
- Assessment of pulses (by palpation and Doppler flow), sensation, and motor strength determines limb viability. Patients are then classified based on viability of the ischemic limb as follows: viable (stage I), marginally threatened (IIa), immediately threatened (IIb), and irreversibly damaged (III).
- Endovascular thrombolysis is most appropriate for patients with a viable or marginally threatened limb (I and IIa), acute occlusion (less than 2 weeks duration), and a history strongly suggestive of arterial or graft thrombosis.
- Surgical revascularization is preferred for patients with an immediately threatened limb (IIb), occlusion of more than 2 weeks' duration, proximal occlusion (suprainguinal), and embolic occlusion.

INTRODUCTION

Acute limb ischemia is a medical emergency with significant morbidity and mortality. The incidence is estimated to be 1.5 cases per 10,000 persons per year.[1] Rapid diagnosis is essential because timely treatment needs to be initiated to restore blood flow to the extremity. This is a time-sensitive condition, and the diagnosis is primarily

There are no commercial or financial conflicts of interest or copyright constraints to report. There are no funding sources for the author. This work has not been published elsewhere and is not under review elsewhere.

[a] Department of Emergency Medicine, University of Wisconsin School of Medicine and Public Health, 600 Highland Avenue, Madison, WI 53792, USA; [b] Emergency Department, Beloit Memorial Hospital, 1969 W Hart Road, Beloit, WI 53511, USA
* 6709 Century Avenue, #204, Middleton, WI 53562.
E-mail address: santistevanja@gmail.com

Emerg Med Clin N Am 35 (2017) 889–909
http://dx.doi.org/10.1016/j.emc.2017.07.006
emed.theclinics.com

clinical. An emergency physician must make the diagnosis and urgently involve the vascular surgeon for definitive management to prevent loss of life or limb.

DEFINITIONS

It is important for an emergency physician to distinguish between acute versus chronic limb ischemia. Chronic limb ischemia is most commonly caused by peripheral arterial disease (PAD) and gradually worsens over time, leading to progressive symptoms, known as claudication. PAD includes a broad variety of disorders that cause progressive stenosis or occlusion of arteries, most commonly atherosclerosis.[2–4]

Claudication is defined as fatigue, discomfort, or pain occurring in a specific limb muscle group during effort. Symptoms of claudication are a result of exercise-induced ischemia. Patients with claudication have sufficient blood flow to the limb so that symptoms are absent at rest. During exertion when there is increased demand for oxygen, blood flow is inadequate to meet metabolic demands, and therefore the limb suffers from muscular fatigue or pain.

Chronic ischemia from PAD can progress to the degree of causing compromised limb viability, known as critical limb ischemia (CLI). CLI is defined as limb pain that occurs at rest or impending limb loss caused by severe compromise of blood flow to the extremity.[2,5] CLI may be the result of acute or chronic ischemia and is usually caused by progressive obstructive PAD but can also be caused by embolic disease, vasculitis, and thrombosis in situ related to hypercoagulable states, popliteal entrapment, vasospasm, compartment syndrome, or trauma. Patients with CLI have resting perfusion that is inadequate to sustain metabolic demands of the distal tissue bed, causing pain at rest or loss of tissue, such as skin ulceration or gangrene.

ALI occurs when there is sudden decrease in limb perfusion that threatens limb viability, with "acute" defined as within 2 weeks of the onset of symptoms.[5] ALI can be the result of thrombotic, embolic, inflammatory, traumatic, anatomic, or iatrogenic causes. Whereas claudication reoccurs with walking set distances and abates after 2 minutes to 5 minutes of rest, acute ischemia occurs abruptly and is not relieved by rest.

Chronic ischemia induces the development of collateral blood vessels and results in skin changes secondary to progressive ischemia. Patients with preexisting occlusive PAD and claudication can also present with ALI; however, because there has been time for collateral vessels to develop, they may have milder symptoms than patients with minimal or no preexisting PAD.[2] Patients with normal underlying vasculature who develop acute ischemia have greater threat to limb viability because there has been insufficient time for new blood vessel growth to compensate for sudden loss of perfusion (**Table 1**).[1,2]

RISK FACTORS

The most common cause of PAD is atherosclerosis. Risk factors for atherosclerosis include cigarette smoking, diabetes, dyslipidemia, hypertension, family history, and hyperhomocysteinemia.[6–13]

Disorders of collagen formation and vascular inflammation (vasculitis) may also lead to PAD by causing loss of structural integrity and dilation of the arteries. Disorders of collagen formation include Marfan and Ehlers-Danlos syndromes. Vasculitis can affect any arterial bed; for example, the aorta and its first-order and second-order branches may be involved in Takayasu disease, Behçet syndrome, and relapsing polychondritis[14,15]; medium-sized vessels are the target of polyarteritis nodosa, temporal arteritis, Wegener granulomatosis, Churg-Strauss syndrome, and Kawasaki disease[16–18]; and

Table 1
Chronic versus acute limb ischemia

	Claudication	Acute Limb Ischemia
Onset of symptoms	Occurs with physical activity, gradually worsens over time	Occurs suddenly
Pain relieved with rest	Yes	No
Pathophysiology	Progressive stenosis of peripheral arteries	Sudden occlusion of a peripheral artery
Most common causes	Atherosclerosis	Thrombosis or embolism
Skin findings	Changes associated with chronic vascular disease (hair loss, shiny skin)	May be normal (embolic occlusion) or show changes of vascular disease (thrombotic occlusion)

radiation-associated arteritis can affect any size of vessels. Thromboangiitis obliterans, or Buerger disease, is an arterial obliterative and thrombotic disease that is observed in young patients who smoke—it behaves like a vasculitis and can affect arteries of all sizes.[19–21]

Prothrombotic diseases may predispose patients to limb ischemia and can be caused by abnormalities in the clotting system (eg, protein C, protein S, or antithrombin III deficiencies; factor V Leiden or prothrombin mutations; and hyperhomocysteinemia); the presence of a lupus anticoagulant or anticardiolipin antibody; and the prothrombotic state associated with malignancies, inflammatory bowel disease, and heparin-induced thrombocytopenia (HIT).[8,22,23]

Vasospastic diseases (ie, those causing pathologic vasoconstriction) may also predispose a patient to limb ischemia and can affect any muscular vessel in the body. Migraine headache, Prinzmetal angina, Raynaud syndrome, and ergot toxicity are all examples of vasospastic syndromes.[24,25] In the extremities, vasospasm may occur as a primary event (Raynaud syndrome) or secondary to an underlying disease process such as scleroderma or systemic lupus erythematosus, medications, or in the advent of trauma.

PATHOPHYSIOLOGY

CLI results when there is insufficient oxygenated blood to meet the metabolic demand of the tissues. The longer the limb is without oxygen, the greater the likelihood of cell death and irreversible damage. The tissues most sensitive to ischemia are peripheral nerves, skin, and subcutaneous tissues, followed by skeletal muscle. Animal studies have shown that cell damage results approximately 3 hours after acute ischemia, and complete cell death results by 6 hours.[26] In humans, however, the ability of a limb to tolerate ischemia varies because not all ischemic insults are complete due to the presence of preexisting collateral vessels.[27]

Traditionally, it has been taught that a patient with acute arterial occlusion has approximately 6 hours before irreversible damage occurs; however, the time frame varies depending on the presence and degree of collateral vessels.[28] Therefore, the old belief that salvage is possible if reperfusion occurs within 4 hours to 6 hours is not accurate. Patients without well-formed collateral circulation can suffer significant tissue loss at shorter time intervals.

Ischemia causes depletion of oxygen to tissues, leading to inability of cells to perform mitochondrial oxidative phosphorylation. The cell shifts energy metabolism from aerobic to anaerobic process, producing lactic acid. Progressive ischemia causes depletion of energy-rich ATP, leading to leakage of extracellular calcium into the muscle cells. This ultimately results in dysfunction and cell death. Reperfusion injury occurs on restoration of blood flow to the ischemic limb. Ischemic tissue in the limb produces oxygen free radicals. These free radicals trigger peroxidation of membrane lipids, leading to increased capillary permeability and filtration causing swelling, associated with compartment syndrome. Inflammation results and leukocyte-activated platelets cause platelet aggregation and activation of the complement system. This results in occlusion of the reperfused vessels, exhibiting the no-reflow phenomenon.[29] Byproducts of cell death are released into the systemic circulation and include potassium, phosphate, myoglobin, creatine kinase, and thromboplastin. Resulting hyperkalemia, hyperphosphatemia, metabolic acidosis, and myoglobinemia can lead to rhabdomyolysis, cardiac dysrhythmia, multiorgan failure, disseminated intravascular coagulation, and death.[30]

Etiologies of Acute Limb Ischemia

ALI arises when a rapid decrease in limb perfusion threatens tissue viability. Severity depends on location and extent of arterial obstruction and the presence of capacity of collateral arteries to perfuse the limb. Severity may also be influenced by variables of systemic perfusion, such as cardiac output and peripheral vascular resistance.[2] Acute ischemia is most often due to thrombosis within a diseased artery with thromboemboli being the second most common cause of ALI.[31]

Thrombotic limb ischemia occurs in patients with underlying PAD. Atherosclerotic plaques within the arteries cause progressive narrowing of the vessel associated with symptoms of claudication. Complete arterial obstruction can occur when a vulnerable plaque ruptures and a thrombus forms. Thrombotic occlusion is the most common cause of ALI (80%–85%).[31,32] Arterial thrombosis superimposed on a stenotic atherosclerotic plaque commonly occurs in the superficial femoral artery, although occlusion can occur anywhere from the aorta to digital arteries. Thrombosis may also occur in arterial aneurysms (particularly in the popliteal artery) and in bypass grafts, previously normal limb artery in patients with thrombophilic conditions, and secondary to compression, as seen with popliteal artery compression syndrome, or secondary to trauma, as seen with knee dislocation. Once thrombosis occurs, the thrombus tends to propagate proximally in the artery, and the resultant low-flow state of blood distal to the thrombus encourages distal thrombus propagation, which supports the rationale for systemic anticoagulation.[2]

Embolic limb ischemia is less common (14%–15%).[31,32] Most emboli are generated in the heart, with atrial fibrillation associated with two-thirds of all peripheral emboli.[33] The second most common source is a mural thrombus in the ventricle after recent myocardial infarction (MI) (20% of limb emboli).[33] These emboli form due to poor cardiac wall motion leading to stagnant blood in the cardiac chambers and clot formation. Other sources of emboli include atrial myxoma, vegetation from valve leaflets, thrombi formation on prosthetic valves, thrombi formation in the walls of arterial aneurysms, and atherosclerotic plaques in the proximal vessels. Smaller atheroemboli are produced from plaque fragmentation, resulting in obstruction of the microcirculation and ischemia to the toes and hands peripherally (blue toe syndrome). Additionally, paradoxic emboli occur when a venous clot passes from the right to the left side of the heart through a shunt, such as a patent foramen ovale (PFO) or atrial septal defect (ASD).

If an embolism affects an artery, which has not been conditioned by collaterals, the resulting ischemia is severe. Arterial embolism, therefore, is more likely than arterial thrombosis to cause severe, limb-threatening ischemia.[2,34,35] Arterial emboli typically lodge at the branch points in the arteries where the caliber decreases: 34% at the common femoral artery, 14.2% at the popliteal artery, 13.6% at the common iliac artery, and 9.1% at the aortic bifurcation.[34,36] Embolism to the aortoiliac bifurcation may produce bilateral lower limb ischemia, which has a high mortality rate and can be associated with paraplegia.[37,38]

Aortic dissection may lead to limb ischemia via propagation resulting in the false lumen extending across a branch point for an artery where the false lumen occludes blood flow to the involved artery. Traumatic vessel injury secondary to invasive catheters, intravascular balloons, surgery, and intra-arterial drug injection are other potential causes of ALI. Rare causes of arterial thrombosis include popliteal entrapment, cystic adventitial disease, and repetitive trauma.

PRESENTATION

The clinical features of ALI are colloquially known as the Six Ps: pain, pallor, paralysis, pulselessness, paresthesias, and poikilothermia.[1,2,5,39] The diagnosis cannot be excluded, however, if all of these features are absent. Additionally, patients with chronic peripheral vascular disease often have a well-developed collateral blood supply, resulting in more subtle symptoms.[28,35] Differentiation of thrombotic versus embolic cause can be difficult and is clinically impossible in 10% to 15% of cases.[40] In general, sudden-onset development of ischemic symptoms in a patient who was previously asymptomatic is most consistent with embolus, and sudden worsening symptoms in a patient with a history of chronic ischemia and claudication is more indicative of arterial thrombosis (**Table 2**).[2]

Table 2
Differentiating embolic versus thrombotic presentations of acute limb ischemia

	Embolism	Thrombosis
History		
Onset of pain	Rapid onset of symptoms	Sudden worsening of claudication symptoms
Past medical history	No known PAD history ± atrial fibrillation, recent MI, valvular disease	Known history of PAD ± coronary artery disease, cerebrovascular disease
Prior vascular surgery	Usually none	Often yes
Physical examination		
Appearance	Mottled, distinct demarcation	Bluish, no distinct demarcation
Temperature	Cold	Cool
Neurologic	Paralysis	Paresthesias
Contralateral limb	Normal	Abnormal pulse examination, hair loss, shiny skin, thickened nails
Most common cause	Cardiac thromboemboli	Plaque rupture
Most common ischemic class	Immediately threatened (IIb)	Marginally threatened (IIa)

Data from Henke PK. Contemporary management of acute limb ischemia: factors associated with amputation and in-hospital mortality. Semin Vasc Surg 2009;22:34–40; and Fukuda I, Chiyoya M, Taniguchi S, et al. Acute limb ischemia: contemporary approach. Gen Thorac Cardiovasc Surg 2015;63:540–8.

Pain is typically the first symptom of ALI, most often distal to the site of obstruction.[2,28] The pain of lower extremity ischemia is often localized to the forefoot and gradually increases in severity, progressing proximally with increased duration of ischemia, eventually extending above the ankle.[2] As ischemia progresses to the degree of neurologic damage, the pain may begin to subside.[2,39]

Numbness or paresthesias are common complaints associated with persistent limb ischemia and reflect early nerve dysfunction.[39] The anterior compartment of the lower leg is most sensitive to ischemia, and therefore patients often first complain of sensory loss over the dorsum of the foot as the earliest neurologic manifestation.[39] As ischemia progresses, anesthesia and paralysis become more prominent and are signs of impending loss of limb viability.

It is important for an emergency physician to determine whether a patient has a history of claudication or arterial interventions or arterial or aortic aneurysm and whether there is an established diagnosis of heart disease with particular reference to prior or recent MI, atrial fibrillation, PFO or ASD, or ventricular dysfunction.[2] The patient should also be evaluated for concurrent diseases and risk factors for PAD, such as hyperlipidemia, hypertension, and tobacco use.

DIAGNOSIS

Differential Diagnosis

The differential diagnosis of ALI includes conditions that mimic arterial occlusion, nonatherosclerotic causes of arterial occlusion, and differentiation of ALI secondary to thrombosis versus embolism.

Conditions that mimic arterial occlusion include low cardiac output (especially when superimposed on chronic lower extremity PAD), acute deep vein thrombosis (DVT), (especially when associated with features of phlegmasia cerulea dolens), chronic peripheral neuropathy (diabetic neuropathy), or acute compressive peripheral neuropathy (compartment syndrome).[1,2] Acute DVT and peripheral neuropathy should be distinguished from acute arterial occlusion by palpable pulses, unless chronic arterial occlusive disease or vasospasm exists. In chronic peripheral neuropathy, skin temperature is normal, which is unusual for ALI. DVT may present with cyanosis and coolness (phlegmasia cerulean dolens), and pulses may be difficult to palpate if significant edema exists. Edema does not occur, however, with acute arterial occlusion unless diagnosis is delayed and swelling begins to develop.[2] Compartment syndrome may present with cool, pale, pulseless limb and tense muscle compartments, which are absent in acute ischemia. Potential causes of nonischemic limb pain include acute gout, spontaneous venous hemorrhage, or traumatic soft tissue injury.[1,2]

Nonatherosclerotic causes of arterial occlusion include arterial trauma, vasospasm, vasculitis, hypercoagulable states, aortic dissection, and external arterial compression, such as with popliteal cyst. A history of recent arterial catheterization may suggest direct arterial trauma or arterial dissection as the cause of acute ischemia. Aortic dissection should be suspected in patients with tearing chest pain with radiation to the back and should be strongly considered in patients with unilateral or bilateral iliac occlusion.[5] Popliteal cysts and popliteal entrapment syndrome should be considered in younger patients with absent atherosclerotic risk factors.[5]

Physical examination may demonstrate skin pallor early after onset of ischemia, but over time, cyanosis develops.[2] Coolness of the painful limb when the other extremity is warm is a typical finding.[2,28,34] Patients with embolic occlusion are more likely to have a cold limb with mottled skin, whereas patients with thrombosis are more likely to have cool skin (owing to collateral blood vessels) and a bluish discoloration (indicative of chronic ischemia).[28] There may be an abrupt line of transition in temperature or color, more commonly in embolic occlusion.[28] Capillary refill is variable and dependent on environmental and interobserver factors, but in general, capillary refill is slower or absent in ALI.[2]

Some patients with sensory loss describe numbness or paresthesias. Sensory deficits may be subtle in the early phase of ALI. Light touch 2-point discrimination, vibratory perception, and proprioception are usually lost before perception of deep pain and pressure.[2] Motor deficits indicate advanced, limb-threatening ischemia. In acute ischemia, the more distal portion of the limb is affected first. More proximal muscles produce foot movement at the ankle, whereas the intrinsic muscles of the foot produce toe movement.[2] Therefore, detection of early motor weakness requires testing toe movement (eg, extension of the great toe) in comparison with the contralateral foot. Persistent pain, sensory loss, and toe muscle weakness are among the most important findings that identify a patient with threatened limb loss. Muscle rigor, tenderness, paralysis, and pain on passive movement are signs of advanced ischemia (**Box 1**).[2,5,41]

Classification

Classification of ALI by severity is important because evaluation and treatment modality depend on the degree of ischemic tissue damage and the prognosis for limb salvage. The degree of severity is determined by physical examination, specifically evaluating for sensory and motor deficits and the presence of arterial or venous flow signals using a handheld Doppler device.[41] Physical examination findings categorize patients as follows: stage I, viable; stage IIa, marginally threatened; stage IIb, immediately threatened; and stage III, irreversible (**Table 3**).[41]

Viable (I) suggests there is no immediate threat to the limb. Patients in this category have no sensory loss or muscle weakness and have audible arterial and Doppler flow. Marginally threatened (IIa) implies mild to moderate threat to limb viability, which is salvageable if revascularized soon. Patients in this category have no or minimal sensory loss (usually in the toes if present) but no muscle weakness. The arterial Doppler signals may be inaudible or weak, but venous Doppler signal is audible. Both stages I and IIa allow time for vascular imaging. In contrast; immediately threatened (IIb) suggests that the limb is salvageable only with immediate revascularization; thus, intervention should not be delayed for imaging. Patients in this category have sensory loss involving more than the toes. In addition there is mild to moderate muscle weakness. Arterial Doppler signals are usually inaudible, but venous Doppler signals are still audible. Irreversible (III) applies to patients with advanced ischemia in which there is major loss of tissue (gangrene) or permanent nerve damage. These are usually inevitable, regardless of attempts at revascularization. Patients with stage III ischemia have profound sensory loss and muscle weakness, generally with paralysis and possible rigor. Arterial and venous Doppler signals are inaudible. Patients in this category generally do not require vascular imaging and go on to have limb amputation. Revascularization, however, may be attempted in some cases to permit healing of the limb stump or to allow amputation at a more distal level.[39] A note of caution should be made regarding patients with level III ischemia. Occasionally, patients who present soon after onset of acute ischemia may have a salvageable limb if revascularization occurs immediately, that is, within 1 hour to 2 hours.[5,41] This is an exception to the rule, and most of these exceptional cases are due to embolic occlusion with dramatic onset and early presentation along with profound ischemic symptoms. Regardless of a patient's classification of severity, treatment should begin with heparin to prevent further clot extension, whereas additional evaluation and treatment decisions are made in conjunction with vascular surgery.[41]

Box 1
Important elements of the medical history and the differential diagnosis for acute limb ischemia

History of present illness

Location, timing, and onset of symptoms

Increasing or decreasing severity

Associated neurologic symptoms (numbness, tingling, and weakness)

Recent symptoms of claudication

Recent traumatic injuries or other inciting events (injections)

Other associated symptoms (swelling, redness, fevers/chills, chest pain, and shortness of breath)

Medical history

Vascular disease (coronary artery disease, peripheral arterial disease, cerebrovascular disease, vasculitis, and aortic or arterial aneurysm)

Cardiac disease (atrial fibrillation or other dysrhythmias, recent MI, valvular heart disease, PFO, or ASD)

Tobacco use

Diabetes mellitus

Hypertension

Hyperlipidemia

Clotting disorder

Prior interventions, including vascular grafts to the aorta or extremities

Differential diagnosis

Ischemic causes
- Thrombotic arterial occlusion secondary to atherosclerosis
- Embolic arterial occlusion
- Arterial trauma
- Arterial vasospasm
- Aortic dissection
- Spontaneous thrombotic occlusion secondary to hypercoagulable state
- Arterial compression secondary to compartment syndrome, phlegmasia cerulea dolens, popliteal cyst, knee dislocation

Nonischemic causes
- Deep venous thrombosis
- Neuropathy
- Acute gout
- Cellulitis
- Musculoskeletal trauma
- Spontaneous venous hemorrhage

Data from Hirsch AT, Haskal ZJ, Hertzer NR, et al. ACC/AHA 2005 Practice Guidelines for the management of patients with peripheral arterial disease (lower extremity, renal, mesenteric, and abdominal aortic): a collaborative report from the American Association for Vascular Surgery/Society for Vascular Surgery, Society for Cardiovascular Angiography and Interventions, Society for Vascular Medicine and Biology, Society of Interventional Radiology, and the ACC/AHA Task Force on Practice Guidelines (Writing Committee to Develop Guidelines for the Management of Patients With Peripheral Arterial Disease): endorsed by the American Association of Cardiovascular and Pulmonary Rehabilitation; National Heart, Lung, and Blood Institute; Society for Vascular Nursing; TransAtlantic Inter-Society Consensus; and Vascular Disease Foundation. Circulation 2006;113:e463–654; and Norgren L, Hiatt WR, Dormandy JA, et al. Inter-society consensus for the management of peripheral arterial disease (TASC II). J Vasc Surg 2007;45(Suppl S):S5–67.

Table 3
Stages of acute limb ischemia

Category	Description/Prognosis	Sensory Loss	Muscle Weakness	Arterial Doppler	Venous Doppler
Viable (I)	Not immediately threatened	None	None	Audible	Audible
Marginally threatened (IIa)	Salvageable if promptly threatened	Minimal (toes) or none	None	Often inaudible	Audible
Immediately threatened (IIb)	Salvageable with immediate revascularization	Extends beyond toes; pain at rest	Mild to moderate	Usually inaudible	Audible
Irreversible damage (III)	Major tissue loss or permanent nerve damage inevitable	Profound, anesthetic	Profound, paralysis or rigor	Inaudible	Inaudible

From Rutherford RB. Clinical staging of acute limb ischemia as the basis for choice of revascularization method: when and how to intervene. Semin Vasc Surg 2009;22:5–9.

Diagnostic Tests

Patients presenting with signs and symptoms of ALI should first undergo pulse evaluation. Often, patients have a palpable pulse in the contralateral unaffected limb and absent pulse by palpation in the affected limb. If pulses are not readily palpable, a hand-held Doppler device should be used to confirm the presence of dorsalis pedis, posterior tibial, popliteal, or femoral artery signals of the lower extremity or the radial, ulnar, brachial, or axillary artery signals in the upper extremity.[39] If arterial Doppler flow is present, then an ankle-brachial index (ABI) or wrist-brachial index (WBI) should be obtained.[1]

For the lower extremity, an ABI is the ratio of systolic blood pressure of the foot (with the cuff just above the malleolus) to the highest brachial pressure in either arm. A normal ABI is 0.91 to 1.3. A normal test excludes occlusive arterial disease.[42,43] Patients with chronic obstructive vascular disease have an ABI less than or equal to 0.9 (95% specific and 100% sensitive for lesions with $\geq$50% occlusion).[44] An ABI greater than 1.4 can be seen in patients with a noncompressible artery due to severe calcification.[3] Values from 0.4 to 0.9 represent some degree of stenosis often associated with claudication.[45] An ABI less than 0.4 represents CLI, and heparin should be initiated and vascular surgery consult should be obtained. If a patient does not have palpable pulses or audible arterial Doppler signal, then an ABI cannot be calculated, and the patient should be treated immediately with heparin and vascular surgery consult should be obtained.

Other diagnostic tests should include coagulation panel, electrolyte panel, and total creatine kinase (CK). Blood type and screen should be ordered in anticipation for surgery or thrombolysis and possible resultant bleeding complications. If concerned about acute MI resulting in embolus, then obtain ECG and troponin. ECG and cardiac monitoring may also detect dysrhythmia resulting in embolus (atrial fibrillation). Echocardiogram may identify intracardiac thrombus, valvular disease, or structural cardiac defects, such as left ventricular (LV) aneurysm or intracardiac shunts. These investigations, however, should not delay treatment of ALI.

Vascular Imaging

Clinical evaluation is the most useful tool to make the diagnosis of ALI. If suspected based on history and physical examination, a vascular surgeon should be consulted prior to performing confirmatory imaging. The time required to obtain imaging should be weighed against the urgency for revascularization, and the decision for the type of imaging should be made in conjunction with a vascular surgeon. Patients should be anticoagulated prior to imaging and monitored during imaging for progression of ischemia.

Patients with viable and marginally threatened limbs (I, IIa) can undergo further imaging studies to guide therapeutic decisions.[41] Classically, patients with an immediately threatened limb (IIb) have been taken directly to the operating room (OR); however, if imaging does not delay revascularization, it may be appropriate to obtain imaging studies prior to revascularization (**Fig. 1**).[41]

Imaging modalities include noninvasive duplex ultrasonography, multidetector helical (CT angiography), magnetic resonance angiography (MRA), and catheter-based conventional angiography. The appropriate image depends on local resources, the time required to obtain testing, and local radiologic expertise. For patients with acute on chronic ischemia, or occlusion of a prior revascularization, prior vascular imaging studies should be obtained if possible for comparison.

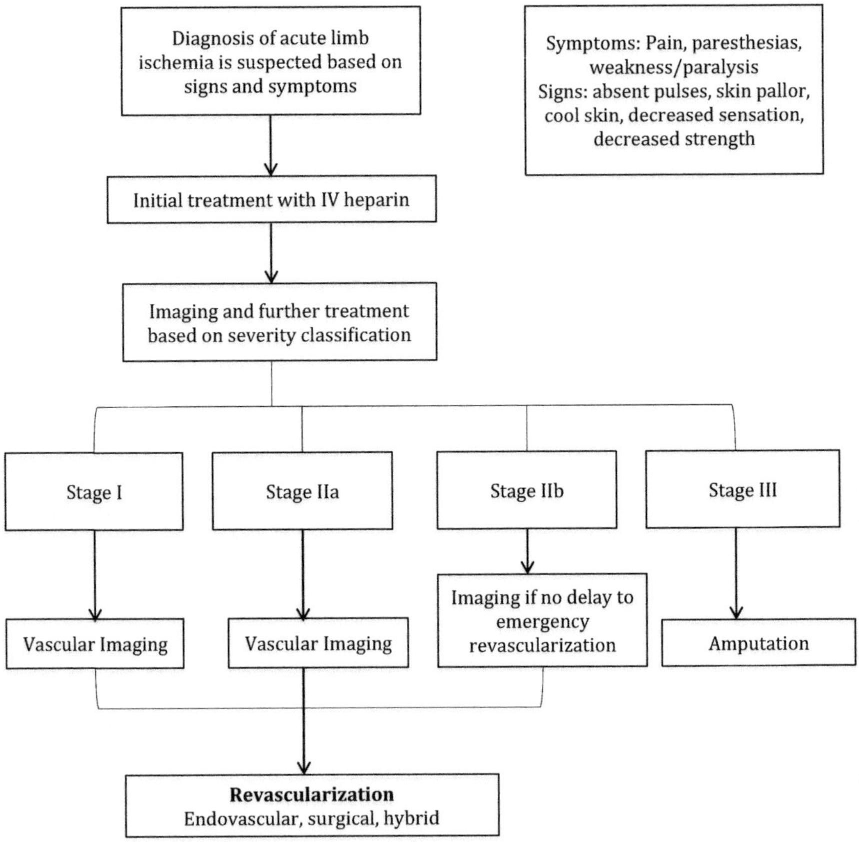

Fig. 1. Management of ALI. (*Data from* Creager MA, Kaufman JA, Conte MS. Clinical practice. Acute limb ischemia. N Engl J Med 2012;366:2198–206; and Rutherford RB. Clinical staging of acute limb ischemia as the basis for choice of revascularization method: when and how to intervene. Semin Vasc Surg 2009;22:5–9.)

Duplex ultrasound is accurate for detecting complete or incomplete obstruction in the common femoral, superficial femoral, and popliteal vessels, and in patients with previous bypass grafts. The sensitivity for ultrasound decreases when occlusion is located at or below the calf level.[46,47] For the upper extremity, duplex ultrasound has high sensitivity for detecting obstruction in the axillary, subclavian, and brachial arteries.[2,48]

Angiography is usually required for planning of surgical intervention, the gold standard of which is catheter-based, digital subtraction aortography. This has the advantage of being performed on the OR table before and during surgery. CT angiography is readily available in the emergency department and has sensitivity similar to aortography.[49] CTA for the detection of occlusion has shown excellent accuracy with sensitivities and specificities of 94% and 100%, respectively.[50] MRI has similar sensitivity and specificity but is less available and more time consuming.[51,52]

CTA has advantages compared with catheter angiography, including creation of 3-D images, which can be freely rotated in space to evaluate for other areas of stenosis and identification of collateral vessels.[49,50,53] CTA can identify atherosclerotic plaques, collateral arteries, and distal arterial patency and also images the surrounding vasculature identifying aneurysms and popliteal entrapment, which may not be detected on catheter angiography.[54] CTA can detect ALI secondary to aortic dissection.

CTA has potential advantages over MRA. Patients with pacemakers or defibrillators that are not compatible with magnetic resonance machines may be imaged safely with CTA. Scan times are significantly faster with CTA than with MRA. Claustrophobia is far less of a problem with CTA. CTA does have potential disadvantages, however, including use of iodinated contrast, which may be nephrotoxic in patients with azotemia or underlying renal disease. It also requires ionizing radiation, although radiation doses may be less than with catheter-based angiography[55] (**Fig 2**).

MANAGEMENT

Initial Management

The goals of treatment are preservation of limb and life, restoration of blood flow, and prevention of recurrent thrombosis or embolism. When the diagnosis is suspected based on history and physical examination, the patient should receive an IV heparin bolus followed by a continuous heparin infusion.[2,5,28,56] Current practice is to administer IV unfractionated heparin with 80 U/kg to 150 U/kg bolus followed by infusion of 18 U/kg/h to achieve therapeutic heparin level and activated partial thromboplastin time at 2 to 2.5 times baseline. If the patient has a known history of HIT or an antithrombin III deficiency, alternative agents, such as direct thrombin inhibitors (lepirudin or argatroban), can be used.[57] The exception to anticoagulation is patients with active bleeding. The goal of systemic anticoagulation is to prevent propagation of thrombus and to inhibit thrombosis distally in the arterial and venous systems due to low flow and stasis.[39,58] The decision to administer heparin should not be delayed while waiting for vascular surgery consultation or diagnostic imaging.

Aspirin should also be administered. The patient should be placed in dependent position to increase perfusion pressure to the limb, and the limb should be kept warm.[2] Adequate pain control is paramount, and resuscitation with IV crystalloid fluids in the hypovolemic patient is advised. It may be beneficial to use normal saline and avoid potassium-containing fluids until serum potassium levels and renal function have been determined. Hypoxic patients should receive supplemental oxygen. Patients presenting in acute heart failure and dysrhythmias should be treated promptly to improve limb perfusion.

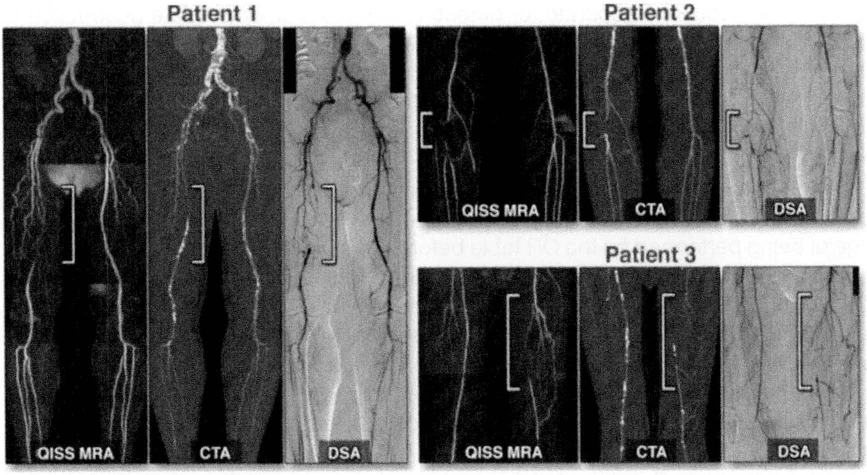

Fig. 2. Accuracy of noncontrast quiescent-interval single-shot lower-extremity MR angiography versus CT angiography for diagnosis of peripheral artery disease. representative case examples corresponding quiescent-interval single-shot MRA (QISS MRA), CTA, and digital subtraction angiography (DSA) images in 3 different patients with PAD. Patient 1 is a 75-year-old man with complete occlusion of the right superficial femoral artery (brackets). Although the massive calcification limits the evaluation of luminal stenosis with CTA, QISS-MRA provides close to identical angiographic assessment compared with DSA. Patient 2 is a 71-year-old man with right infrapopliteal occlusion (brackets) and subsequent extensive collateral circulation visualized by all 3 techniques. Patient 3 is a 63-year-old man with proximal occlusion of the left superficial femoral artery reconstituting distally via collaterals from the profunda femoral artery (brackets). (*From* Varga-Szemes A, Wichmann JL, Schoepf UJ, et al. Accuracy of noncontrast quiescent-interval single-shot lower extremity MR angiography vs CT angiography for diagnosis of peripheral artery disease: comparison with digital subtraction angiography. JACC Cardiovasc Imaging 2017. http://dx.doi.org/10.1016/j.jcmg.2016.09.030.)

Assessment of limb viability must be performed and vascular surgery consultation obtained to develop a plan for immediate revascularization. Options for reperfusion of limb ischemia include endovascular and surgical therapies. The potential for limb salvage, duration of ischemia, medical comorbidities, and arterial anatomy are critical factors in determining the method of revascularization.[2] It is important for the emergency physician to have some understanding of the methods used and the factors that may exclude certain therapies.

Endovascular Therapies

Endovascular therapy involves the use of medications (thrombolytics), mechanical devices, or both, to restore blood flow to the ischemic limb. During endovascular therapy, a guide wire is used to bypass the occlusion with a catheter, which allows for direct delivery of a thrombolytic agent into the thrombus.

Thrombolytic agents (eg, alteplase, reteplase, and tenecteplase) convert plasminogen to plasmin, which degrades the fibrin clot. These agents may be given systemically (intravenous) or locally via catheter-directed therapy. Systemic infusions of thrombolytic agents have been shown to have poor efficacy and increased adverse event rates compared with intra-arterial, catheter-directed thrombolysis.[37] As a result, catheter-directed thrombolysis has replaced systemic thrombolysis.

During catheter-directed thrombolysis, the thrombolytic agent is infused over a period of 24 hours to 48 hours.[59,60] Patients with profound ischemia who may not tolerate such a prolonged procedure are not candidates for catheter-directed thrombolysis.[61] Major bleeding occurs in 6% to 9% of patients, including intracranial hemorrhage in less than 3%.[62] Factors associated with an increased risk of bleeding include the intensity and duration of thrombolytic therapy, the presence of hypertension, patient age greater than 80 years, and thrombocytopenia.[63,64]

Endovascular thrombolysis is most appropriate for patients with a history strongly suggestive of arterial or graft thrombosis.[28] Patients with a nonviable limb (stage III), bypass graft with suspected infection, or contraindication to thrombolysis (history of intracranial hemorrhage, recent major surgery, or intracranial neoplasm or active bleeding) are not candidates for catheter-directed thrombolysis. Catheter-directed thrombolysis may have a role in treating occlusion of bypass grafts and may also be an option for poor surgical candidates or occlusion in small arteries that are not accessible with surgery.[65] Endovascular treatment with thrombolysis is also contraindicated in patients with infective endocarditis, tumor emboli, and mural or floating thrombi in the LV or left atrium.

Several percutaneous mechanical devices exist that can perform aspiration, fragmentation, and ultrasonography-assisted fibrinolysis, which can be used independently or in combination with catheter-directed thrombolysis. Data comparing these devices with pharmacologic thrombolysis alone are, however, lacking.

Surgical Intervention

Surgical approaches to ALI include thromboembolectomy with a balloon catheter, bypass surgery, and surgical adjuncts, such as endarterectomy, patch angioplasty, and intraoperative thrombolysis. Often, these techniques are used in combination to achieve restoration of blood flow.

The cause of occlusion (thrombotic vs embolic) and the individual anatomic features determine the type of surgical strategy used. Patients with thrombotic occlusion and underlying severe vascular disease often require thrombectomy followed by surgical endarterectomy. Patients with embolic occlusion may undergo surgery to expose the affected artery, followed by balloon catheter thromboembolectomy.[66] Patients with severe systemic comorbidities may not be candidates for a surgical approach.

Endovascular Versus Surgical Revascularization

Several studies have compared endovascular versus surgical approaches to revascularization of ALI. The Rochester study showed improved outcomes for catheter-directed thrombolysis compared with surgical embolectomy.[67] The STILE study[61] and the TOPAS study[32] demonstrated the same or better outcomes in the embolectomy group; however, endovascular thrombolysis is associated with higher rates of major hemorrhage compared with surgery.[68]

In general, catheter-directed thrombolysis is preferred for patients with viable or marginally threatened limb (I and IIa), recent occlusion (no more than 2 weeks duration), and thrombosis of a synthetic graft or an occluded stent.[5,69,70] Surgical intervention is preferred for patients with an immediately threatened limb (IIb) or symptoms of occlusion for more than 2 weeks. Additionally, surgery may be preferred for patients with traumatic causes of ischemia and suprainguinal occlusion (absent femoral pulse) as in the case of large embolus in the proximal common iliac artery or distal aorta.[5] The use of hybrid procedures, which combine surgical and endovascular options, can be performed in select circumstances.[71]

Long-term Management

Patients are often managed on long-term anticoagulation after endovascular or surgical intervention for ALI. The type of therapy depends on the initial cause of limb ischemia. Oral anticoagulation is indicated for patients with thrombosis of native artery associated with thrombophilia or those with cardiac embolism. These patients have traditionally been treated with warfarin. The novel oral anticoagulants (such as dabigatran or rivaroxaban) may be considered in patients with atrial fibrillation and resultant embolism; however, the efficacy of these medications for patients with peripheral-artery thrombosis is not known.

Long-term antiplatelet therapy is indicated when the cause of ALI is thrombosis superimposed on an atherosclerotic plaque to reduce the risk of MI, stroke, and vascular death.[72–74] Aspirin, in daily doses of 75 mg to 325 mg, is recommended.[2] Clopidogrel (75 mg per day) is an accepted alternative antiplatelet therapy to aspirin.[2,72] The combination of aspirin and clopidogrel may be considered in patients with atherosclerotic PAD who are not at increased bleeding risk but who are high perceived cardiovascular risk.[75,76]

COMPLICATIONS

Compartment Syndrome

Muscles in the extremities are arranged into compartments surrounded by fascia. Reperfusion of ischemic muscles can produce profound edema and increased compartmental pressure, leading to compartment syndrome; 20% of patients with ALI who undergo reperfusion develop compartment syndrome.[34]

Clinical manifestations include severe pain, tense muscle compartments, pain with passive movement, and eventually neurologic compromise (paresthesias and paralysis) followed by arterial compression (pulselessness). Capillary blood flow becomes compromised when compartmental pressures increase to within 25 mm Hg to 30 mm Hg of mean arterial pressures.[77] Fasciotomy is indicated if the delta pressure, or diastolic blood pressure minus the compartment pressure, is greater than 30 mm Hg.[78,79] Compartment syndrome most often occurs in the lower leg, which includes anterior, lateral, deep, and posterior compartments, but the thigh, buttock, and the forearm can also be affected by compartment syndrome.

Reperfusion Injury

Reperfusion results in release of products of cell death, including potassium, phosphate, and myoglobin. Metabolic abnormalities and kidney injury associated with these metabolic may require emergent treatment and the severity of these derangements depends on the extent and duration of limb ischemia. Additionally, the effects of reperfusion injury seem more pronounced in the absence of heparin anticoagulation.[80]

Hyperkalemia can cause life-threatening cardiac dysrhythmia and cardiac arrest. ECG changes associated with hyperkalemia included peaked T-waves, loss of P-waves, widening of QRS complexes, and sine wave. Hyperkalemia should be treated aggressively in the presence of ECG changes. This may include multiple modalities, including IV calcium to stabilize the cardiac membrane and IV insulin (given along with dextrose to prevent hypoglycemia), continuous nebulized albuterol, and IV sodium bicarbonate for transcellular shift.

Myoglobinemia and rhabdomyolysis manifest as elevated serum muscle enzymes (creatine kinase), red to brown urine due to myoglobinuria, and acute renal failure. Peak serum CK levels depend on the amount of muscle breakdown in the involved extremity. Aggressive saline hydration is the main therapy for rhabdomyolysis, with goal urine output of 3 mL/kg/h.

PROGNOSIS

Despite medical and surgical advances, the morbidity, mortality, and rates of limb loss from acute lower extremity ischemia remain high. Mortality rates for ALI range from 15% to 20%.[5,81] Approximately one-third of deaths related to ALI are due to metabolic complications associated with revascularization, namely acidosis and hyperkalemia.[82]

The prognosis of patients with lower extremity PAD is characterized by increased risk for cardiovascular ischemic events due to concomitant coronary artery and cerebrovascular disease.[9,83–85] Patients with atherosclerotic PAD have an annual mortality rate of 4% to 6%.[86–88] These patients have an increased risk of MI and 2-fold to 6-fold increase risk of death due to coronary artery disease events.[89–91] The 1-year mortality rate in patients with CLI is approximately 25% and may be as high as 45% in those who have undergone amputation.[92–94] Observational studies have found that the risk of death, MI, and amputation is substantially greater in those individuals with PAD who continue to smoke than in those who stop smoking.[95–97]

For patients presenting with ALI, the prognosis for the limb depends on the extent of the underlying arterial disease, the acuity of ischemia, and the rapidity of restoring perfusion. The amputation rate has been found to be proportional to the interval between onset of ischemia and reperfusion (6% if within 12 hours, 12% within 13–24 hours, and 20% after 24 hours).[98] Amputation, the majority above the knee, occurs in 10% to 15% of patients during hospitalization for CLI.[99,100]

Fasciotomy is required in up to 25% of patients.[99] Additionally, the rate of limb salvage is lower when ischemia is due to thrombosis compared to embolism.[81] For patients with chronic arterial occlusive disease who have continued progression of symptoms to CLI as demonstrated by pain at rest or gangrene, the prognosis of the limb is poor. For patients with acute occlusive events, such as sudden embolic occlusion without underlying arterial disease, the prognosis of the limb depends on the rapidity of revascularization prior to the onset of permanent muscular and nerve damage produced by ischemia.

DISPOSITION

All patients with ALI requiring surgical intervention should be admitted to the hospital or transferred to a facility with vascular surgery capabilities. Patients found to have chronic arterial disease without immediate threat to limb viability can be discharged home with follow-up with a vascular surgeon for further care. These patients should be instructed to return if they experience sudden worsening of symptoms. Other nonsurgical management of chronic obstructive arterial disease should focus on smoking cessation, exercise, and pharmacotherapy. Aspirin should be prescribed (75–100 mg daily) if there are no contraindications to reduce the risk of MI, stroke, or vascular death.[2]

SUMMARY

ALI requires prompt diagnosis by the emergency physician. If suspected based on history and physical examination, heparin should be administered and vascular surgery consulted. Patients with a viable or marginally threatened limb (I and IIa) can undergo vascular imaging. If the limb is immediately threatened (stage IIb), patients should undergo immediate revascularization, and imaging may be obtained if it does not delay revascularization. If the limb is irreversibly damaged (stage III), patients likely require amputation. The decision for endovascular thrombolysis or standard surgery depends on the etiology, duration, and location of vascular occlusion.

REFERENCES

1. Creager MA, Kaufman JA, Conte MS. Clinical practice. Acute limb ischemia. N Engl J Med 2012;366:2198–206.
2. Hirsch AT, Haskal ZJ, Hertzer NR, et al. ACC/AHA 2005 Practice Guidelines for the management of patients with peripheral arterial disease (lower extremity, renal, mesenteric, and abdominal aortic): a collaborative report from the American Association for Vascular Surgery/Society for Vascular Surgery, Society for Cardiovascular Angiography and Interventions, Society for Vascular Medicine and Biology, Society of Interventional Radiology, and the ACC/AHA Task Force on Practice Guidelines (Writing Committee to Develop Guidelines for the Management of Patients With Peripheral Arterial Disease): endorsed by the American Association of Cardiovascular and Pulmonary Rehabilitation; National Heart, Lung, and Blood Institute; Society for Vascular Nursing; TransAtlantic Inter-Society Consensus; and Vascular Disease Foundation. Circulation 2006; 113:e463–654.
3. Rooke TW, Hirsch AT, Misra S, et al. 2011 ACCF/AHA Focused Update of the Guideline for the Management of Patients With Peripheral Artery Disease (updating the 2005 guideline): a report of the American College of Cardiology Foundation/American Heart Association Task Force on Practice Guidelines. J Am Coll Cardiol 2011;58:2020–45.
4. Layden J, Michaels J, Bermingham S, et al. Diagnosis and management of lower limb peripheral arterial disease: summary of NICE guidance. BMJ 2012; 345:e4947.
5. Norgren L, Hiatt WR, Dormandy JA, et al. Inter-society consensus for the management of peripheral arterial disease (TASC II). J Vasc Surg 2007;45(Suppl S): S5–67.
6. Ross R. Cellular and molecular studies of atherogenesis. Atherosclerosis 1997; 131(Suppl):S3–4.
7. Fowkes FG, Housley E, Riemersma RA, et al. Smoking, lipids, glucose intolerance, and blood pressure as risk factors for peripheral atherosclerosis compared with ischemic heart disease in the Edinburgh Artery Study. Am J Epidemiol 1992;135:331–40.
8. Taylor LM Jr, DeFrang RD, Harris EJ Jr, et al. The association of elevated plasma homocyst(e)ine with progression of symptomatic peripheral arterial disease. J Vasc Surg 1991;13:128–36.
9. Criqui MH, Denenberg JO, Langer RD, et al. The epidemiology of peripheral arterial disease: importance of identifying the population at risk. Vasc Med 1997;2:221–6.
10. Kannel WB, McGee DL. Update on some epidemiologic features of intermittent claudication: the Framingham Study. J Am Geriatr Soc 1985;33:13–8.
11. Bowlin SJ, Medalie JH, Flocke SA, et al. Epidemiology of intermittent claudication in middle-aged men. Am J Epidemiol 1994;140:418–30.
12. Cole CW, Hill GB, Farzad E, et al. Cigarette smoking and peripheral arterial occlusive disease. Surgery 1993;114:753–6 [discussion: 6–7].

13. Powell JT, Edwards RJ, Worrell PC, et al. Risk factors associated with the development of peripheral arterial disease in smokers: a case-control study. Atherosclerosis 1997;129:41–8.
14. Johnston SL, Lock RJ, Gompels MM. Takayasu arteritis: a review. J Clin Pathol 2002;55:481–6.
15. Cid MC, Font C, Coll-Vinent B, et al. Large vessel vasculitides. Curr Opin Rheumatol 1998;10:18–28.
16. Salvarani C, Macchioni L, Olivieri I, et al. Diagnosis and management of polymyalgia rheumatica/giant cell arteritis. BioDrugs 1998;9:25–32.
17. Langford CA, Sneller MC. New developments in the treatment of Wegener's granulomatosis, polyarteritis nodosa, microscopic polyangiitis, and Churg-Strauss syndrome. Curr Opin Rheumatol 1997;9:26–30.
18. Barron KS. Kawasaki disease: etiology, pathogenesis, and treatment. Cleve Clin J Med 2002;69(Suppl 2):Sii69–78.
19. Olin JW. Thromboangiitis obliterans (Buerger's disease). N Engl J Med 2000; 343:864–9.
20. Szuba A, Cooke JP. Thromboangiitis obliterans. An update on Buerger's disease. West J Med 1998;168:255–60.
21. Aqel MB, Olin JW. Thromboangiitis obliterans (Buerger's disease). Vasc Med 1997;2:61–6.
22. Lee R. Factor V Leiden: a clinical review. Am J Med Sci 2001;322:88–102.
23. Linkins LA, Dans AL, Moores LK, et al. Treatment and prevention of heparin-induced thrombocytopenia: Antithrombotic Therapy and Prevention of Thrombosis, 9th ed: American College of Chest Physicians Evidence-Based Clinical Practice Guidelines. Chest 2012;141:e495S–530S.
24. Fraenkel L. Raynaud's phenomenon: epidemiology and risk factors. Curr Rheumatol Rep 2002;4:123–8.
25. Belch JJ, Ho M. Pharmacotherapy of Raynaud's phenomenon. Drugs 1996;52: 682–95.
26. Lindsay TF, Liauw S, Romaschin AD, et al. The effect of ischemia/reperfusion on adenine nucleotide metabolism and xanthine oxidase production in skeletal muscle. J Vasc Surg 1990;12:8–15.
27. Adiseshiah M, Round JM, Jones DA. Reperfusion injury in skeletal muscle: a prospective study in patients with acute limb ischaemia and claudicants treated by revascularization. Br J Surg 1992;79:1026–9.
28. Henke PK. Contemporary management of acute limb ischemia: factors associated with amputation and in-hospital mortality. Semin Vasc Surg 2009;22:34–40.
29. Paaske WP, Sejrsen P. Microvascular function in the peripheral vascular bed during ischaemia and oxygen-free perfusion. Eur J Vasc Endovasc Surg 1995;9:29–37.
30. Abela CB, Homer-Vanniasinkham S. Clinical implications of ischaemia-reperfusion injury. Pathophysiology 2003;9:229–40.
31. Ouriel K, Veith FJ, Sasahara AA. A comparison of recombinant urokinase with vascular surgery as initial treatment for acute arterial occlusion of the legs. Thrombolysis or Peripheral Arterial Surgery (TOPAS) Investigators. N Engl J Med 1998;338:1105–11.
32. Ouriel K, Veith FJ, Sasahara AA. Thrombolysis or peripheral arterial surgery: phase I results. TOPAS Investigators. J Vasc Surg 1996;23:64–73 [discussion: 4–5].
33. Tarnay TJ. Arterial embolism of the extremities. Experience with 62 patients. Arch Surg 1969;99:615–8.

34. Fukuda I, Chiyoya M, Taniguchi S, et al. Acute limb ischemia: contemporary approach. Gen Thorac Cardiovasc Surg 2015;63:540–8.
35. Costantini V, Lenti M. Treatment of acute occlusion of peripheral arteries. Thromb Res 2002;106:V285–94.
36. Haimovici H. Arterial embolism of the extremeities and technique of embolictomy. In: Haimovici H, editor. Vascular surgery: principle and techniques. 2nd edition. Norwalk (CT): Appleton-Century- Crofts; 1984. p. 351–78.
37. Mercer KG, Berridge DC. Saddle embolus–the need for intensive investigation and critical evaluation: a case report. Vasc Surg 2001;35:63–5.
38. Ha JW, Chung N, Chang BC, et al. Aortic saddle embolism. Clin Cardiol 1999;22:229–30.
39. Mitchell ME, Carpenter JP. Overview of acute arterial occlusion of the extremities (acute limb ischemia). UpToDate; 2016. Available at: https://www.uptodate.com/contents/overview-of-acute-arterial-occlusion-of-the-extremities-acute-limb-ischemia?source=search_result&search=acute+limb+ischemia&selectedTitle=1∼91. Accessed August 2, 2017.
40. Dormandy J, Heeck L, Vig S. Acute limb ischemia. Semin Vasc Surg 1999;12:148–53.
41. Rutherford RB. Clinical staging of acute limb ischemia as the basis for choice of revascularization method: when and how to intervene. Semin Vasc Surg 2009;22:5–9.
42. Mitchell E. Noninvasive diagnosis of arterial disease. UpToDate; 2016. Available at: https://www.uptodate.com/contents/noninvasive-diagnosis-of-arterial-disease?source=search_result&search=Noninvasive+diagnosis+of+arterial+disease.&selectedTitle=1∼150. Accessed August 2, 2017.
43. Pascarelli EF, Bertrand CA. Comparison of blood pressures in the arms and legs. N Engl J Med 1964;270:693–8.
44. Mohler ER 3rd. Peripheral arterial disease: identification and implications. Arch Intern Med 2003;163:2306–14.
45. Wolf EA Jr, Sumner DS, Strandness DE Jr. Correlation between nutritive blood flow and pressure in limbs of patients with intermittent claudication. Surg Forum 1972;23:238–9.
46. Sacks D, Robinson ML, Marinelli DL, et al. Peripheral arterial Doppler ultrasonography: diagnostic criteria. J Ultrasound Med 1992;11:95–103.
47. Allard L, Cloutier G, Durand LG, et al. Limitations of ultrasonic duplex scanning for diagnosing lower limb arterial stenoses in the presence of adjacent segment disease. J Vasc Surg 1994;19:650–7.
48. Baxter BT, Blackburn D, Payne K, et al. Noninvasive evaluation of the upper extremity. Surg Clin North Am 1990;70:87–97.
49. Tins B, Oxtoby J, Patel S. Comparison of CT angiography with conventional arterial angiography in aortoiliac occlusive disease. Br J Radiol 2001;74:219–25.
50. Rieker O, Duber C, Schmiedt W, et al. Prospective comparison of CT angiography of the legs with intraarterial digital subtraction angiography. AJR Am J Roentgenol 1996;166:269–76.
51. Baum RA, Rutter CM, Sunshine JH, et al. Multicenter trial to evaluate vascular magnetic resonance angiography of the lower extremity. American College of Radiology Rapid Technology Assessment Group. JAMA 1995;274:875–80.
52. Koelemay MJ, Lijmer JG, Stoker J, et al. Magnetic resonance angiography for the evaluation of lower extremity arterial disease: a meta-analysis. JAMA 2001;285:1338–45.

53. Ota H, Takase K, Igarashi K, et al. MDCT compared with digital subtraction angiography for assessment of lower extremity arterial occlusive disease: importance of reviewing cross-sectional images. AJR Am J Roentgenol 2004;182:201–9.
54. Beregi JP, Djabbari M, Desmoucelle F, et al. Popliteal vascular disease: evaluation with spiral CT angiography. Radiology 1997;203:477–83.
55. Rubin GD, Schmidt AJ, Logan LJ, et al. Multi-detector row CT angiography of lower extremity arterial inflow and runoff: initial experience. Radiology 2001;221:146–58.
56. Alonso-Coello P, Bellmunt S, McGorrian C, et al. Antithrombotic therapy in peripheral artery disease: antithrombotic therapy and prevention of thrombosis, 9th ed: American college of chest physicians evidence-based clinical practice guidelines. Chest 2012;141:e669S–90S.
57. Axelrod DA, Wakefield TW. Future directions in antithrombotic therapy: emphasis on venous thromboembolism. J Am Coll Surg 2001;192:641–51.
58. Jackson MR, Clagett GP. Antithrombotic therapy in peripheral arterial occlusive disease. Chest 2001;119:283s–99s.
59. Morrison HL. Catheter-directed thrombolysis for acute limb ischemia. Semin Intervent Radiol 2006;23:258–69.
60. Rajan DK, Patel NH, Valji K, et al. Quality improvement guidelines for percutaneous management of acute limb ischemia. J Vasc Interv Radiol 2005;16:585–95.
61. Weaver FA, Comerota AJ, Youngblood M, et al. Surgical revascularization versus thrombolysis for nonembolic lower extremity native artery occlusions: results of a prospective randomized trial. The STILE investigators. surgery versus thrombolysis for ischemia of the lower extremity. J Vasc Surg 1996;24:513–21 [discussion: 21–3].
62. van den Berg JC. Thrombolysis for acute arterial occlusion. J Vasc Surg 2010;52:512–5.
63. Agle SC, McNally MM, Powell CS, et al. The association of periprocedural hypertension and adverse outcomes in patients undergoing catheter-directed thrombolysis. Ann Vasc Surg 2010;24:609–14.
64. Kuoppala M, Akeson J, Svensson P, et al. Risk factors for haemorrhage during local intra-arterial thrombolysis for lower limb ischaemia. J Thromb Thrombolysis 2011;31:226–32.
65. Belkin M, Donaldson MC, Whittemore AD, et al. Observations on the use of thrombolytic agents for thrombotic occlusion of infrainguinal vein grafts. J Vasc Surg 1990;11:289–94 [discussion: 95–6].
66. Fogarty TJ, Cranley JJ, Krause RJ, et al. A method for extraction of arterial emboli and thrombi. Surg Gynecol Obstet 1963;116:241–4.
67. Ouriel K, Shortell CK, DeWeese JA, et al. A comparison of thrombolytic therapy with operative revascularization in the initial treatment of acute peripheral arterial ischemia. J Vasc Surg 1994;19:1021–30.
68. Berridge DC, Gregson RH, Hopkinson BR, et al. Randomized trial of intra-arterial recombinant tissue plasminogen activator, intravenous recombinant tissue plasminogen activator and intra-arterial streptokinase in peripheral arterial thrombolysis. Br J Surg 1991;78:988–95.
69. Kessel DO, Berridge DC, Robertson I. Infusion techniques for peripheral arterial thrombolysis. Cochrane Database Syst Rev 2004;(1):CD000985.

70. Comerota AJ, Gravett MH. Do randomized trials of thrombolysis versus open revascularization still apply to current management: what has changed? Semin Vasc Surg 2009;22:41–6.
71. Setacci C, De Donato G, Setacci F, et al. Hybrid procedures for acute limb ischemia. J Cardiovasc Surg (Torino) 2012;53:133–43.
72. CAPRIE Steering Committee. A randomised, blinded, trial of clopidogrel versus aspirin in patients at risk of ischaemic events (CAPRIE). Lancet 1996;348: 1329–39.
73. Antithrombotic Trialists' Collaboration. Collaborative meta-analysis of randomised trials of antiplatelet therapy for prevention of death, myocardial infarction, and stroke in high risk patients. BMJ 2002;324:71–86.
74. Catalano M, Born G, Peto R. Prevention of serious vascular events by aspirin amongst patients with peripheral arterial disease: randomized, double-blind trial. J Intern Med 2007;261:276–84.
75. Bhatt DL, Fox KA, Hacke W, et al. Clopidogrel and aspirin versus aspirin alone for the prevention of atherothrombotic events. N Engl J Med 2006;354:1706–17.
76. Cacoub PP, Bhatt DL, Steg PG, et al. Patients with peripheral arterial disease in the CHARISMA trial. Eur Heart J 2009;30:192–201.
77. Reneman RS, Slaaf DW, Lindbom L, et al. Muscle blood flow disturbances produced by simultaneously elevated venous and total muscle tissue pressure. Microvasc Res 1980;20:307–18.
78. McQueen MM, Court-Brown CM. Compartment monitoring in tibial fractures. The pressure threshold for decompression. J Bone Joint Surg Br 1996;78: 99–104.
79. Ovre S, Hvaal K, Holm I, et al. Compartment pressure in nailed tibial fractures. A threshold of 30 mmHg for decompression gives 29% fasciotomies. Arch Orthop Trauma Surg 1998;118:29–31.
80. Hobson RW 2nd, Neville R, Watanabe B, et al. Role of heparin in reducing skeletal muscle infarction in ischemia-reperfusion. Microcirc Endothelium Lymphatics 1989;5:259–76.
81. Kuukasjarvi P, Salenius JP. Perioperative outcome of acute lower limb ischaemia on the basis of the national vascular registry. The Finnvasc Study Group. Eur J Vasc Surg 1994;8:578–83.
82. Haimovici H. Muscular, renal, and metabolic complications of acute arterial occlusions: myonephropathic-metabolic syndrome. Surgery 1979;85:461–8.
83. Smith GD, Shipley MJ, Rose G. Intermittent claudication, heart disease risk factors, and mortality. The Whitehall Study. Circulation 1990;82:1925–31.
84. Simons PC, Algra A, Eikelboom BC, et al. Carotid artery stenosis in patients with peripheral arterial disease: the SMART study. SMART study group. J Vasc Surg 1999;30:519–25.
85. Ness J, Aronow WS. Prevalence of coexistence of coronary artery disease, ischemic stroke, and peripheral arterial disease in older persons, mean age 80 years, in an academic hospital-based geriatrics practice. J Am Geriatr Soc 1999;47:1255–6.
86. Criqui MH, Langer RD, Fronek A, et al. Mortality over a period of 10 years in patients with peripheral arterial disease. N Engl J Med 1992;326:381–6.
87. McKenna M, Wolfson S, Kuller L. The ratio of ankle and arm arterial pressure as an independent predictor of mortality. Atherosclerosis 1991;87:119–28.
88. McDermott MM, Feinglass J, Slavensky R, et al. The ankle-brachial index as a predictor of survival in patients with peripheral vascular disease. J Gen Intern Med 1994;9:445–9.

89. Leng GC, Lee AJ, Fowkes FG, et al. Incidence, natural history and cardiovascular events in symptomatic and asymptomatic peripheral arterial disease in the general population. Int J Epidemiol 1996;25:1172–81.
90. Kornitzer M, Dramaix M, Sobolski J, et al. Ankle/arm pressure index in asymptomatic middle-aged males: an independent predictor of ten-year coronary heart disease mortality. Angiology 1995;46:211–9.
91. Newman AB, Sutton-Tyrrell K, Vogt MT, et al. Morbidity and mortality in hypertensive adults with a low ankle/arm blood pressure index. JAMA 1993;270:487–9.
92. Luther M. The influence of arterial reconstructive surgery on the outcome of critical leg ischaemia. Eur J Vasc Surg 1994;8:682–9.
93. Dormandy J, Heeck L, Vig S. The fate of patients with critical leg ischemia. Semin Vasc Surg 1999;12:142–7.
94. Weitz JI, Byrne J, Clagett GP, et al. Diagnosis and treatment of chronic arterial insufficiency of the lower extremities: a critical review. Circulation 1996;94:3026–49.
95. Faulkner KW, House AK, Castleden WM. The effect of cessation of smoking on the accumulative survival rates of patients with symptomatic peripheral vascular disease. Med J Aust 1983;1:217–9.
96. Lassila R, Lepantalo M. Cigarette smoking and the outcome after lower limb arterial surgery. Acta Chir Scand 1988;154:635–40.
97. Jonason T, Bergstrom R. Cessation of smoking in patients with intermittent claudication. Effects on the risk of peripheral vascular complications, myocardial infarction and mortality. Acta Med Scand 1987;221:253–60.
98. Bergqvist D, Troeng T, Elfstrom J, et al. Auditing surgical outcome: ten years with the Swedish Vascular Registry–Swedvasc. The Steering Committee of Swedvasc. Eur J Surg Suppl 1998;(581):3–8.
99. Eliason JL, Wainess RM, Proctor MC, et al. A national and single institutional experience in the contemporary treatment of acute lower extremity ischemia. Ann Surg 2003;238:382–9 [discussion: 9–90].
100. Earnshaw JJ, Whitman B, Foy C. National audit of thrombolysis for acute leg ischemia (NATALI): clinical factors associated with early outcome. J Vasc Surg 2004;39:1018–25.

Ischemic Stroke

Advances in Diagnosis and Management

Courtney R. Cassella, MD, Andy Jagoda, MD, FACEP*

KEYWORDS

• Acute ischemic stroke • Thrombolysis • Alteplase • Thrombectomy

KEY POINTS

- Tissue plasminogen activator (tPA) (Alteplase) is an treatment approved for treatment of acute ischemic stroke for patients who meet inclusion criteria and who are treated in the appropriate setting.
- The risk of symptomatic hemorrhagic conversion in properly selected patients can be less than 2% with no increase in disability or mortality; conversely, the risk can be greater than 15% in patients with significant comorbidities.
- A decision not to use tPA in the appropriate setting is acceptable, but clinical decision-making must be well supported in the medical record.
- The earlier the treatment for acute ischemic stroke, the better the outcome.
- Exclusion criteria for tPA have been revised: minor strokes, severe strokes, age, and seizures must be placed in context of risk/benefit.

INTRODUCTION

The 3 broad categories of stroke are ischemic (87%), hemorrhagic (10%), and subarachnoid hemorrhage (3%).[1,2] The specific definition is brain, spinal cord, or retinal cell death secondary to infarction. Of ischemic strokes, 60% are thrombotic, and 40% are embolic. The brain in ischemic stroke has a core infarct area and ischemic penumbra. The penumbra represents an area that may be salvaged with prompt reperfusion. The neurologic deficit can be devastating, and stroke remains the leading cause of disability and fourth most common cause of death in the United States.[2]

In the United States, approximately 795,000 people suffer a stroke annually, 77% of which are new strokes and 23% are recurrent.[2] The lifetime risk of stroke from age 55 to 75 years is 20% in women and 15% in men.[3] Approximately 10% of patients with an

Disclosure Statement: Dr A. Jagoda is on the Executive Committee of the Brain Attack Coalition; he has indirectly received honorariums from Vindico, a medical education company, which received an educational grant from Genentech.
Mount Sinai Department of Emergency Medicine, Icahn School of Medicine at Mount Sinai, One Gustave Levy Place, Box 1620, New York, NY 10128, USA
* Corresponding author.
E-mail address: Andy.Jagoda@mssm.edu

Emerg Med Clin N Am 35 (2017) 911–930
http://dx.doi.org/10.1016/j.emc.2017.07.007
emed.theclinics.com

acute ischemic stroke (AIS) die within 1 year, and 20% to 25% of patients remain severely disabled.[4–7]

There have been advances in prevention, diagnosis, and therapy over the past 22 years since the National Institute of Neurologic Disorders and Stroke (NINDS) trial was published demonstrating a higher likelihood of having a favorable clinical outcome at 3 months when tPA (Alteplase) was administered versus placebo.[1] Since then, several other studies and data base analyses have supported the benefit of tPA within the appropriate time window,[4–7] and its use is recommended by all major societies, including the American College of Emergency Physicians, the American Stroke Association (ASA), and the American Academy of Neurology.[8–11] This review provides a summary of guideline recommendations with a primary focus on the advances in thrombolytic inclusion/exclusion criteria, diagnostic neuroimaging, and management of large vessel occlusion (LVO).

STROKE ASSESSMENT AND DIFFERENTIAL DIAGNOSIS

The assessment for stroke often starts with prehospital measures by emergency medical services (EMS). Activation of EMS is recommended by the ASA based on evidence showing activation improves door-to-needle times, and thus may be related to improved outcomes (Class I; Level B evidence, see "Applying Classification of Recommendations and Level of Evidence" at reference 12 for grading scheme[11]).[12,13] As EMS plays a crucial role in stroke timelines, the emergency physician (EP) must be aware of prehospital history, assessment tools, and interventions.

The prehospital history emphasizes time of symptom onset, history of diabetes, prior stroke, seizures, hypoglycemia, hypertension, and atrial fibrillation. Additional history aids in the assessment for tPA eligibility, including medications such as antiplatelet/anticoagulants, surgeries within the past 3 months, and head or other major trauma.

The history is performed in conjunction with assessment tools for stroke. In the prehospital setting, the 2 most commonly used tools are the Los Angeles (LAPSS)[14] and Cincinnati Prehospital Stroke Screen (CPSS)[15] (Class I; Level B evidence[11]). Both screens activate stroke notification if any point is abnormal. The LAPSS includes asymmetry of facial smile/grimace, grip, and arm strength/drift. The CPSS assesses for unilateral facial droop, unilateral arm drift, and slurred speech. Given advancements in LVO management, Perez de la Ossa and colleagues[16] developed the Rapid Arterial Occlusion Evaluation (RACE) scale as a prehospital tool to assess stroke severity and possibly identify LVO with the premise that patients identified as high risk of LVO are best transferred to a stroke center with endovascular capabilities. The RACE scale was derived from National Institutes of Health Stroke Scale (NIHSS) items that highly correlate with LVO. The scale encompasses 5 items rated in score 0 to 2, including facial palsy, arm motor function, leg motor function, head and gaze deviation, and aphasia or agnosia. In the validation study, a score of $\geq$5 showed sensitivity 0.85, specificity of 0.68, positive predictive value of 0.42, and negative predictive value of 0.94 for LVO.[16] Despite the promising data, further study is warranted to further validate scales for LVO risk stratification.[17]

Focused prehospital measures include standard ABCs, intravenous (IV) access, cardiac monitoring, and correction of hypoglycemia. Given that hypoglycemia can be a stroke mimic, fingerstick glucose should be checked by EMS (Class I; Level B evidence[11]), and if less than 60 mg/dL, the patient should be given 50 mL of 50% dextrose.

On arrival to the emergency department (ED), the EP should perform the history, physical examination, and stabilizing measures. As thrombolysis is a time-sensitive therapy, these measures should be accomplished as part of a coordinated team approach, shown in **Table 1**.[12] History should address signs and symptoms of stroke mimics, discussed in **Box 1**.

The ED stroke assessment encompasses the standardized NIHSS.[18] This scale, which ranges from 0 to 42, assists in categorizing stroke into "mild" (1–5), "moderate" (6 and 13), and "severe" (>13). Lower scores are associated with a smaller risk of hemorrhagic conversion after tPA and overall better outcomes. "Mild" strokes can still be associated with significant disability, and the score alone should not be used as the sole determinate for thrombolytic eligibility. Physical examination may localize the lesion, assisting radiology interpretation, further explored in **Table 2**. The physical examination must also evaluate for signs of head or other body trauma, signs of seizure, dysrhythmia, or stigmata of coagulopathy.

In addition to initial stabilization ensuring brain oxygenation and perfusion, blood glucose assessment and reassessment is fundamental. Diagnostic tests should include an electrocardiogram, imaging, complete blood count, basic metabolic panel, coagulation panel (prothrombin time, partial thromboplastin time, international normalized ratio), and troponin (Class I; Level C evidence[11]). Of these studies, the only result required before tPA is glucose determination. Therapy should not be delayed for coagulation or platelet studies unless there is suspected bleeding abnormality or thrombocytopenia, history of anticoagulation use, or anticoagulation use is uncertain.[11] In retrospective reviews, the rate of unsuspected coagulopathy or thrombocytopenia in ischemic stroke is very low, comprising 0.4% with unsuspected coagulopathy[19] and 0.3% with unsuspected thrombocytopenia.[20]

An essential step before tPA is neuroimaging. Door to imaging times include 25 minutes to initiation of imaging and 45 minutes to interpretation. Commonly, head noncontrast computed tomography (NCCT) is the imaging modality of choice, however MRI is an option. In the case of suspected LVO, advanced imaging using IV contrast should be performed. Additional imaging should not delay the administration of tPA if the patient is eligible (Class I; Level A evidence[11]).

Use of contrast in both MRI and CT is relatively contraindicated in patients with impaired renal function. In computed tomography (CT), contrast can cause contrast-induced nephropathy (CIN), defined as an absolute increase in serum creatinine of greater than 0.5 mg/dL or greater than 25% above baseline within 48 to 72 hours after contrast administration. In patients with no known renal disease, the risk of CIN is approximately 2% with no reported cases needing hemodialysis.[21–23] Therefore, in patients with no known renal disease, practitioners should not wait for serum creatinine measurements before scanning. Interestingly, a study by Davenport and colleagues[24] stratified patients receiving IV contrast by stable estimated glomerular filtration rate (eGFR); contrast was nephrotoxic in patients with eGFR less than

Table 1
Emergency department care timeline

Action	Time
Door to physician	≤10 min
Door to stroke team	≤15 min
Door to computed tomography (CT) initiation	≤25 min
Door to CT interpretation	≤45 min
Door to drug (≥80% compliance)	≤60 min
Door to stroke unit admission	≤3 h

Box 1
Ischemic stroke mimics

Central nervous system (CNS) abscess

CNS tumor

Drug toxicity

Hypertensive encephalopathy

Hypoglycemia/Hyperglycemia

Migraine with aura (complicated migraine)

Seizure with postictal paresis, aphasia, or neglect

Psychogenic

Wernicke encephalopathy

Head trauma

Multiple sclerosis, degenerative neurologic disorders

Intracranial hemorrhage

Systemic infection

Syncope

30 (CKD stage 4–5) and did not appear to be nephrotoxic in adults with eGFR greater than 45 (CKD stage 3A and above). In MRI, contrast in those with eGFR less than 30 is associated with gadolinium-induced nephrogenic systemic fibrosis or dermatosis.

ADVANCES IN INCLUSION AND EXCLUSION CRITERIA

The Food and Drug Administration (FDA) contraindications for tPA were largely based on the 1995 NINDS trial.[1] The derivation of the trial's inclusion and exclusion criteria arose from expert opinion, cardiac literature on thrombolysis, and basic science publications. Controversies over the tPA contraindications led to extensive research culminating in a February 2016 ASA Scientific Statement revising the inclusion and exclusion criteria for AIS (note: this is independent of the FDA-approved package insert inclusion/exclusion criteria).[25]

The benefits of tPA have been published in trials demonstrating improved rates of disability after treatment, based on disability scores.[4,6,7,26] Despite this, many patients do not receive tPA despite presenting within the treatment time window due to an exclusion criterion.[27,28] The changes in the 2016 ASA Statement address these barriers. The FDA approved tPA (Alteplase) for treatment within 3 hours from time of symptom onset, shown in **Table 3**. The extended time window to 4.5 hours is endorsed by all major societies involved in stroke care for patients meeting inclusion criteria after shared decision making on risks and benefits[8–11]; however, use beyond 3 hours is not FDA approved, see **Table 4**.

Modifications in exclusion criteria span 2 broad categories of patients: those at risk of hemorrhage and those with stroke mimics. High risk of hemorrhage includes prior stroke in the preceding 3 months, prior intracranial hemorrhage (ICH), and postsurgical patients. The data are lacking on the specific risks and time relation after these events. In the case of prior ICH, the risk likely corresponds to the volume of encephalomalacia from the previous ICH, if the stroke is in the same vascular territory, and how recently the ICH took place.[25] Nevertheless, studies have found only a handful

Table 2
Stroke syndromes

Distribution	Deficits
Anterior cerebral artery (ACA)	Paratonic rigidity, abulia: lack of initiative Contralateral motor (more commonly lower extremity) Contralateral sensory (more commonly lower extremity) Gait apraxia
Middle cerebral artery (MCA)	Homonymous hemianopia Neglect (nondominant) Aphasia: Wernicke, Broca Contralateral motor (more commonly face and upper extremity, more than lower extremity but can have frank hemiplegia) Contralateral sensory
Penetrating; also known as lacunar	Dysarthria Internal capsule: contralateral pure motor Thalamus: contralateral pure sensory Cerebellar: ipsilateral ataxia
Posterior cerebral artery (PCA)	Occipital cortex (visual): homonymous hemianopia, macula sparing, visual perseverations Cranial nerve (CN) III palsy: paresis of vertical eye movements Alexia without agraphia Cerebral peduncle, midbrain: motor, sensory, choreoathetosis Thalamus: spontaneous pain
Vertebrobasilar	Dizziness, nausea, vomiting, coma CN palsies, diplopia Dysarthria, dysphagia, hiccups Motor deficit crossed sensory deficit: ipsilateral face and contralateral body involvement Limb/gait ataxia
Anterior spinal artery	Caudal medulla (CN XII): tongue deviates ipsilateral Contralateral motor deficit Contralateral proprioception
Posterior inferior cerebellar artery (PICA)	Vertigo, vomiting, nystagmus Ipsilateral Horner syndrome: ptosis, anhidrosis, miosis CN IX-X deficit: dysphagia, hoarseness, decreased gag Contralateral limb and ipsilateral face pain, temperature Ipsilateral ataxia, dysmetria
Anterior inferior cerebellar artery (AICA)	Vertigo, vomiting, nystagmus CN VII deficit: decreased lacrimation CN V: decreased corneal reflex, ipsilateral Horner syndrome Facial motor, pain, and temperature

of patients who were given tPA with prior ICH.[29,30] For prior stroke $\leq$3 months, studies by Karlinski and colleagues[31,32] suggest no increase in symptomatic ICH (sICH) if readministering tPA. Based on these limited data, tPA is still considered potentially harmful in the cases of prior stroke and prior ICH (Class III; Level B evidence).[25] However, for prior stroke $\leq$3 months, the potential risks and benefits

Table 3
Noncontrast CT findings in acute stroke

Imaging Finding	Description
Dense middle cerebral artery (MCA)/MCA dot sign	Increased density in a major cerebral artery Dot: distal MCA branches in the sylvian fissure
Hypodensity of lentiform nucleus	Loss of definition between the putamen and globus pallidus
Insular ribbon sign	Loss of definition of the gray-white interface in the lateral margins of the insula
Loss of gray/white differentiation	Loss of distinction between gray and white matter, especially between the basal ganglia and internal capsule or insular or frontoparietal cortex and underlying white matter
Hypodensity	Cytotoxic edema and increased water content, commonly quantified by increased Hounsfield Units

of tPA should be discussed during the decision-making process (Class I; Level C evidence)[25] (**Tables 5–7**).

Patients with recent major surgery have a risk of surgical site hemorrhage after tPA. There is only Level C evidence, limited population or expert consensus, available. Reviews of off-label use of tPA include small numbers of 3-month postsurgical patients with scattered incidence of systemic hemorrhage.[33,34] Thus, for carefully selected patients at fewer than 14 days after surgery, the risk of surgical site hemorrhage should be weighed against the benefit of treatment (Class IIb; Level C evidence).[25]

Originally, seizure at the beginning of stroke onset, hypoglycemia, and hyperglycemia were exclusion criteria, as these can have presentations that mimic stroke. It is estimated that 6% to 30% of patients presenting as acute stroke are found to have a stroke mimic, and 2% to 4% of patients treated as an acute stroke with tPA have a mimic.[35–38] Fortunately these patients do well with extremely low likelihood of hemorrhage; that is, less than 0.5% (95% confidence interval [CI] 0%–2%).[36–38]

Severe, mild, and rapidly resolving stroke symptoms in the past were listed as exclusion criteria for treatment. Severe strokes, that is, NIHSS greater than 24, were historically contraindicated, as these patients often have poor outcomes and an increased risk of sICH.[39] However, studies have demonstrated that patients with severe strokes have a better functional outcome when treated with tPA.[26,40,41] Additionally, the relative increase in sICH between tPA versus placebo is the same irrespective of stroke severity.[41,42] On the other end of the spectrum, mild stroke is no longer considered an absolute contraindication for treatment in that it can still lead to significant disability, and the risk of sICH is considerably less than the 6.4% composite risk reported for all stroke types combined. For example, a patient with an NIHSS of 2 secondary to a speech deficit can be significantly impaired and consequently disabled unless treated. In one study, 28.3% of patients with mild stroke who did not receive tPA were not discharged home and 28.5% were not able to ambulate.[43] Hence, tPA is recommended based on clinical judgment of disability and not exclusively on the NIHSS. Neurology consultation and discussion of the specific deficits is recommended.

Rapidly improving stoke symptoms were also once used to exclude patients with acute stroke from treatment. However, it has been recognized that strokes can have a stuttering presentation, and there can be periods of improvement followed by rapid deterioration.[44,45] Even with rapid improvement, especially in LVO, patients

Table 4
American Heart Association (AHA) Guidelines Exclusion Criteria less than 3 hours

AHA 2013	Update AHA 2016
Significant head trauma in previous 3 mo	
Prior stroke in previous 3 mo	Removed: The potential for increased risk of symptomatic intracranial hemorrhage is not well established (Class IIB; Level B) however should be weighted against anticipated benefits (Class I; Level C)
Symptoms suggest subarachnoid hemorrhage	Subarachnoid hemorrhage
Arterial puncture at noncompressible site in previous 7 d	
History of previous intracranial hemorrhage	Removed: Warning for recent intracranial hemorrhage
History of intracranial neoplasm	Modified: Contraindicated in intra-axial intracranial neoplasm (Class III; Level C). Probably recommended in extra-axial intracranial neoplasm (Class IIA; Level C)
History of arteriovenous malformation or aneurysm	Modified: Increased risk of intracranial hemorrhage; however, may be considered in severe neurologic deficits and high likelihood of morbidity and mortality (Class IIB; Level C)
Intracranial or intraspinal surgery within 3 mo	
Elevated blood pressure (systolic >185 mm Hg or diastolic >110 mm Hg)	Current severe uncontrolled hypertension No specific values
Active internal bleeding	
Infective endocarditis	
Acute bleeding diathesis	
Platelet count <100,000 mm^3	
Heparin within 48 h with elevated activated partial thromboplastin time	
Use of direct thrombin inhibitors or direct factor Xa inhibitors with elevated laboratory tests	
Current use of anticoagulation with international normalized ratio >1.7 or prothrombin time >15 s	

ata from Jauch EC, Saver JL, Adams HP Jr, et al. Guidelines for the early management of patients vith acute ischemic stroke: a guideline for healthcare professionals from the American Heart ssociation/American Stroke Association. Stroke 2013;44(3):870–947; and Demaerschalk BM, Klein-orfer DO, Adeoye OM, et al. Scientific rationale for the inclusion and exclusion criteria for intra-enous alteplase in acute ischemic stroke: a statement for healthcare professionals from the merican Heart Association/American Stroke Association. Stroke 2016;47(2):581–641.

nay still ultimately deteriorate and have profound disability.[46] Consequently, rapidly nproving deficits are no longer an absolute exclusion; instead, the total clinical pre-entation must be placed in the context of risk for delayed progression.

DVANCES IN DIAGNOSTIC IMAGING

n AIS, neuroimaging is essential, as it may identify the etiology of stroke, location f the lesion, potential stroke mimics, or contraindications to thrombolysis. The

Table 5
American Heart Association (AHA) guidelines exclusion criteria less than 3 h

Relative Exclusion	
AHA 2013	**Update AHA 2016**
Blood glucose concentration <50 mg/dL	Removed: It is reasonable to consider tissue plasminogen activator (tPA) after glycemic management (dextrose) and neurologic reexamination within 15 min
Computed tomography demonstrates multilobar infarction (hypodensity > one-third cerebral hemisphere) AHA 2013 Class III, Level A	Removed: There is insufficient evidence to identify a threshold of hypoattenuation. However, tPA in extensive regions of clear hypoattenuation is not recommended (Class III; Level A)
Minor or rapidly improving stroke symptoms	Removed
Pregnancy	
Seizure at onset with postictal residual neurologic deficits	Removed (Class IIa; Level C)
Major surgery or serious trauma within previous 14 d	Removed: tPA may be considered with risks of bleeding weighted against severity and potential disability (Class IIb; Level C)
Gastrointestinal or urinary tract hemorrhage within previous 21 d	Gastrointestinal or urinary tract hemorrhage
Acute myocardial infarction (MI) within previous 3 mo	Modified: Reasonable if MI was non–ST-elevation MI (STEMI) (Class IIa: Level C) or STEMI involving the right or inferior myocardium (Class IIa; Level C) or STEMI involving left anterior myocardium (Class IIb; Level C)

Data from Jauch EC, Saver JL, Adams HP Jr, et al. Guidelines for the early management of patients with acute ischemic stroke: a guideline for healthcare professionals from the American Heart Association/American Stroke Association. Stroke 2013;44(3):870–947; and Demaerschalk BM, Kleindorfer DO, Adeoye OM, et al. Scientific rationale for the inclusion and exclusion criteria for intravenous alteplase in acute ischemic stroke: a statement for healthcare professionals from the American Heart Association/American Stroke Association. Stroke 2016;47(2):581–641.

2013 ASA Guidelines have a Class I recommendation for obtaining head NCCT imaging in suspected stroke.[11] NCCT offers both logistical and practical advantages as the first neuroimaging modality. Logistically, NCCT has wide availability, rapidity of imaging, and overall fewer contraindications. CT is a fast modality, with a total scan time generally less than 5 minutes, compared with MRI protocols of 10 to 15 minutes not including additional time delays secondary to scanner availability, screening for imaging safety, and ensuring scanner-compatible equipment. Other issues with MRI use include patient claustrophobia and movement artifact. Furthermore, MRI is contraindicated in patients with noncompatible pacemakers, metal implants, or foreign bodies. Practically, NCCT evaluates for stroke mimics such as intracranial mass lesions and contraindications to fibrinolysis, such as intracranial hemorrhage.

Early NCCT findings that indicate AIS include dense middle cerebral artery (MCA)[47]/MCA dot[48] sign, loss of gray and white matter differentiation,[49] insular ribbon sign,[50] hypodensity of lentiform nucleus,[51] and tissue hypodensity.[52] These are discussed in **Table 3** and **Fig. 1**.

Table 6
American Heart Association (AHA) guidelines inclusion and exclusion criteria less than 4.5 h

Inclusion	
Diagnosis of ischemic stroke causing measurable neurological deficit Onset of symptoms within 3.0–4.5 h	
Relative Exclusion	
AHA 2013	Updated AHA 2016
Aged >80 y	Removed: In >80 y tissue plasminogen activator (tPA) is safe and can be as effective as in younger patients (Class IIa, Level B)
Severe stroke (National Institutes of Health Stroke Scale >25)	
Taking an oral anticoagulant regardless of international normalized ratio (INR)	Modified: Taking oral anticoagulation with an INR <1.7 tPA appears safe and may be beneficial (Class IIa; Level B)
History of both diabetes and prior ischemic stroke	Removed: tPA may be as effective as in the 0–3-h window (Class IIb: Level B)

Data from Jauch EC, Saver JL, Adams HP Jr, et al. Guidelines for the early management of patients with acute ischemic stroke: a guideline for healthcare professionals from the American Heart Association/American Stroke Association. Stroke 2013;44(3):870–947; and Demaerschalk BM, Kleindorfer DO, Adeoye OM, et al. Scientific rationale for the inclusion and exclusion criteria for intravenous alteplase in acute ischemic stroke: a statement for healthcare professionals from the American Heart Association/American Stroke Association. Stroke 2016;47(2):581–641.

Numerous studies have been performed to correlate prognosis or probability of stroke with these findings. Of these studies, tissue hypodensity may increase the risk of hemorrhage from fibrinolysis. In particular, tissue hypodensity seen in greater than 33% of the MCA territory correlates with worse outcomes, including increased risk of hemorrhage, and consequently this finding provides a contraindication for thrombolysis.[52,53]

As there is variability in approximation of the one-third MCA rule, the Alberta Stroke Program Early CT Score (ASPECTS) was developed to better quantify early ischemic changes.[54] ASPECTS is determined based on 2 standardized NCCT axial cuts, one at the level of the thalamus and basal ganglion and one at the superior margin of the ganglionic structures; at these 2 levels there are 10 distinct regions. The score is calculated by deducting 1 point for each region that demonstrates early ischemic change such as focal swelling or hypoattenuation. Several studies have used ASPECTS in conjunction with other imaging modalities such as CT angiography (CTA), CT perfusion (CTP), or MRI to predict outcomes of stroke parameters.[55–57] ASPECT scores less than 6 are a relative contraindication to thrombectomy, discussed as follows.[58,59]

Following NCCT, additional imaging is often obtained to evaluate for large-vessel disease or ischemic penumbra. A noninvasive intracranial vascular study is required if contemplating endovascular therapy (Class I; Level A evidence).[59–64] Head CTA is a common adjunct, as the patient is already in the CT suite. CTA has benefits over MRI or Transcranial Doppler (TCD), in that it is widely available, has rapid image acquisition, and includes images of the aorta and neck vessels for endovascular planning.[65] In addition, angiography of the neck may evaluate for carotid dissection and for carotid vessel atherosclerotic disease, a stroke risk factor. MRI may be used to evaluate vasculature; however, CT has far fewer

Table 7
Endovascular therapy trials

Trial (n)	Inclusion	Outcome (Intervention vs Control)
MR CLEAN (500)	<6 h Distal ICA MCA (M1/M2) ACA (A1/A2) NIHSS ≥2	mR, 0–2 @ 90 d: 32.6% vs 19.1% NIHSS @ 24 h: 13 vs 16 NIHSS @ 5–7 d: 8 vs 14 Reperfusion, mTICI 2b/3: 58.7% No significant difference in sICH or death New ischemic CVA in new area: 5.6% vs 0.4%
EXTEND-IA (70)	<6 h Distal ICA MCA (M1/M2) Eligible for IV tPA at 4.5 h CT perfusion mR <2 Ischemic core <70 mL	mR, 0–2 @ 90 d: 71% vs 40% NIHSS @ 24 h: NIHSS @ 5–7 d: Reperfusion, mTICI 2b/3: 86% No significant difference in sICH or death
ESCAPE (316)	<12 h[a] Distal ICA MCA (M1/M2)	mR, 0–2 @ 90 d: 53% vs 29.3% NIHSS @ 24 h: 6 vs 13 NIHSS @ 5–7 d: 2 vs 8 Reperfusion, mTICI 2b/3: 72.4% No significant difference in sICH Mortality 10.4 vs 19% (*P* = .04)
SWIFT PRIME (196)	<6 h Distal ICA M1 MCA	mR, 0–2 @ 90 d: 60% vs 35% Change in NIHSS @ 27 h: −8.5 ± 7.1 vs −3.9 ± 6.2 Reperfusion, mTICI 2b/3: 88% No significant difference in sICH or death
REVASCAT (206)	<8 h[b] M1 MCA ± Distal ICA Received IV tPA <4.5 h, no revascularization after 30 min or contraindications to IV tPA mR <2, NIHSS ≥6 ASPECTS ≥7	mR, 0–2 @ 90 d: 43.7% vs 28.2% NIHSS @ 24 h: 13 vs 16 NIHSS @ 5–7 d: 8 vs 14 Reperfusion, mTICI 2b/3: 65.7% No significant difference in sICH or death

Abbreviations: ACA, anterior cerebral artery; CVA, cerebrovascular accident; ICA, internal carotid artery; IV, intravenous; MCA, middle cerebral artery; mR, modified Rankin; mTICI, modified treatment in cerebral ischemia; NIHSS, National Institutes of Health Stroke Scale; sICH, symptomatic intracranial hemorrhage; tPA, tissue plasminogen activator

[a] Only 15.5% of patients randomized greater than 6 h, not powered to assess therapy separately for this time range.

[b] Only 12.6% of patients randomized greater than 6 h.

contraindications. In addition to the contraindications listed previously in NCCT, contraindications for contrast CT or MRI include allergy to contrast or stage 4 or 5 chronic kidney disease (eGFR <30).[62]

CTP protocols were developed to identify the ischemic penumbra and hence the ideal target for reperfusion. CTP requires postprocessing technology to yield mean transit time (MTT), cerebral blood volume (CBV), and cerebral blood flow (CBF) maps. In an oversimplification, CBV indicates area of core infarct, whereas MTT and CBF delineate the potentially salvable penumbra. An example is shown in **Fig. 2**.

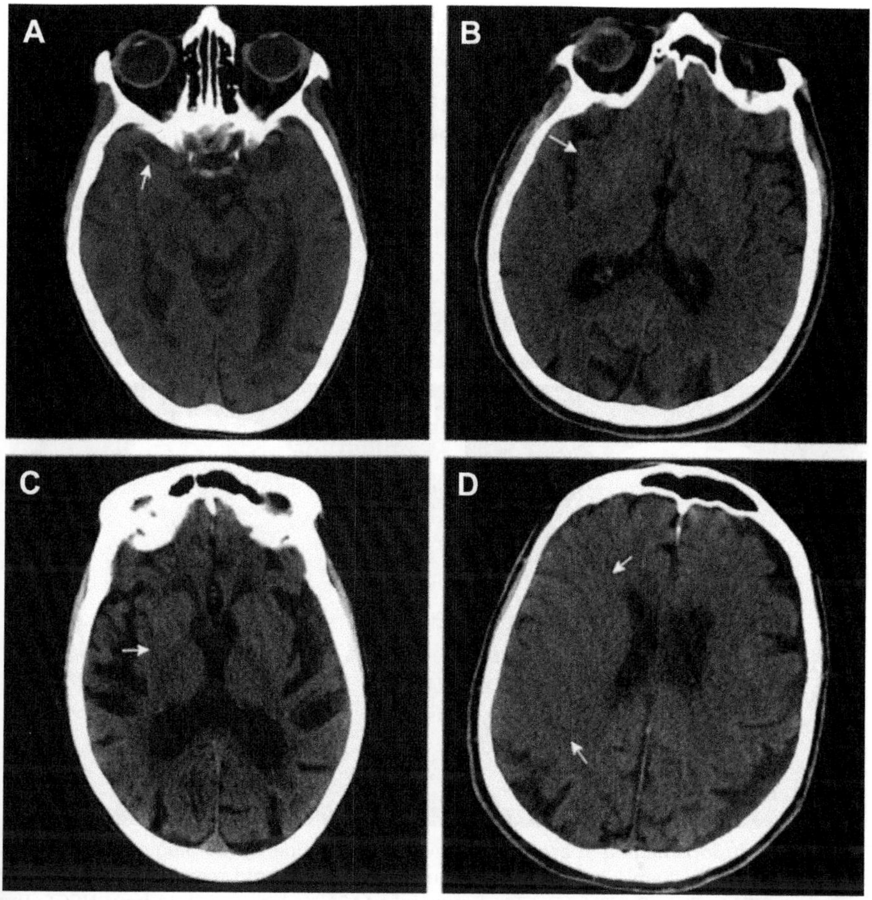

Fig. 1. Early signs (<6 hours) of cerebral infarction on noncontrast head CT. High density in the proximal MCA is thought to represent an acute thrombus lodged in the middle cerebral artery, and is referred to as the "hyperdense MCA sign" (*arrow* in *A*). The presence of edema in the distribution of the lenticulostriate arteries produces loss of the normal striated appearance of the insular cortex or "insular ribbon sign" (*arrow* in *B*) and local hypoattenuation in the basal ganglia, or "obscuration of the lentiform nuclei" (*arrow* in *C*). Loss of gray-white matter differentiation and sulcal effacement (region between the 2 *arrows* in *D*) indicate diffuse cerebral swelling and, of the described signs, carry the poorest clinical prognosis. (*From* Kunst MM, Schaefer PW. Ischemic stroke. Radiol Clin North Am 2011;49(1):126.)

CTP in conjunction with CTA can give valuable information on collateral blood flow and the ischemic penumbra to better identify candidates for reperfusion, although this is still in need of further research.[66,67] A study by Turk and colleagues[68] demonstrated that patients selected for endovascular therapy based on CTP instead of time cutoffs had similar rates of good functional outcome and sICH. The ASA suggests that CTP or MRI perfusion may have a role in reperfusion therapy beyond the window for IV fibrinolysis (Class IIB; Level B evidence).[11] Two thrombectomy trials, EXTEND-IA and SWIFT PRIME, both included CTP exclusion criteria, discussed later in this article.[61,64] Criticisms of CTP predominantly arise from limitations in brain coverage, variations in

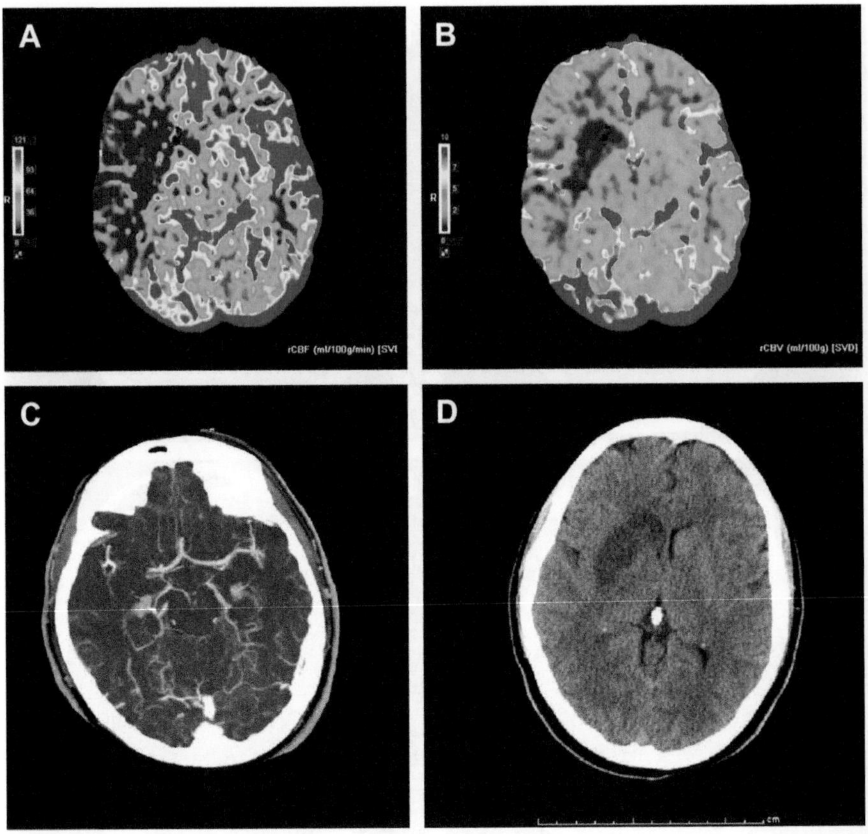

Fig. 2. CT perfusion imaging of acute left MCA infarct. Example of radiological findings in a patient with a right hemisphere stroke who underwent successful recanalization: baseline perfusion CT: (*A*) CBF, (*B*) CBV. (*C*) CTA shows right MCA occlusion; (*D*) 24-hour NCCT. The mismatch between the area of reduced CBV and the area of reduced CBF represents the penumbral zone. The infarct at 24 hours correlates with the area of reduced CBV. (*From* Kawiorski MM, Vicente A, Lourido D, et al. Good Clinical and Radiological Correlation from Standard Perfusion Computed Tomography Accurately Identifies Salvageable Tissue in Ischemic Stroke. J Stroke Cerebrovasc Dis 2016;25(5):1062–9.)

postprocessing methods, and delays in interpretation.[69] Newer-generation whole-brain CT scanners, standardization in software, and increasing experience will potentially address these concerns.

Although CT has many strengths, MRI allows better visualization of brain parenchyma if using diffuse weighted sequences. MRI diffusion has the benefit of better visualization of the posterior fossa and of characterizing small strokes that are often missed on CT, see **Fig. 3**.[70] With the increased resolution, MRI identifies cerebral microbleeds (CMBs). The cause of CMBs is unclear and may represent reperfusion injury or disrupted cerebral autoregulation.[25] Regardless, the Bleeding Risk Analysis in Stroke Imaging Before Thrombolysis (BRASIL) study found no significant difference in sICH in patients with CMBs treated with tPA versus those without CMBs.[71,72]

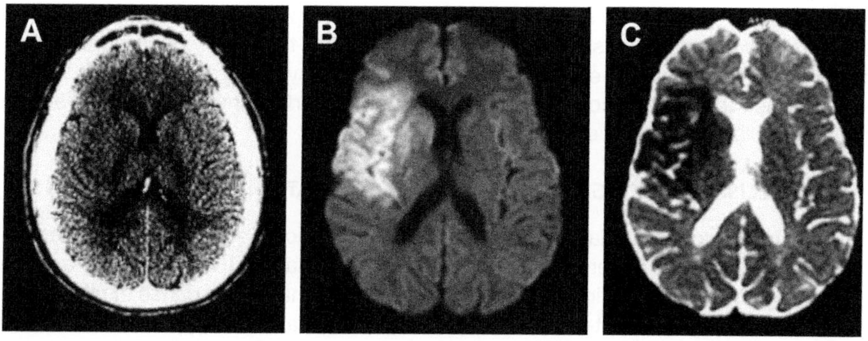

Fig. 3. (*A*) Subtle hypodensity in the right putamen and insula. Concurrent MRI diffusion-weighted (*B*) and apparent diffusion coefficient (*C*) images delineate a larger region of ischemic injury involving the right basal ganglia, insula, and frontal operculum. (*Data from* Yoo AJ, González RG. Clinical applications of diffusion MR imaging for acute ischemic stroke. Neuroimaging Clin N Am 2011;21(1):51–69, vii.)

ADVANCES IN MANAGEMENT OF LARGE VESSEL OCCLUSION

LVO is associated with high rates of morbidity and mortality secondary to the lesion itself and complications such as hemorrhage and edema. Further supporting the need for decisive management of LVO, only 25% to 30% of patients with LVO who receive tPA will recanalize.[73,74] Early studies using angioplasty, stenting, or arterial thrombolytics were promising but showed limited success.[75–81] However, 2015 was a "break-through" year for the use of new-generation stent retriever devices.

Five seminal stent retriever trials changed the landscape of LVO treatment: MR CLEAN,[60] EXTEND-IA,[61] ESCAPE,[62] REVASCAT,[63] and SWIFT PRIME.[64] Study design and characteristics were similar encompassing multicenter, prospective, randomized, open clinical trials. Providers should consider the large number of patients screened in these studies to use these interventions. Most investigated endovascular clot retrieval within a 6-hour window. ESCAPE and REVASCAT extended the interval to 12 hours and 8 hours, respectively; however, the proportions of patients after 6 hours was less than 20% and not powered to assess therapy separately for extended time points. All gave standard dosing intravenous tPA (0.9 mg/kg body-weight) if eligible. All of these studies had some CT imaging criteria to target LVO, predominantly M1 MCA or internal carotid artery (ICA) distribution, although some studies did include M2 MCA and A1/A2 anterior cerebral artery (ACA). Most of these studies used inclusion criteria of age $\geq$18 years, ASPECTS $\geq$6, CTP with core infarct less than 70 mL,[34,36] good prestroke functional status, and/or NIHSS score $\geq$6. Baseline characteristics were typically balanced between intervention and control groups, including a median NIHSS of 17 across all study participants.[56–60]

The 5 trials demonstrated endovascular (EV) therapy promoted recanalization with significant improvement in modified Rankin scores (mRS) with no increase in sICH or mortality, discussed further in **Table 6**. The number needed to treat for endovascular thrombectomy to reduce disability at least one level of mRS is 2.6.[82] Effect improved in specific groups including age older than 80 years (OR 3.68, 95% CI 1.95–6.92), more than 300 minutes after symptom onset (1.76, 1.05–2.97), and those not eligible for tPA (2.43, 1.30–4.55).[82]

Given the significant effect of EV therapy, it is recommended that stroke systems try to improve accessibility to the intervention. This is a challenge that will take time and money to meet. The stent retriever trials occurred at institutions with neuro-interventionalists or systems of care with prompt transfer capabilities. ASA recommends that patients should be transported rapidly to primary or comprehensive stroke centers (Class I; Level A evidence), and regional systems of stroke care should be developed to provide access to centers capable of performing endovascular stroke treatment (Class I; Level A evidence).[59]

SHARED DECISION MAKING AND POTENTIAL COMPLICATIONS FROM TREATMENT

sICH is a major concern related to the use of thrombolytics in AIS. Intracranial hemorrhage is classified as either symptomatic or asymptomatic. sICH is defined as new hemorrhage not seen on prior CT or suspicion of hemorrhage as a cause of neurologic deterioration. The composite risk of sICH from tPA when all stroke types are combined is 6.4% (vs 0.6% in placebo).[7,42] However, risk must be adjusted for stroke type and comorbidities; this is particularly important when engaging patients or their surrogates in the informed consent or shared decision-making (SDM) process. In this discussion, benefits including improved functional outcome and deficits should be weighed against risks, particularly sICH. The discussion should include individualized expectations including but not limited to functional status before stroke and comorbidities. The Totaled Health Risks in Vascular Events (THRIVE) score was developed as a prediction score for ischemic stroke outcomes.[83–86] The THRIVE score assigns 1 point for age 60 to 79 years, 2 points for $\geq$80 years, 2 points for NIHSS score 11 to 20, 4 points for NIHSS $\geq$21, and 1 point each for hypertension, diabetes, and atrial fibrillation. For each increasing point, the odds ratio of sICH increases 1.21.[86] A THRIVE score of 1 is correlated with a 3% incidence of sICH, whereas a THRIVE score of 7 is associated with a 15% incidence. Consequently, understanding the factors linked to risk for sICH is an important component of the SDM process.

If opting to proceed with tPA, the EP should monitor for hemorrhage and angioedema. The EP should discontinue the tPA infusion and obtain an emergency CT scan if there is a change in the patient's level of consciousness or if there is a new severe headache, change in pupil size and reactivity, new nausea and vomiting, or acute hypertension. Although poorly studied, treatments have included reversal as well as consultation for surgical decompression or hematoma evacuation.[11] Replacement of clotting factors or reversal is attempted with cryoprecipitate, fresh frozen plasma, vitamin K, platelet transfusion, recombinant factor VIIa, and aminocaproic acid. A study by Yaghi and colleagues[87] found patients with hematoma expansion had severe hypofibrinogenemia, highlighting the role of cryoprecipitate.

Angioedema, defined as swelling of the tongue, lips, or oropharynx, after intravenous tPA is estimated to occur in 1% to 5% of all patients.[88–90] This reaction is typically mild, transient, and contralateral to the ischemic hemisphere.[89] After administration of tPA, patients should be monitored for angioedema. If symptoms occur, treatment includes IV ranitidine, diphenhydramine, and methylprednisolone.[90]

SUMMARY

tPA (Alteplase) is FDA approved for the treatment of AIS. Outcomes are related to time to treatment, thus emphasizing the importance of rapid EMS activation and transport, and hospital-based stroke teams with protocols that facilitate minimizing "door-to-needle times." Prehospital assessment scales may be used to aid in stroke activation and triage to comprehensive stroke centers. Evaluation and diagnostic studies should be attained rapidly with the goal of "door-to-needle time" within 60 minutes.

Exclusion criteria for thrombolytic therapy has been revised based on analysis of outcomes from large data bases; minor stroke, severe stroke, rapidly improving stroke, advanced age, seizure, history of stroke, history of intracranial hemorrhage, and recent surgery are no longer exclusionary, and risk versus benefit must be taken into consideration. SDM is encouraged when possible. The THRIVE score may help facilitate discussions on the risk of sICH.

Advances in neuroimaging aid in the diagnosis the treatment decisions in AIS. In select patients, CTA head and neck should be performed to assess for LVO and eligibility for endovascular therapy. The ASPECT score and CT perfusion are tools to evaluate extent of infarct and can be incorporated into treatment selection. Endovascular therapy has dramatically improved outcomes from LVOs, and many of these patients are no longer condemned to a life with severe disability. The future holds tremendous promise, and continued advances in our ability to diagnose and treat patients with acute strokes can be anticipated.

REFERENCES

1. The National Institute of Neurological Disorders and Stroke rt-PA Stroke Study Group. Tissue plasminogen activator for acute ischemic stroke. N Engl J Med 1995;333(24):1581–7.
2. Writing Group M, Mozaffarian D, Benjamin EJ, et al. Executive summary: heart disease and stroke statistics–2016 update: a report from the American Heart Association. Circulation 2016;133(4):447–54.
3. Seshadri S, Beiser A, Kelly-Hayes M, et al. The lifetime risk of stroke: estimates from the Framingham Study. Stroke 2006;37(2):345–50.
4. Hacke W, Donnan G, Fieschi C, et al. Association of outcome with early stroke treatment: pooled analysis of ATLANTIS, ECASS, and NINDS rt-PA stroke trials. Lancet 2004;363(9411):768–74.
5. Wahlgren N, Ahmed N, Davalos A, et al. Thrombolysis with alteplase 3-4.5 h after acute ischaemic stroke (SITS-ISTR): an observational study. Lancet 2008; 372(9646):1303–9.
6. Hacke W, Kaste M, Bluhmki E, et al. Thrombolysis with alteplase 3 to 4.5 hours after acute ischemic stroke. N Engl J Med 2008;359(13):1317–29.
7. Wahlgren N, Ahmed N, Davalos A, et al. Thrombolysis with alteplase for acute ischaemic stroke in the Safe Implementation of Thrombolysis in Stroke-Monitoring Study (SITS-MOST): an observational study. Lancet 2007;369(9558):275–82.
8. American College of Emergency Physicians Clinical Policies Subcommittee on Use of Intravenous t PAfIS, Brown MD, Burton JH, Nazarian DJ, et al. Clinical policy: use of intravenous tissue plasminogen activator for the management of acute ischemic stroke in the Emergency Department. Ann Emerg Med 2015;66(3): 322–33.e331.
9. European Stroke Organisation Executive Committee, ESO Writing Committee. Guidelines for management of ischaemic stroke and transient ischaemic attack 2008. Cerebrovasc Dis 2008;25(5):457–507.
10. Holmes M, Davis S, Simpson E. Alteplase for the treatment of acute ischaemic stroke: a NICE single technology appraisal; an evidence review group perspective. Pharmacoeconomics 2015;33(3):225–33.
11. Jauch EC, Saver JL, Adams HP Jr, et al. Guidelines for the early management of patients with acute ischemic stroke: a guideline for healthcare professionals from the American Heart Association/American Stroke Association. Stroke 2013;44(3): 870–947.
12. Abdullah AR, Smith EE, Biddinger PD, et al. Advance hospital notification by EMS in acute stroke is associated with shorter door-to-computed tomography time and

increased likelihood of administration of tissue-plasminogen activator. Prehosp Emerg Care 2008;12(4):426–31.
13. McKinney JS, Mylavarapu K, Lane J, et al. Hospital prenotification of stroke patients by emergency medical services improves stroke time targets. J Stroke Cerebrovasc Dis 2013;22(2):113–8.
14. Kidwell CS, Starkman S, Eckstein M, et al. Identifying stroke in the field. Prospective validation of the Los Angeles prehospital stroke screen (LAPSS). Stroke 2000;31(1):71–6.
15. Kothari RU, Pancioli A, Liu T, et al. Cincinnati Prehospital Stroke Scale: reproducibility and validity. Ann Emerg Med 1999;33(4):373–8.
16. Perez de la Ossa N, Carrera D, Gorchs M, et al. Design and validation of a prehospital stroke scale to predict large arterial occlusion: the rapid arterial occlusion evaluation scale. Stroke 2014;45(1):87–91.
17. Turc G, Maier B, Naggara O, et al. Clinical scales do not reliably identify acute ischemic stroke patients with large-artery occlusion. Stroke 2016;47(6):1466–72.
18. Brott T, Adams HP Jr, Olinger CP, et al. Measurements of acute cerebral infarction: a clinical examination scale. Stroke 1989;20(7):864–70.
19. Rost NS, Masrur S, Pervez MA, et al. Unsuspected coagulopathy rarely prevents IV thrombolysis in acute ischemic stroke. Neurology 2009;73(23):1957–62.
20. Cucchiara BL, Jackson B, Weiner M, et al. Usefulness of checking platelet count before thrombolysis in acute ischemic stroke. Stroke 2007;38(5):1639–40.
21. Dittrich R, Akdeniz S, Kloska SP, et al. Low rate of contrast-induced nephropathy after CT perfusion and CT angiography in acute stroke patients. J Neurol 2007; 254(11):1491–7.
22. Hopyan JJ, Gladstone DJ, Mallia G, et al. Renal safety of CT angiography and perfusion imaging in the emergency evaluation of acute stroke. AJNR Am J Neuroradiol 2008;29(10):1826–30.
23. Krol AL, Dzialowski I, Roy J, et al. Incidence of radiocontrast nephropathy in patients undergoing acute stroke computed tomography angiography. Stroke 2007; 38(8):2364–6.
24. Davenport MS, Khalatbari S, Cohan RH, et al. Contrast material-induced nephrotoxicity and intravenous low-osmolality iodinated contrast material: risk stratification by using estimated glomerular filtration rate. Radiology 2013;268(3):719–28.
25. Demaerschalk BM, Kleindorfer DO, Adeoye OM, et al. Scientific rationale for the inclusion and exclusion criteria for intravenous alteplase in acute ischemic stroke: a statement for healthcare professionals from the American Heart Association/American Stroke Association. Stroke 2016;47(2):581–641.
26. IST-3 collaborative group, Sandercock P, Wardlaw JM, Lindley RI, et al. The benefits and harms of intravenous thrombolysis with recombinant tissue plasminogen activator within 6 h of acute ischaemic stroke (the third international stroke trial [IST-3]): a randomised controlled trial. Lancet 2012;379(9834):2352–63.
27. Kothari R, Jauch E, Broderick J, et al. Acute stroke: delays to presentation and emergency department evaluation. Ann Emerg Med 1999;33(1):3–8.
28. de Los Rios la Rosa F, Khoury J, Kissela BM, et al. Eligibility for intravenous recombinant tissue-type plasminogen activator within a population: the effect of the European Cooperative Acute Stroke Study (ECASS) III Trial. Stroke 2012; 43(6):1591–5.
29. Aleu A, Mellado P, Lichy C, et al. Hemorrhagic complications after off-label thrombolysis for ischemic stroke. Stroke 2007;38(2):417–22.

30. Matz K, Brainin M. Use of intravenous recombinant tissue plasminogen activator in patients outside the defined criteria: safety and feasibility issues. Expert Rev Neurother 2013;13(2):177–85.
31. Karlinski M, Kobayashi A, Czlonkowska A, et al. Intravenous thrombolysis for stroke recurring within 3 months from the previous event. Stroke 2015;46(11): 3184–9.
32. Karlinski M, Kobayashi A, Mikulik R, et al. Intravenous alteplase in ischemic stroke patients not fully adhering to the current drug license in Central and Eastern Europe. Int J Stroke 2012;7(8):615–22.
33. Guillan M, Alonso-Canovas A, Garcia-Caldentey J, et al. Off-label intravenous thrombolysis in acute stroke. Eur J Neurol 2012;19(3):390–4.
34. Meretoja A, Putaala J, Tatlisumak T, et al. Off-label thrombolysis is not associated with poor outcome in patients with stroke. Stroke 2010;41(7):1450–8.
35. Merino JG, Luby M, Benson RT, et al. Predictors of acute stroke mimics in 8187 patients referred to a stroke service. J Stroke Cerebrovasc Dis 2013;22(8): e397–403.
36. Chernyshev OY, Martin-Schild S, Albright KC, et al. Safety of tPA in stroke mimics and neuroimaging-negative cerebral ischemia. Neurology 2010;74(17):1340–5.
37. Tsivgoulis G, Alexandrov AV, Chang J, et al. Safety and outcomes of intravenous thrombolysis in stroke mimics: a 6-year, single-care center study and a pooled analysis of reported series. Stroke 2011;42(6):1771–4.
38. Tsivgoulis G, Zand R, Katsanos AH, et al. Safety of intravenous thrombolysis in stroke mimics: prospective 5-year study and comprehensive meta-analysis. Stroke 2015;46(5):1281–7.
39. Demchuk AM, Tanne D, Hill MD, et al. Predictors of good outcome after intravenous tPA for acute ischemic stroke. Neurology 2001;57(3):474–80.
40. Generalized efficacy of t-PA for acute stroke. Subgroup analysis of the NINDS t-PA Stroke Trial. Stroke 1997;28(11):2119–25.
41. Emberson J, Lees KR, Lyden P, et al. Effect of treatment delay, age, and stroke severity on the effects of intravenous thrombolysis with alteplase for acute ischaemic stroke: a meta-analysis of individual patient data from randomised trials. Lancet 2014;384(9958):1929–35.
42. Whiteley WN, Emberson J, Lees KR, et al. Risk of intracerebral haemorrhage with alteplase after acute ischaemic stroke: a secondary analysis of an individual patient data meta-analysis. Lancet Neurol 2016;15(9):925–33.
43. Smith EE, Fonarow GC, Reeves MJ, et al. Outcomes in mild or rapidly improving stroke not treated with intravenous recombinant tissue-type plasminogen activator: findings from get with the guidelines-stroke. Stroke 2011;42(11):3110–5.
44. Alexandrov AV, Felberg RA, Demchuk AM, et al. Deterioration following spontaneous improvement: sonographic findings in patients with acutely resolving symptoms of cerebral ischemia. Stroke 2000;31(4):915–9.
45. Muengtaweepongsa S, Singh NN, Cruz-Flores S. Pontine warning syndrome: case series and review of literature. J Stroke Cerebrovasc Dis 2010;19(5):353–6.
46. Nedeltchev K, Schwegler B, Haefeli T, et al. Outcome of stroke with mild or rapidly improving symptoms. Stroke 2007;38(9):2531–5.
47. Pressman BD, Tourje EJ, Thompson JR. An early CT sign of ischemic infarction: increased density in a cerebral artery. AJR Am J Roentgenol 1987;149(3):583–6.
48. Barber PA, Demchuk AM, Hudon ME, et al. Hyperdense sylvian fissure MCA "dot" sign: A CT marker of acute ischemia. Stroke 2001;32(1):84–8.

49. Dubey N, Bakshi R, Wasay M, et al. Early computed tomography hypodensity predicts hemorrhage after intravenous tissue plasminogen activator in acute ischemic stroke. J Neuroimaging 2001;11(2):184–8.
50. Truwit CL, Barkovich AJ, Gean-Marton A, et al. Loss of the insular ribbon: another early CT sign of acute middle cerebral artery infarction. Radiology 1990;176(3):801–6.
51. Tomura N, Uemura K, Inugami A, et al. Early CT finding in cerebral infarction: obscuration of the lentiform nucleus. Radiology 1988;168(2):463–7.
52. Marks MP, Holmgren EB, Fox AJ, et al. Evaluation of early computed tomographic findings in acute ischemic stroke. Stroke 1999;30(2):389–92.
53. von Kummer R, Meyding-Lamade U, Forsting M, et al. Sensitivity and prognostic value of early CT in occlusion of the middle cerebral artery trunk. AJNR Am J Neuroradiol 1994;15(1):9–15 [discussion: 16–8].
54. Pexman JH, Barber PA, Hill MD, et al. Use of the Alberta Stroke Program Early CT Score (ASPECTS) for assessing CT scans in patients with acute stroke. AJNR Am J Neuroradiol 2001;22(8):1534–42.
55. Haussen DC, Dehkharghani S, Rangaraju S, et al. Automated CT perfusion ischemic core volume and noncontrast CT ASPECTS: correlation and clinical outcome prediction in large vessel stroke. Stroke 2016;47:2318–22.
56. Kawiorski MM, Martinez-Sanchez P, Garcia-Pastor A, et al. Alberta Stroke Program Early CT Score applied to CT angiography source images is a strong predictor of futile recanalization in acute ischemic stroke. Neuroradiology 2016;58(5):487–93.
57. McTaggart RA, Jovin TG, Lansberg MG, et al. Alberta stroke program early computed tomographic scoring performance in a series of patients undergoing computed tomography and MRI: reader agreement, modality agreement, and outcome prediction. Stroke 2015;46(2):407–12.
58. Yoo AJ, Berkhemer OA, Fransen PS, et al. Effect of baseline Alberta Stroke Program Early CT Score on safety and efficacy of intra-arterial treatment: a subgroup analysis of a randomised phase 3 trial (MR CLEAN). Lancet Neurol 2016;15(7):685–94.
59. Powers WJ, Derdeyn CP, Biller J, et al. 2015 American Heart Association/American Stroke Association focused update of the 2013 guidelines for the early management of patients with acute ischemic stroke regarding endovascular treatment: a guideline for healthcare professionals from the American Heart Association/American Stroke Association. Stroke 2015;46(10):3020–35.
60. Berkhemer OA, Fransen PS, Beumer D, et al. A randomized trial of intraarterial treatment for acute ischemic stroke. N Engl J Med 2015;372(1):11–20.
61. Campbell BC, Mitchell PJ, Kleinig TJ, et al. Endovascular therapy for ischemic stroke with perfusion-imaging selection. N Engl J Med 2015;372(11):1009–18.
62. Goyal M, Demchuk AM, Menon BK, et al. Randomized assessment of rapid endovascular treatment of ischemic stroke. N Engl J Med 2015;372(11):1019–30.
63. Jovin TG, Chamorro A, Cobo E, et al. Thrombectomy within 8 hours after symptom onset in ischemic stroke. N Engl J Med 2015;372(24):2296–306.
64. Saver JL, Goyal M, Bonafe A, et al. Stent-retriever thrombectomy after intravenous t-PA vs. t-PA alone in stroke. N Engl J Med 2015;372(24):2285–95.
65. Demchuk AM, Menon BK, Goyal M. Comparing vessel imaging: noncontrast computed tomography/computed tomographic angiography should be the new minimum standard in acute disabling stroke. Stroke 2016;47(1):273–81.

66. Vagal A, Menon BK, Foster LD, et al. Association between CT angiogram collaterals and CT perfusion in the interventional management of stroke III trial. Stroke 2016;47(2):535–8.
67. van Seeters T, Biessels GJ, Kappelle LJ, et al. The prognostic value of CT angiography and CT perfusion in acute ischemic stroke. Cerebrovasc Dis 2015;40(5–6):258–69.
68. Turk AS, Magarick JA, Frei D, et al. CT perfusion-guided patient selection for endovascular recanalization in acute ischemic stroke: a multicenter study. J Neurointerv Surg 2013;5(6):523–7.
69. Goyal M, Menon BK, Derdeyn CP. Perfusion imaging in acute ischemic stroke: let us improve the science before changing clinical practice. Radiology 2013;266(1):16–21.
70. Leslie-Mazwi TM, Hirsch JA, Falcone GJ, et al. Endovascular stroke treatment outcomes after patient selection based on magnetic resonance imaging and clinical criteria. JAMA Neurol 2016;73(1):43–9.
71. Fiehler J, Albers GW, Boulanger JM, et al. Bleeding Risk Analysis in Stroke Imaging before thromboLysis (BRASIL): pooled analysis of T2*-weighted magnetic resonance imaging data from 570 patients. Stroke 2007;38(10):2738–44.
72. Mettler FA Jr, Huda W, Yoshizumi TT, et al. Effective doses in radiology and diagnostic nuclear medicine: a catalog. Radiology 2008;248(1):254–63.
73. Alexandrov AV, Grotta JC. Arterial reocclusion in stroke patients treated with intravenous tissue plasminogen activator. Neurology 2002;59(6):862–7.
74. Saqqur M, Molina CA, Salam A, et al. Clinical deterioration after intravenous recombinant tissue plasminogen activator treatment: a multicenter transcranial Doppler study. Stroke 2007;38(1):69–74.
75. Dotter CT, Judkins MP. Transluminal treatment of arteriosclerotic obstruction. description of a new technic and a preliminary report of its application. Circulation 1964;30:654–70.
76. Levy EI, Ecker RD, Hanel RA, et al. Acute M2 bifurcation stenting for cerebral infarction: lessons learned from the heart: technical case report. Neurosurgery 2006;58(3):E588 [discussion: E588].
77. Levy EI, Siddiqui AH, Crumlish A, et al. First Food and Drug Administration-approved prospective trial of primary intracranial stenting for acute stroke: SARIS (stent-assisted recanalization in acute ischemic stroke). Stroke 2009;40(11):3552–6.
78. Kelly ME, Furlan AJ, Fiorella D. Recanalization of an acute middle cerebral artery occlusion using a self-expanding, reconstrainable, intracranial microstent as a temporary endovascular bypass. Stroke 2008;39(6):1770–3.
79. Ciccone A, Valvassori L, SYNTHESIS Expansion Investigators. Endovascular treatment for acute ischemic stroke. N Engl J Med 2013;368(25):2433–4.
80. Broderick JP, Palesch YY, Demchuk AM, et al. Endovascular therapy after intravenous t-PA versus t-PA alone for stroke. N Engl J Med 2013;368(10):893–903.
81. Kidwell CS, Jahan R, Gornbein J, et al. A trial of imaging selection and endovascular treatment for ischemic stroke. N Engl J Med 2013;368(10):914–23.
82. Goyal M, Menon BK, van Zwam WH, et al. Endovascular thrombectomy after large-vessel ischaemic stroke: a meta-analysis of individual patient data from five randomised trials. Lancet 2016;387(10029):1723–31.
83. Flint AC, Kamel H, Rao VA, et al. Validation of the Totaled Health Risks In Vascular Events (THRIVE) score for outcome prediction in endovascular stroke treatment. Int J Stroke 2014;9(1):32–9.

84. Kamel H, Patel N, Rao VA, et al. The totaled health risks in vascular events (THRIVE) score predicts ischemic stroke outcomes independent of thrombolytic therapy in the NINDS tPA trial. J Stroke Cerebrovasc Dis 2013;22(7):1111–6.
85. Flint AC, Faigeles BS, Cullen SP, et al. THRIVE score predicts ischemic stroke outcomes and thrombolytic hemorrhage risk in VISTA. Stroke 2013;44(12):3365–9.
86. Flint AC, Gupta R, Smith WS, et al. The THRIVE score predicts symptomatic intracerebral hemorrhage after intravenous tPA administration in SITS-MOST. Int J Stroke 2014;9(6):705–10.
87. Yaghi S, Boehme AK, Dibu J, et al. Treatment and outcome of thrombolysis-related hemorrhage: a multicenter retrospective study. JAMA Neurol 2015;72(12):1451–7.
88. Hill MD, Buchan AM, Canadian Alteplase for Stroke Effectiveness Study Investigators. Thrombolysis for acute ischemic stroke: results of the Canadian Alteplase for Stroke Effectiveness Study. CMAJ 2005;172(10):1307–12.
89. Hill MD, Lye T, Moss H, et al. Hemi-orolingual angioedema and ACE inhibition after alteplase treatment of stroke. Neurology 2003;60(9):1525–7.
90. Hill MD, Barber PA, Takahashi J, et al. Anaphylactoid reactions and angioedema during alteplase treatment of acute ischemic stroke. CMAJ 2000;162(9):1281–4

UNITED STATES POSTAL SERVICE®

Statement of Ownership, Management, and Circulation (All Periodicals Publications Except Requester Publications)

1. Publication Title	2. Publication Number	3. Filing Date
EMERGENCY MEDICINE CLINICS OF NORTH AMERICA	000 – 714	9/18/2017
4. Issue Frequency	5. Number of Issues Published Annually	6. Annual Subscription Price
FEB, MAY, AUG, NOV	4	$323.00

7. Complete Mailing Address of Known Office of Publication (*Not printer*) (*Street, city, county, state, and ZIP+4®*)
ELSEVIER INC.
230 Park Avenue, Suite 800
New York, NY 10169

Contact Person
STEPHEN R. BUSHING
Telephone (*Include area code*)
215-239-3688

8. Complete Mailing Address of Headquarters or General Business Office of Publisher (*Not printer*)
ELSEVIER INC.
230 Park Avenue, Suite 800
New York, NY 10169

9. Full Names and Complete Mailing Addresses of Publisher, Editor, and Managing Editor (*Do not leave blank*)

Publisher (*Name and complete mailing address*)
ADRIANNE BRIGIDO, ELSEVIER INC.
1600 JOHN F KENNEDY BLVD. SUITE 1800
PHILADELPHIA, PA 19103-2899

Editor (*Name and complete mailing address*)
PATRICK MANLEY, ELSEVIER INC.
1600 JOHN F KENNEDY BLVD. SUITE 1800
PHILADELPHIA, PA 19103-2899

Managing Editor (*Name and complete mailing address*)
PATRICK MANLEY, ELSEVIER INC.
1600 JOHN F KENNEDY BLVD. SUITE 1800
PHILADELPHIA, PA 19103-2899

10. Owner (*Do not leave blank. If the publication is owned by a corporation, give the name and address of the corporation immediately followed by the names and addresses of all stockholders owning or holding 1 percent or more of the total amount of stock. If not owned by a corporation, give the names and addresses of the individual owners. If owned by a partnership or other unincorporated firm, give its name and address as well as those of each individual owner. If the publication is published by a nonprofit organization, give its name and address.*)

Full Name	Complete Mailing Address
WHOLLY OWNED SUBSIDIARY OF REED/ELSEVIER, US HOLDINGS	1600 JOHN F KENNEDY BLVD. SUITE 1800 PHILADELPHIA, PA 19103-2899

11. Known Bondholders, Mortgagees, and Other Security Holders Owning or Holding 1 Percent or More of Total Amount of Bonds, Mortgages, or Other Securities. If none, check box ☐ None

Full Name	Complete Mailing Address
N/A	

12. Tax Status (*For completion by nonprofit organizations authorized to mail at nonprofit rates*) (*Check one*)
The purpose, function, and nonprofit status of this organization and the exempt status for federal income tax purposes:
☒ Has Not Changed During Preceding 12 Months
☐ Has Changed During Preceding 12 Months (*Publisher must submit explanation of change with this statement*)

13. Publication Title	14. Issue Date for Circulation Data Below
EMERGENCY MEDICINE CLINICS OF NORTH AMERICA	FEBRUARY 2017

PS Form **3526**, July 2014 *[Page 1 of 4 (see instructions page 4)]* PSN: 7530-01-000-9931 **PRIVACY NOTICE:** See our privacy policy on *www.usps.com.*

15. Extent and Nature of Circulation			Average No. Copies Each Issue During Preceding 12 Months	No. Copies of Single Issue Published Nearest to Filing Date
a. Total Number of Copies (*Net press run*)			522	500
b. Paid Circulation (*By Mail and Outside the Mail*)	(1)	Mailed Outside-County Paid Subscriptions Stated on PS Form 3541 (Include paid distribution above nominal rate, advertiser's proof copies, and exchange copies)	257	248
	(2)	Mailed In-County Paid Subscriptions Stated on PS Form 3541 (*Include paid distribution above nominal rate, advertiser's proof copies, and exchange copies*)	0	0
	(3)	Paid Distribution Outside the Mails Including Sales Through Dealers and Carriers, Street Vendors, Counter Sales, and Other Paid Distribution Outside USPS®	95	62
	(4)	Paid Distribution by Other Classes of Mail Through the USPS (e.g., First-Class Mail®)	0	0
c. Total Paid Distribution [*Sum of 15b (1), (2), (3), and (4)*] ▶			352	310
d. Free or Nominal Rate Distribution (*By Mail and Outside the Mail*)	(1)	Free or Nominal Rate Outside-County Copies included on PS Form 3541	74	75
	(2)	Free or Nominal Rate In-County Copies Included on PS Form 3541	0	0
	(3)	Free or Nominal Rate Copies Mailed at Other Classes Through the USPS (e.g., First-Class Mail)	0	0
	(4)	Free or Nominal Rate Distribution Outside the Mail (*Carriers or other means*)	0	0
e. Total Free or Nominal Rate Distribution (*Sum of 15d (1), (2), (3) and (4)*)			74	75
f. Total Distribution (*Sum of 15c and 15e*) ▶			426	385
g. Copies not Distributed (*See Instructions to Publishers #4 (page #3)*) ▶			96	115
h. Total (*Sum of 15f and g*)			522	500
i. Percent Paid (*15c divided by 15f times 100*) ▶			82.63%	80.52%

* If you are claiming electronic copies, go to line 16 on page 3. If you are not claiming electronic copies, skip to line 17 on page 3.

16. Electronic Copy Circulation	Average No. Copies Each Issue During Preceding 12 Months	No. Copies of Single Issue Published Nearest to Filing Date
a. Paid Electronic Copies ▶	0	0
b. Total Paid Print Copies (Line 15c) + Paid Electronic Copies (Line 16a) ▶	352	310
c. Total Print Distribution (Line 15f) + Paid Electronic Copies (Line 16a) ▶	426	385
d. Percent Paid (Both Print & Electronic Copies) (16b divided by 16c × 100) ▶	82.63%	80.52%

☒ **I certify that 50% of all my distributed copies (electronic and print) are paid above a nominal price.**

17. Publication of Statement of Ownership

☒ If the publication is a general publication, publication of this statement is required. Will be printed in the NOVEMBER 2017 issue of this publication. ☐ Publication not required.

18. Signature and Title of Editor, Publisher, Business Manager, or Owner

Stephen R. Bushing

STEPHEN R. BUSHING - INVENTORY DISTRIBUTION CONTROL MANAGER

Date: 9/18/2017

I certify that all information furnished on this form is true and complete. I understand that anyone who furnishes false or misleading information on this form or who omits material or information requested on the form may be subject to criminal sanctions (including fines and imprisonment) and/or civil sanctions (including civil penalties).

PS Form **3526**, July 2014 *(Page 3 of 4)* **PRIVACY NOTICE:** See our privacy policy on *www.usps.com.*